THE
ALTERNATIVE
HEALTH GUIDE

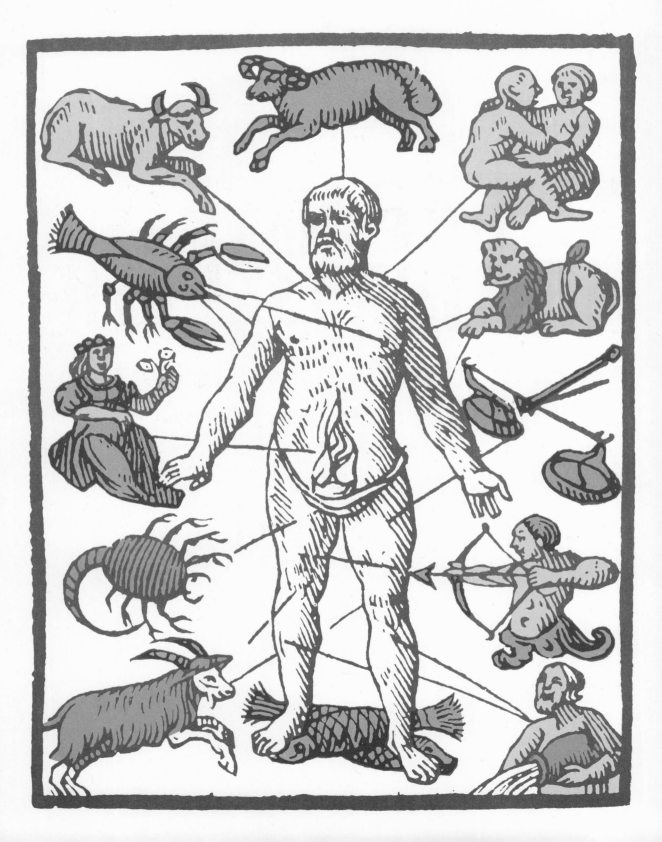

THE ALTERNATIVE HEALTH GUIDE

Brian Inglis & Ruth West

Michael Joseph · London

The Alternative Health Guide
was conceived, edited and designed by
Dorling Kindersley Limited,
9 Henrietta Street, London WC2E 8PS

Project Editor Yvonne McFarlane
Editor Jemima Dunne
Designers Derek Coombes, Gillian Della Casa
Picture Researcher Alisa Lintell

Managing Editor Amy Carroll
Art Director Debbie MacKinnon

First published in Great Britain in 1983 by
Michael Joseph Limited
44 Bedford Square, London WC1B 3DU

Copyright © 1983 Dorling Kindersley Limited
Text copyright © 1983 Brian Inglis and Ruth West

ISBN 0 7181 2185 6

Printed in Italy by A. Mondadori, Verona

Contents

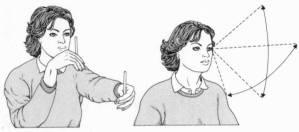

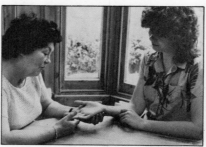

Introduction

Orthodox medicine is experiencing a crisis of confidence. Within the medical profession there is much heart-and-conscience-searching of a kind that the public hears little about, as it surfaces only rarely in the medical journals, and still more infrequently in the lay press.

Patients' discontent has also been mounting. Opinion polls used to put doctors easily at the top of the popularity tables – medicine was the most favoured profession and as many as nine out of ten people were satisfied with their doctors. But by 1980, a survey taken in Britain revealed that the proportion of people who still trusted their general practitioners had fallen from over 50 percent to under 40 percent in a single year.

Natural therapies and the media

At the same time, the media have been displaying an unprecedented interest in unorthodox forms of treatment. In 1960, when Geoffrey Murray compiled a survey of them for the *Spectator* magazine, they were little more than a curiosity, and as they lacked a collective name, the headline was "Fringe Medicine". Although this was not entirely disparaging, it conveyed the impression, with good reason, that the therapies were not taken very seriously. However, over the last 20 years there has been a transformation, and today programmes and articles abound on nature cure, herbalism, homeopathy, osteopathy and chiropractic, hypnotherapy, healing, acupuncture, yoga, and variations on these therapies and techniques. Moreover they are usually serious appraisals rather than the flippant debunkings they used commonly to be.

As for natural therapists themselves, they have been enjoying a spectacular revival of their fortunes. Twenty years ago theirs was largely a hole-and-corner existence: most of them needed part-time jobs to survive. Now, many of them are savouring the novel experience of full appointment books (and a receptionist to keep them) and are charging fees which would be the envy of many an orthodox consultant. The therapies themselves are also proliferating. Some, which in the 1960s had not even been heard of, are now establishing themselves as household names.

Why alternative medicine?

Until little more than 20 years ago, there seemed no serious reason to doubt that medical science was systematically winning the battle against disease. Diagnostic techniques were advancing and one by one the great epidemics had been largely banished. With the discovery of the sulpha drugs, penicillin and the antibiotics, the menace of many common infections appeared to have become a thing of the past. The introduction of cortisone in the treatment of arthritis, and later its derivatives, the steroids, given for the treatment of many other symptoms, promised that

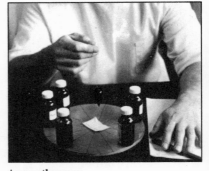

Aromatherapy
Many therapies are now enjoying a revival, aromatherapy, a treatment in which aromatic essences are inhaled, ingested or rubbed into the skin is one. Here a therapist is dowsing to decide which essence to employ in the treatment of his patient.

the "degenerative disorders" – those that are the result of wear and tear – would similarly be eliminated. Moreover with the introduction of the Salk and Sabin vaccines, a new era of immunization procedures dawned and for those diseases which escaped the net, surgery and anesthesia were also improving.

America is one of the most unhealthy nations in the world

In 1959 a warning note was struck by René Dubos, a Professor at the Rockefeller University, New York. Whatever had been happening, he pointed out, it had not made Americans healthier. In almost every respect, they were unhealthier than their fathers and mothers had been. At the very time the wonder drugs had been praised as life-savers for millions, Americans were actually dying younger, on balance, than they had been ten years before.

Since then, there has been further deterioration. In a recent article in *New Realities*, Dr Paavo Airola listed some of the statistics: 30 million Americans suffer from crippling arthritis; 10 million are having treatment for mental illness; one million die annually from heart disease; one thousand die *every day* from cancer, and so on. "Although we have more doctors, more dentists, more and better-equipped hospitals, better drugs and a greater supply of food than any other nation we still are, by far, the sickest nation in the world", Dr Airola concludes.

This is bad news for the western world, as the Americans spend more on health care than any other nation, and indeed have been spending a higher proportion of their national incomes on health every year.

What has gone wrong with orthodox medicine

Dubos put his finger on one of the mistakes which has been made: the assumption that medicine had much to do with the ending of the epidemics. As he showed – and as has since been confirmed by Thomas McKeown in his book *The Role of Medicine* – it was the social reformers in Victorian times, with their campaigns to bring clean water into the cities, to build sewers, to sweep away slums, and to improve standards of diet and hygiene, who were responsible. The antibiotics arrived just in time to speed up this process – and to claim the credit.

Against the degenerative disorders – the chief scourge of our time – drugs have a wretched record. After years of experimenting with cortisone's derivatives – the steroids and their successors, the anti-inflammatory drugs – aspirin remains the best and safest drug in the treatment of chronic arthritis. This is only one of many common disorders which modern drugs have in general failed to help.

Over the past few years critics, both inside and outside the medical profession, have been casting around for an explanation for why orthodox medicine, with all the advantages of modern tech-

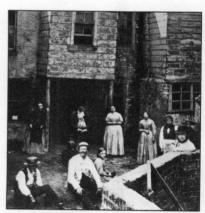

Disease in the nineteenth century
The poverty and appalling living conditions that a large proportion of the population was living under in Victorian England did a great deal to help the spread of "killer" diseases such as consumption.

nology, has failed to combat disease more effectively, and the picture is gradually becoming clearer.

The organic concept of disease

A century ago, it came to be taken for granted that disease is an organic, physical process, caused by pathogens – germs, viruses, toxins and so on. More than that, it came to be assumed that each specific disease had its own specific cause; if the cause could be identified and a cure found for it, that would be that.

Medical students were taught that the mind and the emotions play no part in the disease process. Even mental illness, it was assumed, would eventually be traced to some biochemical malfunctioning. Of course, people might have neurotic or hysterical disorders; but these were not a *real* form of illness. Such patients should be sent packing, told to pull themselves together, and not waste their doctors' time.

Because the new drugs introduced in the 1940s and 1950s appeared to give such spectacular results, the public became largely conditioned to accept this point of view. When a few doctors tried to convince their colleagues of the importance of the psychosomatic element in the disease process, not merely did their colleagues deride them; but "psychosomatic" came to be used by the public as a term of contempt.

The thalidomide tragedy and the Kefauver committee

It was not until the early 1960s that the first serious doubts began to be felt. This came about largely because of the thalidomide tragedy, when hundreds of babies were born deformed because their mothers had taken the drug as a tranquillizer during pregnancy. The Americans were spared it, as the drug had not been licensed by the Federal Drug Authority. However, the report published by the US Senate Committee under Senator Kefauver showed that it was only the most serious of a number of instances of lethal side-effects which were leading to the hasty withdrawal of new drugs from the market. The report by the Kefauver committee also criticized the medical profession for over-prescribing and mis-prescribing on the strength of the drug companies' promotion. Still, over-prescribing and mis-prescribing were mistakes which, it was assumed, the medical profession could take action to prevent in future. The danger from unforseen side-effects could also be prevented by the more rigorous testing procedures, monitored by government agencies set up for that purpose. It is only now coming to be realized that the medical profession is incapable of imposing the necessary discipline upon its members, and that the testing procedures, however rigorous, cannot always detect dangerous side-effects early enough to prevent serious casualties when things go wrong.

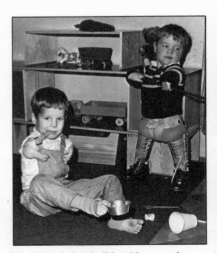

Victims of the thalidomide tragedy
These are two out of several hundred physically and/or mentally handicapped children, all victims of a sedative given to pregnant mothers which was originally declared to be "outstandingly safe".

Disease is dictated by personality and lifestyle

Research over the past 20 years has been revealing that the scientific theories upon which modern medicine has been built are quite simply fallacious. Disease is *not* an organic process; germs, viruses and toxins play a part, but it is a relatively minor one.

Just how minor a part has been exposed by research into heart disease and cancer. It is now clear that these diseases have no single cause, but, there *are* a number of "risk factors" mainly to do with our lifestyles. For example we are more at risk if we smoke heavily and if we eat excessive amounts of animal fat. Research is also beginning to show that some personality types are more susceptible than others and that people are most at risk when exposed to certain kinds of stress – retirement, redundancy, bereavement and so on. It is as if our personalities dictate the type of disorders we are most likely to suffer from (heart disease or cancer for example); our lifestyles decide the level of risk (our vulnerability); and stress precipitates the outcome – the disease.

As recently as 10 years ago, this interpretation would have been rejected outright by the medical profession. Now, it is surprising how many doctors are willing to admit the importance of a patient's lifestyle, personality, diet and so on, in the maintenance of health.

Orthodox practitioners can be a threat to health

The trouble is that the profession is not geared to handle such matters. People do not as a rule go to their doctors unless and until they have something the matter with them, and most doctors give them short shrift if they come when they do *not* have something the matter with them. Of course there are physical check-ups which healthy people can take; but the very fact that they have concentrated on checking upon peoples' physical condition has made them largely a waste of time and money.

Doctors have continued to treat physical symptoms with physical remedies, and with progressively less success. The toll of side-effects from drugs too has been growing. As a result Ivan Illich claimed in his *Medical Nemesis* that the medical establishment had become a major threat to health: "The disabling impact of professional control over medicine has reached the proportions of an epidemic". This was backed up with a mass of evidence which the medical profession was unable to refute.

The bleak fact is that the profession as it stands cannot change its ways, certainly not fast enough to meet the public's need. It is largely self-governing, and the ruling "establishment" consists not, as is commonly thought, of the professional trade unions such as the British and American Medical Associations but – in Britain – of the Royal Colleges. These colleges are controlled by specialists, and the specialists control medical education and they are not going to throw up their hands and say, sorry, we realise that Illich is right, and that we ought to hand over power to somebody else. Certainly, the general practitioners would not be able to take over. They have been conditioned to think in terms of treating whatever physical symptoms their patients have (and mental and emotional problems too) with the latest drugs.

As long ago as 1937 Lord Horder, surveying the future of medicine, pointed out that it would be necessary for the family doctor to concentrate on preventive medicine. "If it is advanced that the doctor's training has not, up till now, fitted him for work of this sort then the sooner it does so fit him the better", Horder argued. "Inevitably the doctor's work in future will be more and more educational and less curative. More and more will he deal with physiology and psychology, less and less with pathology. He will spend this time keeping the fit fit, rather than trying to make the unfit fit". Far from any attention being paid to this proposal, medical students' training became progressively more hospital-bound. The medical students who were to become GPs were, until very recently, given hardly any training in general practice. Even now, their training does not effectively begin, save in a few hospitals, until after their medical student days.

The revival of alternative medicine

As recently as 20 years ago it seemed inconceivable that old-fashioned, outmoded forms of treatment, practised by "quacks" would survive much longer. There were still some practitioners of nature cure, a few herbalists, a few hypnotherapists; and there were many spiritual healers, though they were not, as a rule, professionals. But the only branch which enjoyed any standing in the public mind was osteopathy.

The idea that it might revive took a little longer to impinge upon the United States than it did in Europe. This was unusual, as America had, as a rule, been in the vanguard. Yet this was perhaps predictable, as American laws against the practice of therapies by people who had no medical qualifications tended to be more severe than in Britain. In 1965, however, Dubos remarked upon "the increase in the popularity of what has been called 'fringe medicine'". Whether or not it had therapeutic validity, he argued, was irrelevant: "its popularity points to the failure of the present bio-medical science to satisfy large human needs".

One branch of medical science, had remained to some extent independent of conventional medicine, particularly in the United States: psychology. It was through research by psychologists that the first breach was made in orthodoxy's walls in the late 1960s.

New theories from the East

Briefly, the impetus came partly from eastern teachings, formerly vaguely known as "yoga" and regarded as esoteric, which were

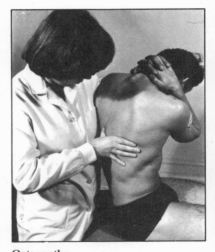

Osteopathy
Osteopathy is based on the principle that the structure and function of the body are entirely dependant upon each other; if for any reason the structure is out of alignment the person may fall ill.

brought to the West by the Maharishi Mahesh Yogi; partly from the development of the "counter culture" with its roots in western California; and partly (and most unexpectedly) from the laboratory work of clinical psychologists who had had little but scorn for either the counter-culture or yoga. Take care of the mind, the implications eventually were seen to be, and the body will take care of itself – except that during the process of learning how to take care of the mind, the body might have a part to play.

The power of the mind over the body

What the new research showed was *why* organic-style medicine, dinned into every medical student, was quite simply wrong. Of our two nervous systems, voluntary and autonomic, the voluntary system enables us to make our bodies do what we want them to do, at our bidding, while the autonomic system regulates those functions which continue automatically, without our having to pay attention to them – heartbeat, blood pressure, temperature, visceral responses and so on. So automatically did this system work, in fact, that students were taught that it cannot be controlled by any mental process. It was known that the various functions could be influenced, temporarily, in many ways, such as by taking exercise, or even by thought processes. But our "homeostat" then ensures that they revert to their former condition.

The new research, both with laboratory animals and with humans, demonstrated that this belief was nonsense. Our homeostats are perfectly capable of responding to the mind's instructions, if ways are found to transmit them. Stories about the ability of yogis to cover their pulse rates, and to go for hours without perceptible breathing, turned out not to be myths after all – as some yogis were able to demonstrate, in laboratory conditions. Nor did these changes last only for as long as attention was concentrated upon them. By the application of techniques of relaxation and meditation, it proved possible for individuals to bring down their blood pressure and keep it down.

Acupuncture – another nail in the coffin of orthodoxy

The next shock to orthodoxy's system came in the early 1970s. Of all the forms of medicine practised in the world, the one which had excited most derision in orthodox medical circles had been acupuncture. Both the theory (that there is a vital force, coursing through the body along "meridians"), and the practice (sticking needles into patients to get the forces flowing), seemed plain daft. But when eminent American physicians, invited to witness acupuncture in China by Chairman Mao, returned after their visit, they had to admit, with embarrassment, that they had been impressed by what they had seen: acupuncture worked.

Orthodoxy's final humiliation came in the mid-1970s, when the discovery of the endorphins and enkephalins (chemical

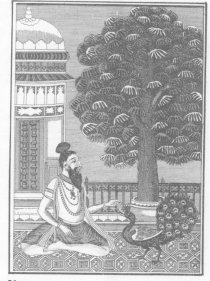

Yoga
A philosophy embracing all aspects of human life, yoga originated in the East over 6,000 years ago. This eighteenth century print depicts a yogi sitting in the classic Lotus *position.*

messengers doing the mind's bidding) showed how by applied concentration, patients could *treat* the body through the mind.

The development of complementary medicine
The reason why people are leaving their doctors and trying unconventional forms of therapy, in short, is not because they have been seduced by way-out, occultist ideas. They are simply becoming disenchanted with orthodox medicine. The proportion of people who have switched to therapists who are not medically qualified is small, but it is growing, according to a survey conducted by Dr Stephen Fulder and Dr Robin Munro for the Threshold Foundation, at a rate of 10 to 15 percent annually.

Fulder and Munro have called their survey *The Status of Complementary Medicine in the United Kingdom* – "complementary" being a term that some practitioners are anxious to popularize in place of "alternative", the idea being that the unconventional therapies should complement, rather than provide an alternative to, orthodox medicine. We have preferred the term "natural" therapies as it has a broader scope, bringing in a range of psychological therapies, for example, which do not find a place in Fulder and Munro's study. There is a very real sense, too, in which much unconventional medicine is *not* complementary, as it is based on theories rejected by medical science.

Natural therapies and orthodox medicine
There have even been many signs lately that the medical profession is taking unorthodox practices more seriously. The *Lancet* has recently run an editorial urging the need for research projects designed to compare conventional with unconventional forms of treatment; with sciatica, for example, doctors must ensure that their patients are kept under their general supervision "but, with this proviso, there need be no prior conditions about which sciatica treatment method has to come up to the standards of the other. Let the best man win – and the patient reap the benefit".

In the winter of 1981, too, the British Postgraduate Medical Federation staged a symposium at the Charing Cross Hospital at which half those present were from the medical profession and its auxiliaries, half from the other camp; and the following summer the annual conference of the Trainee General Practitioners devoted a session to listening to lectures on homeopathy, osteopathy and other such therapies.

In the United States there has been a very rapid development of psychological therapies; but about other therapies it is impossible to generalize, because the legal position varies so much between different states. In general, orthodoxy is being challenged throughout the western world. Our aim has been to try to present as clear a picture as is possible of what has been emerging – whether to complement, or to replace, orthodox methods.

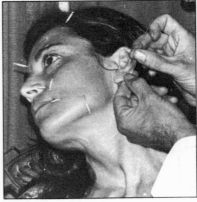

Acupuncture
Although known to the West for centuries, probably through reports brought by traders on the Silk Road as early as 1,000 BC, its reintroduction in recent times has had an astonishing impact on the medical profession.

The
THERAPIES

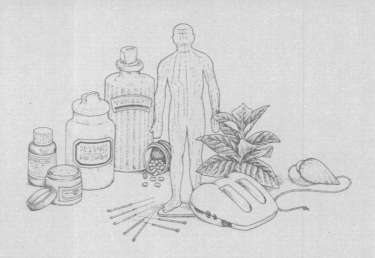

Introduction

For ease of reference, we have divided up the natural therapies into different categories – physical, psychological, paranormal – and sub-categories, and treated each therapy as a separate discipline. But in practice, we must emphasize the distinctions between therapies, and even between categories, are rapidly breaking down. People who have never thought of going to what they have regarded as a "fringe" practitioner understandably assume, when they contemplate taking this step, that if they want to have, say, acupuncture, they should seek out an acupuncturist. But they may find that the acupuncturist in their neighbourhood originally qualified – and may describe himself or herself – as a naturopath, or an osteopath (or both), and may even prescribe herbal or homeopathic remedies, or yoga – and so on.

The structure of each therapy

We have aimed to provide each therapy with: first, a brief explanation of what it is about; second, an examination of its origins (history and development); third, "procedure" – what you can expect if you decide to take the therapy; fourth, research evidence, where available; fifth, suitable cases for that type of treatment. Lastly, where applicable, there is a self-help section.

Some therapies, however, do not fit this pattern, and with several we have omitted the "research" section because such research as has been undertaken does not reach acceptable standards. This is not necessarily the fault of the practitioners of that therapy; the type of research project upon which orthodox medicine now largely relies (controlled trials with two groups of patients, one getting the new drug and the other an old one or a placebo), is not always relevant.

We have concentrated here on the established therapies. The rate of change is now so rapid, however, that we cannot hope to predict what the scene will be like in five years time, and we may well have omitted some newcomers which will turn out to be valuable additions to the company – perhaps included some which will sink without trace. We have omitted certain categories of therapy: one being those systems of medicine, such as Ayurveda, which although established in the East has not taken root in the West; another consists of what have come to be described as the "New Religious Movements" – Scientology, est, Insight and so on. Unquestionably they can produce startling changes in the converts, but they are not, strictly speaking, therapies.

Although we have not, we hope, been too uncritical, it is impossible in a survey of this kind, adequately to assess the relative value of the different therapies. Insofar as all of them rely to some extent, and many to a considerable extent, on their ability to win patients' confidence, the value of any particular therapy must depend to some degree, usually to a considerable degree, on what you bring to it.

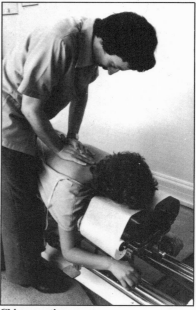

Chiropractic
A method of manipulation derived from similar roots as osteopathy, chiropractic also aims not to deal directly with symptoms but to find any misalignment in the spine itself and correct it manually.

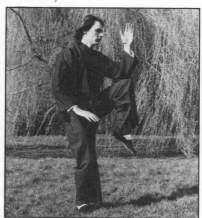

T'ai chi chuan
The ancient Chinese art of T'ai chi works on the principle fundamental to all oriental therapies – to harmonize the body forces in order to encourage chi *energy to flow.*

The holistic principle

Before we go on to look at the individual therapies there is one further point which needs to be emphasized. The initial tendency of people who for one reason or another decide they would like to try out a natural therapy is to think in terms of which one is suitable for their particular symptom or disorder but this is an approach which most natural therapists deplore.

If you ring up to find if they can treat your symptoms, they may say "come along, and we'll see"; but as a rule they will be saying to themselves, "we do not treat your symptoms, but we may be able to help *you*". Symptoms can only be taken as a rough guide to the real nature of your illness.

Holism and the medical profession

Confronted with this, doctors often point out that as medical students, they, too, were continually adjured to think in these holistic terms. The real difference is that the course which orthodox medicine has followed has made this difficult.

General practitioners, with their surgeries full of waiting patients, claim that they simply do not have the time to give their full attention to patients as people, and that even if they had, many of them would be surprised, even irritated, if questioned about, say, their diet or their love life. Patients come to their doctors for tonics or tranquillizers, not for analysis.

How far the medical profession has moved away from the holistic concept of medicine can best be illustrated by the fact that in 1978, a small group of American doctors got together to found the American Holistic Medical Association: such a move would hardly have been necessary if American medicine had already been holistic. Moreover an editorial in the *Journal of the American Medical Association* a few months later made it clear that its readers were unlikely to know anything about holism, bu suggesting it was time they studied the subject.

The temptation to specialize

Although it is fair to say that natural therapists in general pay considerably more attention to the patient as a whole, it has also to be admitted that they, too, are under the temptation to backslide if, say, they win a big reputation for treating a particular type of disorder. So although the great majority regard themselves as believers in holistic medicine, not all of them practise it.

It is consequently impossible to know in advance what to expect when you decide to try any form of natural medicine; but this only emphasizes the need for a different attitude of mind. It is not just a matter of switching from your doctor to an acupuncturist or an osteopath. It is a matter of learning to take more responsibility for your own health; finding out more about diet, how to cope with stressful situations, and so on.

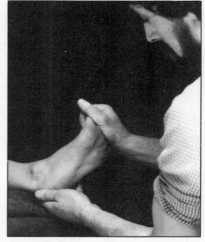

Reflexology
A technique of foot massage, reflexology, is used as a means of rebalancing the body in order to help the subject maintain a state of good health.

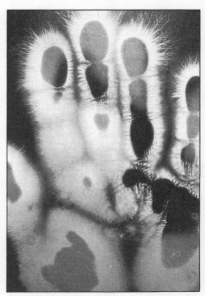

Kirlian photography
Used to photograph the "aura" coming from the hand, Kirlian prints can help with disease diagnosis.

PHYSICAL THERAPIES

"Physical", most of the therapists who practice nature cure, herbalism and the rest will tell you, is today a misnomer. The distinction between physical, psychological and psychic has been breaking down: holism is now king; it should no longer be a matter for surprise if an acupuncturist recommends a course of meditation, or a homeopath employs radionics in diagnosis.

NATURE CURE

The oldest form of medicine, paradoxically, is one in which medicine is not supposed to play a part. The principle of nature cure is precisely what its name implies – that if left to her own devices, nature cures. And, better still, nature can preserve health.

Aspects of nature cure

We no longer live close to nature. We live in towns and villages and often lead unnatural lives in many other respects. Nature cure is inevitably something of a compromise, designed to keep us as healthy as possible in the circumstances in which we find ourselves. Its best-known form is *Naturopathy* (pages 18 to 22). For centuries this has had links with water cure or *Hydrotherapy* (see pages 22 to 27), which must therefore be treated as naturopathy's partner. In addition, there have arisen a great number of therapeutic aids which fall into the nature cure category: *Diets* of various kinds, including those which are designed to put back essential nutrients, such as vitamins, which may be lacking in our daily food (see pages 28 to 37); *Air ionization* (see pages 38 to 39), intended to perform a similar function for the air we breathe; and the *Bates method of eyesight training* (see pages 40 to 42) which aims to enable us to dispense with glasses.

It is generally believed that animals in the wild are basically healthy. They may be preyed on by predators and exploited by parasites, but they know instinctively what is good for them, and what is not good for them.

The instinct for health

How effective this natural instinct is was described by Lord Ritchie-Calder in *Medicine and Man*. An animal suffering from a deficiency "will trek great distances to find a salt lake, or vegetation containing the trace elements it lacks". Sheep, it has been found, will eat the kind of grass which is right for them "before turning to other pastures which would satisfy their hunger but lack the subtler medical requirements". Most remarkable of all, when cattle were dying of a mysterious epidemic in the South African veldt, one group saved themselves by eating bark and herbage of a tree "in the trunk of which there was a single copper nail". The epidemic, it was found, had been caused by a deficiency of the necessary minute traces of copper.

Health, then, is an evolutionary expedient. The concept of the "survival of the fittest" includes "fitness" in the colloquial sense of the term – the healthiest. The instinct for health is built-in, but there is a catch: we humans have lost access to instinct. Reason has taken over, or so we like to think. We do not leave it to instinct to tell us when to eat, what to eat, and how much to eat, nor how much fresh air and exercise to take. Those decisions are made either deliberately or through force of habit.

The purists' standpoint

Believers in nature cure assume that we fall ill because we have blocked instinct off and therefore cannot listen to its promptings, or that we hear them, but take no action because we do not think far enough ahead to worry about the damage we are gradually doing to our systems. If we do decide to listen, however, and cannot tune in to instinct, the next best thing we can do is to adopt a lifestyle modelled as closely as possible on nature's. This means that we should eat only natural food, enjoy fresh air and exercise whenever possible, and shun the bad habits such as smoking, drinking, and eating processed foods.

In time, they believe we will find instinct beginning to come through again, as if we have liberated ourselves from the bondage imposed by our former captors – tobacco, sugar, and the rest. Then we will not need to stick to a regime any longer. We will be able to eat and drink what we like, because what we like will be what's good for us.

This, however, is the purist standpoint, and very few purists remain. The majority of practitioners of nature cure take the view that living as we do in a society which encourages us, with every device known to the advertising industry, to poison ourselves with cigarettes, alcohol and junk food, it may be necessary to offer us actual treatments to set us back on the road to health.

"Natural therapy works more effectively when certain auxiliary forms of treatment are added", Dr E.K. Lederman argues in the introduction to his book on the subject. "Homeopathic medicine enhances the response to stimuli administered by the natural therapist. Manipulation (especially of the spine) and massage give patients further help in recovering from the strains of living, and acupuncture is a means of restoring a healthy equilibrium to the various disturbed functions".

We will be considering homeopathy, manipulation and the others in separate sections, in their own right, but if you go to a naturopath you are likely to find that these techniques are also used as an adjunct to nature cure.

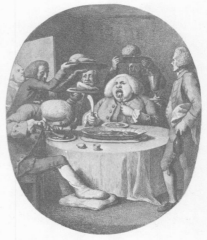

Diet in nature cure
Overeating and excessive drinking have long been known to be detrimental to health but both have been considered to be signs of affluence (as shown here in this cartoon of the eighteenth century poet Samuel Johnson and his companion Boswell). This attitude prevails today in many cases, most notably the "business lunch". An important principle of nature cure, however, is that given the right balance of food and exercise we will remain healthy.

Naturism

There is one form of "straight" nature cure that deserves to be mentioned here, though it is not, strictly speaking, a therapy so much as a way of life (or a way of gaining more pleasure from a holiday, or a day off work), with implications for health.

More commonly known, until recently, as "nudists", naturists have lately achieved recognition of a kind that even a decade ago would have been regarded as out of the question. Every year, more areas are opened to them, in towns as well as on and around beaches. The basic premise of the naturist is that the body is capable of adjusting to a surprisingly large range of changes in temperature, and ought not to be fettered by clothing unnecessarily. Our faces and hands, after all, do not ordinarily require to be covered up; and the rest of us would not require clothing either, if convention had not demanded it. Going about naked, they also believe, is healthier and more hygienic than using the range of unnecessary and often ridiculous garments which habit, or fashion, dictates.

Naturopathy

In *Everybody's Guide to Nature Cure*, published in 1936, Harry Benjamin laid down what he believed were naturopathy's fundamental principles. They still hold today.

The three main principles

The first, most fundamental principle, according to Benjamin, (his italics) is, "*that all forms of disease* are due to the *same cause*, namely, the accumulation in the system of waste materials and bodily refuse, which has been steadily piling up in the body of the individual concerned through years of wrong habits of living". It follows that "the only way in which disease *can be cured* is by the introduction of methods which will enable the system to throw off these toxic accumulations which are daily clogging the wheels of the human machine".

Second, "the body is always striving for the ultimate good of the individual". It follows that the symptoms of all acute diseases, from colds to typhoid, "are nothing more than self-initiated attempts on the part of the body to throw off the accumulations of waste material (some of them hereditary) which are interfering with its proper functioning". By striving to suppress such symptoms, orthodox treatment merely drives them underground, to return another day.

Benjamin's third principle is that "the body contains within itself the power to bring about a return to that condition of normal well-being known as health, provided the right methods are employed to enable it to do so".

Restoring the body's own power

Benjamin's principles are still accepted, though some naturopaths feel that the accumulation of waste material may itself be symptomatic of more complex disorders, psychological rather than dietary. There are differences, too, over how best to set about restoring the power which the body contains within itself. What are the "right methods" to enable it to recover?

Benjamin proposed five: fasting; scientific dieting; hydrotherapy; general body-building and hygienic measures; and psychotherapy. All of these pose questions. Does fasting imply taking no food of any kind? If so, for how long? If not, what nourishment is permitted? No two naturopaths agree on what constitutes a "scientific" diet. Some set little store by hydrotherapy. There are a bewildering variety of body-building and hygienic measures. And as for psychotherapy, the term covers a multitude of different and sometimes contradictory procedures.

With naturopathy, in short, a great deal will depend on the views of the particular naturopath you happen to consult. All that we can do here is to give you an idea of the kind of advice and treatment you are likely to be offered.

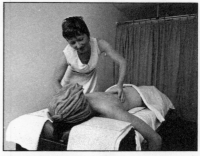

Massage in health farms
Massage is one of the oldest forms of medicine, dating back in western civilization at least as far as the ancient Greeks. Although it lost its popularity for some time, it is now gaining again and is a technique often used at health farms to promote relaxation.

Procedure

Nature cure is usually obtained in one of two different forms: either through an appointment with a naturopath, who will prescribe whatever therapies he or she thinks you require; or, as naturopaths are few in number, by staying at one of the naturopathic establishments, colloquially known as "health farms".

A first visit to a naturopath invariably begins with the taking of your case history, a process which is unlikely to last less than half an hour. Naturopaths make a careful examination of each new patient, to some extent along the same lines as a GP would, but with less emphasis on actual tests and more on sensory impressions of how you look, your posture, breathing, colour and so on.

Detoxification by fasting

It is highly probable that the first phase of treatment will include dietary modification: perhaps fasting. Fasting, the British naturopath Leon Chaitow has observed, "is the oldest therapeutic method known to man. Primitive people instinctively stop eating when not feeling well, in the same way as an animal that is ill will lie quietly, drinking as much as is needed, and eating nothing, until health returns".

Actually starving for a few days, taking no nourishment at all, may be recommended, but quite commonly, fruit or vegetable juice is permitted and even encouraged. A few naturopaths believe in an occasional "drying out" spell – setting aside certain days a week, for three weeks, in which no liquid is to be taken at all. Patients are advised to wash out their mouths with water whenever they need to overcome thirst.

The unpleasant side of fasting

The duration of the fast is determined by the assessment of your needs, and by your reaction to it. The initial reaction, naturopaths always warn, can be (and commonly is) extremely unpleasant: halitosis, diarrhea, vomiting and headache. These symptoms are seen as the effect of your body expelling its accumulated poisons, consequently they should be welcomed, however unbearable they may seem at the time.

Soon, usually within a couple of days, they disappear. At the same time, the pangs of hunger diminish. But eventually your appetite will come back, as Dr E.K. Ledermann recalls: "the tongue clears, and your breath becomes sweet; then the fast can be broken". But the fast should not simply be regarded as a period of physical clean-out. "It can be a turning point in your attitude towards values; you can recognize and correct your tendency to overeat, to rely on alcohol, smoking and coffee", Ledermann urges. "This can be the time when you come to accept responsibility for your health".

When the initial fast is over, there ceases to be any consistent naturopathic policy, partly because of the belief that you must learn to be guided by whatever is right for you, and partly because naturopaths have differing ideas about what should, and what should not, be considered "natural". Some are vegans, some vegetarians (see page 32). Others allow meat and wine in moderation. But all advocate a balanced diet, fresh air and exercise.

Dietary fads and fancies

All naturopaths have their own dietary fads and fancies, and patients have their likes and dislikes to be accounted for. But a general line has been provided in a pamphlet issued by the Friends of the Healing Research Trust, which recommends the 60/20/20 diet: 60 percent raw foods, 20 percent carbohydrates, 20 percent protein, leaving it up to the individual how they are taken. Items to be avoided include refined carbohydrates (white sugar, white bread, cakes, sweets, etc); stimulants, including tea and coffee as well as alcohol; milk in quantity; condiments; fatty and salted meat; and all tinned and packaged foods containing preservatives. For all these, there are natural alternatives: wholemeal flour, herb teas, yoghurt, lean meat, fish, chicken, and so on. This may be said to constitute the kind of diet which you are likely to be recommended to try by a naturopath.

"Dieting" however, in the sense the term is most commonly used, can be a quite different matter, and we have thought it best to put it in a different section (see pages 28 to 37).

The psychological aspects

In the past few years, naturopaths have begun to take more of an interest in the psychological aspects of natural therapy – not that they ever completely ignored them. Half a century ago, Henry Lindlahr, one of the pioneers who revived nature cure between the wars, speaking of the struggle between the healing force of nature and the germs and poisons against which it had to contend, wrote that in this conflict, "mind plays the same role as the commander of an army".

In a sense, though, Lindlahr thought of the mind much as Marshal Kutuzov did of his role in Tolstoy's epic novel *War and Peace* – not as intervening to direct the course of the battle, but as displaying confidence in the outcome. The mind "must have absolute faith in the superiority of nature's healing forces", Lindlahr argued. "If the mind becomes frightened by the inflammatory and febrile symptoms, and pictures to itself in darkest colours their dreadful consequences, these confused and distracted thought vibrations are conveyed instantaneously to the millions of little soldiers fighting in the affected parts". The mind, in other words, is required to subordinate itself to the vital force which nature provides, and which can, by itself, promote health so long as we do not allow our worries and cares to undermine it.

Contemporary naturopaths, however, are usually more conscious of the difficulty people have in leaving things to nature, when psychosocial problems, ranging from fears about redundancy to family rows, may make it hard for patients to avoid disruptive worries and cares. They are consequently more inclined to recommend some technique of relaxation or, where they realize it is required, psychotherapy.

Health farms

The alternative method of undertaking nature cure, booking in to a "health farm", provides, in principle, for the same kind of treatment that you would obtain from a naturopath, but usually on a distinctly plusher scale, as these places often resemble luxury hotels. The naturopath in charge may have become an administrator, and the treatments will often be provided by specialists in osteopathy, massage and so on.

The health farms started in the period between the wars imposed a spartan regime, with an initial period of fasting, followed by a spell on fruit juice and salads, along with fresh air and exercise; and they had some striking successes. Today's health farms tend to be less exacting. Inevitably they have come to cater for the people who can best afford them, and they are apt to

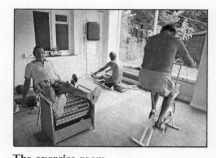

The exercise room
At health farms vigorous exercise is taken as part of a controlled personal regime, combined with a planned diet as well as any required specialist treatments. Frequently, exercise is taken using machines, the body's muscles working against springs and pulleys.

be expensive. Those who can afford them are frequently business or professional men and women who are not interested in nature cure *per se*, but simply want to recover from the assaults made on their systems by expense-account lunches and cocktail parties, or to lose weight, or both. For some, weight loss is both the main objective and the only method by which the success of the course is judged – three weeks or a month used to be the standard length of stay, but many health farms now run single-week courses.

Hydrotherapy

Although fasting and dieting are the staples of nature cure, they have long been supplemented by the use of water, in a variety of ways. Hydrotherapy may be prescribed by a naturopath or obtained at health hydros, spas, and establishments which provide thalassotherapy (sea-water therapy), sauna baths, or Turkish baths.

Origins

It is not known when "taking the waters" first came to be regarded as a way of promoting or restoring good health, but there is no doubt when it first became a recognized form of medical treatment. Hydrotherapy was certainly an integral part of the lifestyle of the Romans and Greeks in classical times. They brought pure mountain water into their towns in aqueducts, to drink or to bathe in. And wherever they went, they founded watering places where the local springs were considered to have health-giving properties.

There was some debate in Roman times as to whether lying around in steam baths was good for the rheumatics and other disorders, as Pliny insisted, or whether it was simply self-indulgence, which was Horace's view. The argument has continued up to the present day, with hydrotherapy sometimes finding favour with orthodoxy, sometimes suffering from neglect – as it has over the past century. In Britain, therefore, it has come to be regarded as part of the alternative medical scene.

Procedure

The waters can be taken in many different ways, internally or externally. The same water may be recommended for both purposes, either because it is known to be pure or because it is full of health-giving impurities, usually minerals, such as sodium, calcium, zinc, and many more.

Let us give nature some chance to work; she understands her business better than we. I have allowed colds, gouty discharges, looseness of bowels, palpitations, headaches and other ailments to grow old in me and die their natural death; they have left me when I have half-inured myself to their company. One can exorcize them better by courtesy than by defiance.

Michel Eyquem de Montaigne (1533–92)
Essay on Experience

In a few places, though not in Britain, geysers gush up through snow-covered ground, offering both, free.

Taking the waters

Water can be used as a stimulant or as a relaxant, as a medium in which to exercise or one in which to rest. It can be drunk for pleasure or as an unpalatable medicine (the Bath waters, Dickens' Sam Weller remarked, had "a very strong flavour of warm flatirons"). In his *About Nature Cure*, Alan Hoyle lists some applications which you may encounter (and with experience, use yourself). These include alternate hot and cold foot baths; packs, in which a wet sheet is wrapped around the body to lower the surface temperature; compresses for sprains, bruises, swellings or inflammations; fomentations; steam inhalations; hip or sitz baths and Epsom salts baths.

Spas

Even after the fall of the Roman Empire, some of the places where its legions had found solace in the water continued to exploit it. And one of them, Spa, in Belgium, was to give its name to the institution which has survived ever since, though it has not always flourished. It was to Spa that Peter the Great of Russia went in

The baths of Titus, Rome
Baths were an essential part of Roman daily life – one of the first buildings to be erected in a new town. They comprised several different rooms which could include hot, tepid, cool and steam baths as well as an oiling chamber where massage would take place.

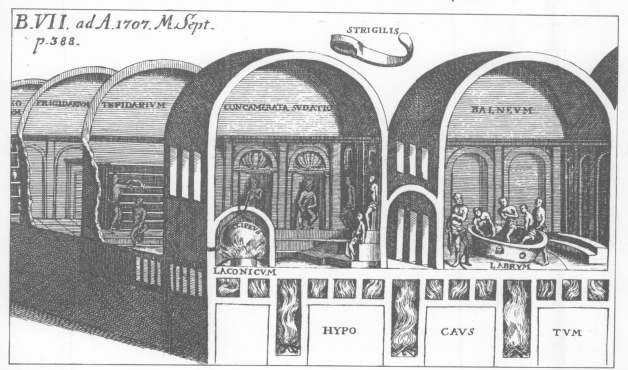

1717 for a cure (a plaque there still testifies to the fact that he felt much the better for it). By that time, however, Bath, in southwest England, was in the process of becoming the most famous of spas, thanks to Beau Nash, the English gambler and dandy, who used his formidable public relations talents to make it fashionable in the eighteenth century.

How far do spas owe their custom to the virtues of their medicinal springs, and how far to the pleasures of high society? "The bath", Daniel Defoe wrote in 1722, "is more of a sport and diversion than a physical prescription for health, and the town is taken up in raffling, gaming, visiting and, in a word, all sorts of gallantry and levity". Whatever the reasons, spas remained fashionable in Britain until the outbreak of the First World War. By that time, however, they were being severely criticized in medical circles as insanitary, as well as of no proven therapeutic value. And ever since, most doctors have been inclined to tell patients that anything the waters can do, drugs can do better, though there are now some signs of a change of heart.

The introduction in 1948 of a National Health Service was a setback to British spas, and for a while, they could not offer their services free. In some other European countries, however, treatment at a spa can be obtained through government health insurance policies, which has led to a great increase in the number of trade union members taking advantage of their facilities. Many spas offer a wide variety of therapeutic opportunities. German spas, for example offer: early morning warm-up exercises, swimming, massage, sun-bathing, loofah-baths, herbal wraps, yoga and even facials.

Health hydros

The first hydrotherapy establishment was founded by Vincent Priessnitz early in the nineteenth century, at Grafenburg in Bohemia. A formidable character, Priessnitz imposed strict discipline on his patients, insisting that they take ice-cold baths, sluices and douches, making them lie around wrapped up in damp sheets, and telling them to drink as much of the local water as they could. Similar institutions were set up in Austria later in the century by the Dominican, Father Kneipp, and by Dr Gully at Malvern in England (this institution was patronized by, among others, Charles Darwin).

Kneipp came to believe that water is capable of curing every curable disease, by dissolving the diseased matter and enabling it to be expelled from the body. But, he added, it is important that it is correctly applied – and how to apply it correctly has remained in contention.

Nowadays, hydros are not, as a rule, distinguishable from health farms – many of which call themselves hydros, and all of which employ water cures of various kinds.

Salt-water treatments

"Of all the medicaments provided by nature, sea-water is the last to have come within the field of modern medicine", the German physician, Heinz Graupner, wrote in his book *Adventures in Healing*. This struck him as strange: "the sea has always fascinated man. He has entrusted himself to it, he has feared it, he has swum in it for his pleasure and has lain on its sunny shores" – yet without realizing its remarkable healing properties. Only in the last few years has the full range of its medicinal content been analyzed by chemists, who have found that the salts in our blood serum are closely linked to those in the sea.

Thalassotherapy

Hot and cold baths of sea-water were quite common at coastal resorts in Victorian times, and recently they have been revived, but in a much more sophisticated form. The term thalassotherapy derives from the Greek word *thalassa* meaning sea (still remembered as the word Xenophon heard shouted with joy by his troops when, after their 1,500-mile march, they saw the Black Sea). Establishments which provide thalassotherapy have been springing up around the continent of Europe (though not as yet to any notable extent in Britain) to provide a holiday in which the usual seaside ingredients – swimming, sunbathing, walking, beach games – are supplemented, or in the case of more seriously ill people, supplanted by a regime of salt-water treatments, These include drinking the water, inhaling it in the form of a fine spray, being sprayed and sluiced by jets of it, having massage in it, and taking a variety of baths (some accompanied by mud packs or seaweed compresses) including a bubble bath of an unfamiliar kind, the large bubbles coming up from underneath, subjecting the body to what feels like a bombardment of tennis balls.

Sauna baths

The principle of a sauna bath is similar to that of a Turkish bath: the bathers sit around in a room heated by birch logs to a high temperature for as long as they can bear, before dashing out to roll in snow, or swim in an icy lake. There may also be what is described as "massage" with the aid of birch twigs or pine needles; this produces a sensation not unlike being caressed with a bunch of stinging nettles.

Twenty-five years ago, sauna baths were still regarded as an eccentric habit indulged in only by the Finns. Now, as Donald Law laments in his *Guide to Alternative Medicine*, "there are many establishments which purport to be saunas but which are far from it". That is putting it mildly. Many of them are in effect brothels, and most are clip joints.

Still, people who can obtain the real thing (even if heating by electricity has to be substituted for the birch logs) find saunas

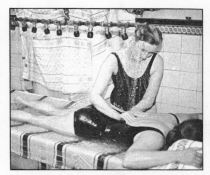

A thalassotherapy treatment
During this thalassotherapy treatment, the patient is being massaged. She is lying in a shallow bed of sea water and more is sprayed on to her back from the jets above.

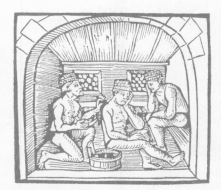

A medieval sauna
Sauna baths have been popular in parts of Scandinavia for hundreds of years. This contemporary woodcut shows what they were like in medieval Denmark.

extremely invigorating. Donald Law says that the temperature should be not less than 38°C (100°F) but can be considerably higher, for those who can bear it. The sitting should be five minutes for beginners, more for initiates. A swim or shower afterwards is deemed essential.

The Finns take a sauna bath for aches and pains, respiratory troubles, indigestion, and much else besides. Saunas are not recommended for people with heart conditions.

Turkish baths

Fashionable for so long, the Turkish bath has recently been losing ground to the sauna in terms of popularity. It served much the same purpose, but had come to be used chiefly – apart from habitués – by people who found it a good way to cure a hangover or a pleasant way, in some establishments, to achieve the relaxation desirable for a good night's sleep before a difficult day's work. Nowadays there are few Turkish baths to be found in our cities and towns.

Leamington Spa
In the therapeutic pool – 2.5 sq. metres (26 sq. ft.) with a depth varying from 76 cm (2 ft. 6 ins.) to 137 cm (4 ft. 6 ins.) – patients are treated individually with appropriate exercises. The pool, kept at 36°C (97°F), is supplemented by a whirlpool bath and Vichy massage douche.

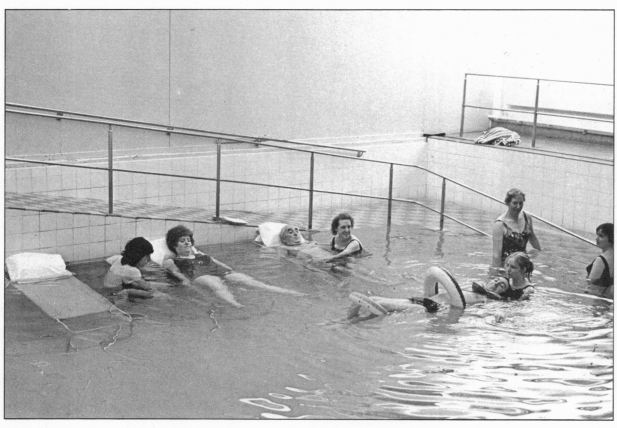

Research

Little research has been done into nature cure as such, nor is it easy to think of ways in which it could be done. But a great deal of modern research into diseases has indirectly, and sometimes directly, vindicated the claims of the naturopaths.

The most striking example has been the epidemiological research into heart disease, originating at Framingham, Massachusetts, and since continued and expanded in countries all over the world. This has shown the importance of diet, exercise, of avoiding harmful habits such as smoking, and cultivating a quiet mind; there is now evidence that those who follow these principles are least at risk of having heart attacks.

From time to time, the naturopaths enjoy unexpected testimonials from researchers in other fields. For example, towards the end of the nineteenth century an Austrian professor, Wilhelm Winternitz, claimed that he had conclusively proved that the use of minerals of any kind in spa water (or bathwater) was futile. The human hide, he believed he had shown, is so constructed that it keeps them out. This view remained unchallenged for many years, but it has recently been shown to be fallacious.

In 1981, the *New Scientist* described research in Australia by Professor W. R. Walker and Dr M. Whitehouse, using "fat-soluble copper salicylate solutions". These, they found, "can penetrate the skin, and they have been shown to be strikingly effective" against artificially induced arthritis. It turns out that they are "powerful anti-inflammatory agents, proving to be excellent when used on arthritis and rheumatism sufferers and on people damaging themselves at sports".

Ruefully, the *New Scientist* comments, "there must be something satisfying about finding that there may be truth in old wives remedies as wearing a copper bracelet"; and increasingly, research has been demonstrating that drugs, too, can be delivered "percutaneously" sometimes with positive advantages, particularly for people who are sensitive to injections. "By giving drugs through the skin", Professor Arnold Beckett of Chelsea College, London, has observed, "we can reduce the problems of high dosage and unpleasant side effects".

Suitable cases/Self-help

Naturopaths maintain that anybody and everybody can benefit from going through a course of treatment at a health farm. That way people can learn the basic elements of nature cure which can be carried on thereafter, for life.

They also constantly emphasize that nature cure *is* self help. All they as practitioners can do is to advise their patients what to do, and it is then up to them to decide whether to take that advice.

Diets

Diets are not necessarily embarked upon for therapeutic purposes. People may eat in certain ways, or eat only certain kinds of food for a variety of reasons – chief among them being habit, conditioned by upbringing and convention. Obviously, personal likes and dislikes also play a big part. Religious beliefs are of importance in some communities, and moral attitudes have been taking their place in others (as in the case of vegetarianism when it arises out of a revulsion against the slaughter of animals).

Origins

Our loss of that instinct which tells wild animals what they can usefully and safely eat led inevitably to the development in tribal communities of what we now regard as folklore about food. This was later to become intertwined with religious doctrine, as displayed in the regulations imposed on the Israelites in the Old Testament. Dieting in the therapeutic sense was first introduced in classical Greece, featuring extensively in the writings of Hippocrates in the fifth century BC, and has played some part in both conventional and natural medicine ever since.

In modern times, when the medical profession came to identify disease with the depredations of germs and viruses, however, diet ceased to seem of much importance. What people ate was their own affair. The general assumption was that although over-indulgence could be unhealthy, there was nothing much wrong with the prevailing dietary pattern.

Recently, however, there has been a growing acceptance of the need to regulate diet for health reasons. Some kinds of food have been named as risk factors in connection with specific disorders; others, notably foods high in vitamins and fibre, have found favour as preventives. In general, there is a wider recognition of the importance of diet in the preservation of health. But there are considerable divergences of opinion about what to do (and what not to do) to obtain the best results.

The dangers of saturated fat

Governments are, in fact, intervening to influence people's diet these days, and often in harmful ways. The first realization of the extent of this intervention and its dangers came from the investigation at Framingham in Massachusetts into risk factors in connection with heart disease (see *Circulatory disorders*, pages 320 to 322), with the discovery that the consumption of "saturated" fats (mostly found in animal fat and dairy products) was high on the list, a finding later confirmed in many other affluent societies. Yet farmers were being encouraged, through government subsidies, to produce more meat, milk and butter.

In Britain, for example, an attempt by the Department of

A few years ago, an experiment was described before the McGovern Select Committee on Human Needs. One group of rats was fed one of the new popular breakfast cereals. A control group was fed the ground-up boxes that the cereals came in. The rats that were fed the boxes lived significantly longer than the rats that were fed the cereal.

Lawrence Le Shan
The Mechanic and the Gardener

Health to encourage people to eat less animal fat was promptly countered by the Minister for Agriculture, who secured an increase in the subsidy for butter manufacture. As the farm lobby is backed by electors whose votes may be decisive in a general election, the chance of any government adopting more energetic policies to encourage lower consumption of animal fats is small.

In recent years, too, there has been a massive increase in the quantity of sugar products and of junk food consumed, as well as of food containing preservatives or colouring matter, or both. Although government regulating agencies have provided the public with some protection where there has been a direct threat to health, they have not been able to halt the trend towards less nourishing meals.

Relating social background to disease

The dangers to health of an unbalanced diet are also increased by the fact that broadly speaking, the less well-off people are, the less balanced their diet. But the medical profession has been unable to come to grips with the problems posed by the belated recognition of the importance of diet in providing protection from diseases, in particular, heart disease, and by the erosion of nutritional standards through the spread of junk food and processed food.

The case for fibre

Another disturbing example of the inability of the medical profession to recognize the importance of diet has been the generally contemptuous attitude to dietary fibre, "roughage", as for a time it was colloquially known. The need for it had always been stressed by naturopaths, the most commonly recommended form being bran. Doctors, on the other hand, held to the belief that what sick patients need, particularly if they have any form of digestive upset, is a bland diet based on "slops" such as bread and milk. "Roughage" was held in contempt by the medical profession because it appeared to be simply waste matter, indigestible stuff which the body evacuated. Research into its role in digestion has revealed that this was a mistake. The colon, Colin Tudge of the *New Scientist* has recalled, "in classic texts featured merely as a sewer", but "is now known to absorb a variety of materials and is crucially involved in many metabolic processes", fibre playing an important part in both. Fibre appears to provide some protection against a number of disorders.

When the reasons for dietary fibre loss are recalled, the tendency is to blame the replacement of wholemeal flour by white flour. But nutritionists point out that there is another foodstuff which has also had serious consequences. "Sugar, as we know it, is the epitome of a fibre-depleted food", Ken Heaton of the University of Bristol has observed; and this applied to brown as well as to white sugar. As a result of getting rid of the fibrous part (the cane), sugar is taken in concentrated form, a form to which the body is not well-adapted, and which also lends itself to promoting addiction. "So let's keep sugar in the front of our minds when we are thinking about fibre", Heaton advises. For our dental protection and for our energy requirements, he suggests, the answer should be "chew it or eschew it".

Naturopaths and nutrition

Members of the medical profession rarely keep in touch with what is going on outside their ranks, and as a result, they have been largely unaware that the results of recent research into the nutritional aspects of health and illness merely confirm what natural therapists have been arguing all along. "Some of the well-tried naturopathic measures have in recent years been subjected to controlled trials, found effective, and hailed as new medical discoveries," the acupuncturist and naturopath Roger Newman-Turner has observed. "Fasting, high-fibre diets and the dangers of refined carbohydrates have all come under the scrutiny of medical researchers who have had facilities at their disposal beyond the reach of any naturopathic practitioner". This work has been valuable corroboration of established methods of treatment.

Even among themselves, however, naturopaths often have different notions of what constitutes a properly balanced, healthy diet. And outside naturopathy the number of diets which have been recommended, some of them for a time becoming fashionable, is legion.

For simplicity, diets can be divided into four categories: religious, ethical, supplementary, and weight-reducing.

Religious and ethical diets

The Mosaic dietary regulations as laid down in the Old Testament, were extremely rigorous, though some of them are still observed today by orthodox Jews. Christians have gradually shed them, except for a few remnants such as the practice of giving up certain kinds of food or drink for Lent, and the proscription against eating meat on Fridays, which was lifted by Pope John XXIII. The dietary laws of Muhammed, which were spelt out in the *Koran* and which borrowed heavily from Mosaic law, also proscribe the consumption of alcoholic drinks, and the laws governing various religious communities in India and the Far East also have their own particular prohibitions. Although in their origins most of the prohibitions were probably based on health-care precautions, diets of this kind hardly fall within our terms of reference here.

Macrobiotics

Diets based on ethical beliefs present a difficulty, as health-care and ethics tend to be confused, as they are in the case of

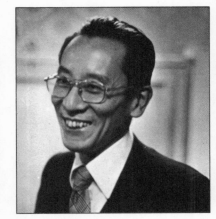

Michio Kushi
A renowned authority on macrobiotics and oriental medicine, Kushi is the director of the East-West Foundation with branches in London, Paris, Boston and Amsterdam.

Yin and yang classification of foods

Practitioners of macrobiotics classify all foods as more *yin* or more *yang* and feel that the dietary requirements of each one of us, while fitting into a general pattern for a particular environment (a *yang* environment is hot and dry, a *yin* one, cold and wet), vary considerably. Thus, in a more yang environment, we should aim to become more yin, and vice versa, and we do this by increasing more *yin* or *yang* food, as appropriate.

In the winter vegetal energy descends into the roots of plants, the leaves die and the plant becomes more yang; plants which grow at this time are drier and can be kept for quite a long time without spoiling. In the summer, the yang time of year, the plants are more watery and therefore perishable; these plants provide the cooling effect required in the summer months. In order for this to be effective, however, all food eaten should be in season in whichever hemisphere we are in at the time.

In addition, physically active (*yang*) people will tend to need more *yang* food, while the mentally active will need more *yin* – each person having different, individual needs.

YIN FOODS
- Grow in a hot, dry (*yang*) environment
- Contain more water
- Grow taller, softer, juicier
- Have a stronger smell
- Tend to be hot, aromatic

YANG FOODS
- Grow in a cold, wet (*yin*) environment
- Are drier, shorter, harder (stems, roots, seeds etc)
- Tend to be sour, salty

macrobiotics, which became fashionable in the West for a time following a campaign by George Ohsawa from Japan who preached his gospel throughout Europe and North America in the 1950s.

Diet, Ohsawa argued, should be based on balancing yin-type foods with yang-type foods (see above, and page 119). When they are not in balance, his belief is, we fall ill. The balance can be restored by finding whether we should be taking more (or less) yin, or more (or less) yang food. But the decision-taking is a complex precess, as it is not just the composition of the foodstuffs which has to be considered, but also their colour and texture and how and where they have been cultivated which can influence their yin/yang standing. Different individuals, too, have different yin/yang requirements, so that what is yin for you may be yang for your companion at the dinner table. And the actual cooking process can also make changes. For example, the yin characteristics are preserved by using small amounts of salt and cooking the food quickly.

There was also a spiritual side to the campaign to win adherents to macrobiotics, including an element of asceticism which brought the diet up against orthodox nutritionists. The American Medical Association denounced it as "one of the most dangerous dietary regimes". In this view they were not entirely at odds with macrobiotic purists, who viewed the proliferation of macrobiotic restaurants and macrobiotic food-peddlers with much the same suspicion as a purist astrologer regards horoscopes in the daily papers as a travesty of the real thing. The "real thing", however, is so demanding that few people stick to it for long.

Vegetarian diets

Of the other moral or ethical dietary regimes, vegetarianism appears to be gradually attracting more converts.

The British Vegetarian Society was founded in 1847, but at the time, and for the best part of a century, its members were regarded as acting on ethical principles rather than on any firm conviction that a vegetable diet was healthier. And when Bernard Shaw, the leading advocate of vegetarianism, had to have liver injections to stay alive, meat eaters tended complacently to take it as proof that plant foods are deficient in some essentials.

Recently, however, evidence that vegetarians are not deprived of any essential nutrients has been accumulating; and the same even applies to vegans.

Vegetarians accept that the break with flesh-eating ought not to be too drastic, in view of the risk that our bodies, which evolution has committed to an omniverous diet, may find it hard to adapt. Dairy products, eggs (so long as they are free-range) and, in some cases, fish are usually allowed.

Veganism

Vegans, however, whose organization dates only from the Second World War, base their diet on *ahimsa*, non-violence or dynamic harmlessness", and will not use any produce of animal origin. Although their diet has been criticized on the grounds of nutritional deficiencies, recent research suggests that it is adequate so long as it contains sufficient vitamin B12; vegans are more likely to suffer from a deficiency of B12 since this vitamin is only available from animal sources. It is also now widely believed that vegan diets are not unhealthy where children are concerned.

The findings of a research project carried out by investigators from Queen Elizabeth College, London and published recently in the *Journal of Human Nutrition*, show that children on a vegan diet are not necessarily at a disadvantage compared to those who are omnivorous (as had been suggested), though they tended to be slightly lighter and shorter. The report emphasized, however, that the few cases of malnutrition that had been found were in families when the parents lacked knowledge of vitamin requirements as publicized by the Vegan Society.

Dietary supplements

The chief nutritional supplements are vitamins – substances essential to life which our bodies cannot manufacture, and which must therefore be present in our diet, or added to it if they are not. Their importance became evident when in the eighteenth century the Scottish physician James Lind showed that the way to prevent scurvy on sailing vessels was to give each member of the crew a tot of lemon or lime juice, though it was not until two centuries later that vitamins as such were identified and vitamin C was credited as the preventive substance in scurvy.

Megavitamin therapy

Although the medical profession has accepted the need to ensure an adequate minimum vitamin intake, controversy has continued over what that minimum ought to be – and also what the maximum, if any, ought to be. Over the past decade, it has centred upon the merits, or defects, of what has become known as megavitamin therapy. This is the better-known name for what Dr Linus Pauling originally called "orthomolecular psychiatry", and is based on his belief that schizophrenia could be the consequence of vitamin deficiency. This was in the late 1960s and he has since widened his theory to include other illnesses, in particular cancer.

"I believe that it is possible by rather simple means, essentially nutritional, to increase the length of life expectancy for young and middle-aged people (and to some extent, perhaps, old people too) by about 20 years", Pauling has recently claimed. "Not only can the life expectancy be increased, I believe, but also the length of the period of well-being can be increased by the same amount, or perhaps even a little longer".

Megavitamin therapy consists of giving doses of vitamins to patients in appropriate amounts; what is "appropriate" being related to the individual patient's needs which, Pauling argues, are often much greater than has been realized. Megavitamin therapy should only be tried under professional supervision, following a proper diagnosis.

Vitamin C

Although Pauling's honours include two Nobel prizes (for chemistry in 1954 and for peace in 1963), the US Medal of Science and the French Pasteur Medal, they have not been sufficient to save him from being derided as a crank for his beliefs. But gradually it is coming to be accepted that there is more to vitamin C, at least, than has been recognized – as speakers made clear at a conference on the subject organized by the pharmaceutical company, Roche, in the spring of 1981.

What they did *not* succeed in making clear is precisely what vitamin C consists of. "Ascorbic acid" sounds like a description, but as one of the contributors to the discussion admitted, nearly 50 years after its chemical identification it "remains a mystery, a source of intense debate, and a scientific challenge".

Whatever it is, among evidence in its favour produced at the conference was the report by Professor J.W.T. Dickerson of the University of Surrey that cancer patients have an exceptionally high vitamin C requirement. This, as Geoff Watts, the BBC's commentator on health matters, observed, "is what Linus Pauling, doyen of the vitamin lobby, has been saying all along". And Thomas Irvin, a surgeon at the Royal Devon and Exeter Hospital, reported that after categorizing some 60 patients on the basis of the severity of the operations they had just had, he had found that the more severe they were, the greater the fall in blood levels of vitamin C.

These investigations confirm what Pauling has been preaching. When, in 1971, he surmised that with the proper use of vitamin C, the mortality rate from cancer could be reduced by 10 percent, it was on the basis of the vitamin's usefulness in promoting the healing of wounds. By fortifying the tissues, he argued, it would enable them to offer a better resistance to the spread of cancer cells. He has since come to the conclusion that this one in ten figure was too low. The incidence of cancer, he now believes, could be cut by half by appropriate megavitamin therapy.

Pauling's insistence that the vitamin dose must be related to the needs of the individual has often been disregarded, however, particularly in the United States, where vitamin supplements have become big business – much to the dismay of the Food and Drug Administration, who fear that people may be unwittingly swallowing excessive quantities, which could be a danger to health.

What is a balanced diet?

The upsurge of interest in supplementary dieting, with minerals as well as vitamins, has also begun to lead to problems in Britain, as a recent letter in *Here's Health* magazine has revealed. "When no fewer than 56 advertisements appear in one issue for every sort of pill under the sun providing the individual with what they claim to be the necessary", the writer complained, "you defeat the object of naturalness, when surely a good, balanced diet is far healthier and financially more prudent than pill-popping of any sort?"

The magazine's editor was able to counter by pointing out that few people knew how to maintain a well-balanced diet; there is not even any clearly established agreement on what constitutes such a balance. (Even if people do buy the correct ingredients, more often than not, they prepare or cook them in such a way that all valuable vitamins and minerals are lost). Different individuals, too, have different requirements, and so on. (For guidance in choosing which foods should be combined to make a balanced diet, see the chart on *Food group systems*, opposite.) But just as the editor of an orthodox medical journal is not in a position to slam the products of the drug companies whose advertisements alone keep it profitable, so that the intended message of a magazine dedicated to serving natural therapies may be blurred.

Food group systems

A system of "food groups" has been devised by nutritionists to help make it easier to choose a balanced diet. For the system to work, you must eat some food from each group daily and drink at least three to five glasses of water or fluids. The chart outlined below allows you to choose from different foods within each group and receive the same vital nourishment.

Food	Minimum daily requirement	Nourishment provided	Comments
High protein Meat, fish, poultry, game, offal, eggs, cheese, nuts, legumes	*2 servings* (each item = 1 serving) 3 oz meat, fish or poultry; 2 eggs; 4 oz cooked, dried beans, peas or lentils; 4 tbs peanut butter	Protein; fat; iron; A, D, B vitamins	Meat, fish and poultry have the highest concentration of high-quality protein; grains and nuts contain incomplete proteins.
Milk products Milk, cream, yoghurt, ice cream, cheese	*2 servings* (each item = 1 serving) 5 fl oz milk or yoghurt; 12 oz cottage cheese; 1 oz hard cheese	Protein; fat; calcium; D, A, B2 vitamins	Cream and cream cheese provide many calories and therefore energy, but they are low in protein; they are very high in animal fat.
Green/yellow vegetables Cabbage, kohlrabi, kale, mustard greens, spinach, brussel sprouts, green beans, celery, lettuce	*4 servings from among the 3 groups* (each item = 1 serving) 4 oz raw or cooked vegetables	Minerals including calcium, chlorine, chromium, cobalt, copper, manganese, potassium, sodium	All fruit and vegetables provide roughage and water.
Citrus fruits Tomatoes, oranges, grapefruit, strawberries, lemons, melons, papayas	6 fl oz juice; 1 orange; $\frac{1}{2}$ grapefruit; $\frac{1}{4}$ melon; 2 oz strawberries	Vitamin C	
Other fruits and vegetables Potatoes, beets, corn, carrots, cauliflower, apples, bananas, pineapples, apricots	1 large potato; 1 corn on the cob; 1 apple or banana; 4 oz cooked, canned or frozen cauliflower, carrots, peaches or pineapple	Carbohydrates; A, B, C vitamins	
Bread, four and cereals Bread, biscuits, noodles, rice, breakfast cereals, oatmeal	*4 servings* (each item = 1 serving) 1 slice of bread; 2 in biscuit; 1 oz breakfast cereal; 4 oz cooked cereal, rice, noodles or spaghetti	Protein; carbohydrates; B vitamin; iron, calcium	Whole-grain cereals and unpolished grains provide fibre. Avoid foods with refined flours or sugar as they provide few nutrients and many calories
Fats Butter, margarine, vegetable oils, fish oils, animal fats	1 or 2 tablespoons	A, D vitamins	There is more vitamin D in margarine than in butter. Both provide many calories; butter is also high in animal fat.

Weight-reducing diets

The largest proportion of people dieting at any given time is likely to be the weight-reducing, or fat-removing, brigade. Literally hundreds of diets have been worked out to enable the process to be conducted as quickly and effortlessly as possible. To recount them all would fill volumes, and in any case, they are not, strictly speaking, a form of natural therapy. Natural therapists, in fact, regard many of them, particularly the faddy, crash diets with a certain amount of suspicion.

One golden rule, in this connection, was prescribed nearly 2,500 years ago, in the aphorisms which were collected in the Hippocratic treatises. Discussing what to give patients who are unwell, the writer agreed that putting on weight would be dangerous, but insisted that dieting must not be taken to the point when the body becomes very thin: it should be brought "only to a condition which will naturally continue unchanged, whatever that may be". Our bodies, in other words, have, or would have, if we let them, a natural weight, a condition of equilibrium. Our aim should be to find it, and stick to it.

Checking your weight

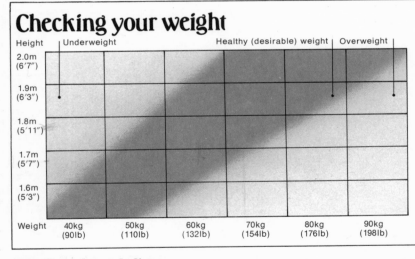

In order to find the healthy "desirable" weight for your height, first find your height on the left of the chart, then run your finger across the chart to your present weight. The dark band in the centre indicates the healthy weight. If yours is towards the edge of this dark band this may indicate that you are slightly below or above average weight in proportion to your height.

Appetite and metabolism

Appetite, naturopaths argue, is the clue. If appetite gets the saliva and the gastric juices working, massive amounts can be digested without difficulty. It is not the amount of food we eat, but our capacity to metabolize it which matters.

But the appetite must be natural. Aperitifs can artificially stimulate it, if it is jaded; they do not assist metabolism. The prospect of eating a sweet may be mouth-watering, but this is a conditioned reflex, an addiction, as the sweet will contain no nutrient worth having.

Food must be appetizing

It follows that any diet which does not appeal to your appetite, or worse, which deliberately sets out to dampen it down, is a bad diet. There is no point in eating raw carrots if you happen to loathe raw carrots, a point emphasized by Dr Ralph Bircher of the celebrated Bircher-Benner clinic near Zurich. The diet there has been kept austere, on fairly rigid naturopathic principles; the emphasis is on raw foods, with no meat, sugar products, alcohol, or coffee. Nevertheless, Dr Bircher has always insisted that it is not enough for a diet to be health-giving and close to nature: "it must also be more attractive than even the *haute cuisine* of the old school otherwise conversion will never be complete".

To some extent this is a matter of breaking with conditioning and with addiction. As anybody who has stopped taking two spoonfuls of sugar in each cup of tea or coffee or who has reduced salt intake will know, the initial stages can be difficult, but the time soon comes when an accidentally sweetened cup or over-salted food is pushed aside with distaste, even with revulsion. But allowing for a spell of getting rid of addictions, the best diet you are likely to find for yourself is one which offers the kind of meals you look forward to. Too often, dieting is presented as a form of self-restraint, which in turn can easily slide into a form of mortification of the flesh. But if appetite is to be aroused, much will depend on the content of the meals and how they are planned, prepared, cooked (if they are cooked), and presented.

Self-help

Dieting is fundamentally a matter of self-help, using the advice given in connection with natural therapies, coupled with any form of autosuggestion which will help, say, to get rid of an addiction to sugar-based food. But there are one or two "don'ts". There is little point in buying any of the gadgets promoted as weight reducers, as, for example, those that are supposed to massage off surplus fat. Some of them are electrically operated; others require muscle power. The common denominator is that they are all useless for the purpose they are intended to serve, though they may be fun to play around with. Surplus fat cannot be got rid of in this way. Nor can "reducing creams" perform any more success-fully. The only weight loss that such methods might bring about would be through the exercise involved. But this would be so slight as not to show up on the bathroom scales.

It is possible to lose weight by taking purgatives, but it is foolish to use them for that purpose. They create an artificial form of diarrhea, moving the food through faster than nature intended, and preventing it from being properly assimilated – a procedure that is hardly more sensible than it would be to reduce weight by taking pills to induce vomiting.

Ionization therapy

Air ionization therapy involves the use of special machines which artificially produce negatively charged air particles or ions.

Most air molecules are neither positively nor negatively charged (pure mountain air, for example contains only about 4,000 in every two million, million, million); those which do carry a charge are described as ionized. Ions are necessary for good health, but they should be in balance or negatively charged. Positively charged ions, it has been found, endanger health. These days most people live in places where negative ions are in short supply (in towns and cities where they are eliminated by smoke, dust and fumes) or where they are positively charged (as they can be in buildings with central heating systems) and need to be artificially boosted).

Origins

The effect of electricity (or certain winds) on health has long been the subject of comment by people who are weather-sensitive, who find they become depressed or suffer from headaches when there is "thunder in the air". With winds, whole populations may be affected. But although the hypothesis that there is a connection between the loss of some essential ingredient in the air and ill-health had been put forward earlier, it was not until the 1970s that proof was presented of the benefits of air ionization, when a paper by Professor A.P. Kreuger of the University of California established that it is possible to utilize negative ions to kill off bacteria. Since then, research projects in many countries have confirmed ionization's value as a form of (or adjunct to) treatment for a wide range of disorders.

Procedure

Air ionizers are available from specialist shops or from health centres. They come in various models and sizes, the commonest resembling a small portable transistor radio. They are portable, and can be used either for prevention of illness (for example in a car or a room where a meeting is being held, to counteract the "fug") and in the treatment of particular disorders.

Research

It has been possible to demonstrate the effects of ionization in controlled trials by comparing the performance of subjects in conditions where the air was positively ionized, negatively ionized and normal. One such trial was carried out in the Human Biology and Health Department of the University of Surrey, where the performance of 45 subjects carrying out standard tests was measured.

‘ The cause of many human ills, you see, is the ions. So says one Roger Wasmer of the US firm Alpha-Omega (and a more sincere fellow never sold a used car); the positive ions in air pollution ("particulants", as Wasmer calls them) are what cause people to become sick, tired and emotional . . .

More than three million Americans are even now paid up and awaiting delivery of Wasmer's box. He just cannot turn them out quickly enough to meet the demand for fresh air. The largest veterans' hospital in the US has one in each recovery room. Greyhound plans to install one in each of its coaches. And employees at a government office in Holland, Michigan, are so fond of the generators' influence that they threatened to walk out if a scientist proceeded with a controlled study of the boxes, which would have entailed turning half of them off. ’

Lois Wingerson
New Scientist (14 May 1981)

The performance of the subjects doing the tests in normal air conditions rose in the morning and afternoon, and declined in the evening, as expected. The same was true of subjects exposed to positively ionized air, except that their performance worsened more dramatically. But subjects exposed to negative ions maintained a high level of performance throughout the afternoon and evening – a result which, the investigators admitted, had not been what they had expected.

Air ionizers may also be used in the treatment of specific illnesses. For *Respiratory disorders* (see also pages 325 to 326), an ionizer can be placed on a table by the bedside. Following a trial with 3,000 patients in a Cologne clinic, Dr K.H. Schultz has reported that in the under 20 age group, over 80 percent of the patients reported complete relief, and a further 15 percent were considerably relieved. In the older age groups half obtained total relief, and only one in ten patients reported that the ionization had no beneficial effect.

No adverse side effects have yet been reported in connection with air ionization therapy – provided, of course, that the machine is in order. After a two-month trial at the Hebrew University in Jerusalem, where a group were exposed to negative ions for 16 hours daily and regular checks made; no harmful results were observed.

As a consequence, the US Food and Drug Administration has approved air ionizers as medical devices for the treatment of allergies, hay fever, and other common respiratory disorders.

Suitable cases

Surveying the evidence at a recent conference on ionization in London, C.A. Laws claimed that enough research had been carried out to remove any doubts about its beneficial effects and emphasized that "the processes are all natural ones carried out by our bodies in response to a trigger designed for that purpose. We are not imposing foreign processes". It follows that the kind of disorders which respond to nature cure in its other forms are likely to respond to ionization; many people without any particular disorder claim a sense of general well-being after exposure to negative ions.

For prevention, its value is likely to be greatest for people who live or work in conditions where the air is polluted by dust, smoke or other ion-removers. In treatment it has been most commonly used to combat respiratory disorders such as hay fever, asthma, and catarrh and for giving relief to patients with severe burns. Ionization has also been found to be of use to patients suffering from headache and hypertension. Respiratory disorders in particular, however, have been found to respond well to regular overnight treatment.

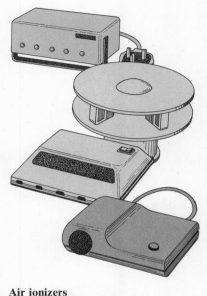

Air ionizers
Used to restore the balance of positive and negative ions in the atmosphere, helping everything from headaches to bronchitis. They are available in a number of different sizes and shapes; small ones can be installed in cars, larger ones are suitable for open-plan offices. Those shown here are for average room with a range of about 3–6 m (10–20 ft).

Bates eyesight training

It used to be believed – and to some extent it is still commonly assumed – that eyesight is a genetic endowment, which gradually deteriorates with age, and that this is a process which we can do nothing effective to delay. Further, actual diseases of the eye, such as glaucoma, can be treated, but there is no cure for sight which is failing from natural causes.

Naturopaths challenge this assumption. They believe that a balanced diet, in particular, can contribute to improving poor eyesight. They also advocate exercises which, they claim, can in some cases enable the wearer of glasses to dispense with them. These exercises are usually derived from the method propounded 60 years ago by Dr William H. Bates.

Origins

Bates was a Cornell graduate who became an eye specialist, and an instructor in opthalmology at the New York Postgraduate Medical School. Becoming dissatisfied with orthodox theory and practice, he gave up this appointment in order to find time to experiment, and in 1919 he published *Better Eyesight Without Glasses*, which was destined to become a bestseller in America – as was Harry Benjamin's description of the method for British readers, published 10 years later. Since then a number of new editions of the book, with revisions, have appeared, but Bates' basic principles remain unaltered.

Procedure

The Bates method has now been in use during a sufficiently long period for some of its practitioners to develop ideas of their own. Patients are usually seen intensively at first and then less frequently as treatment progresses. The aim is to get results right from the first session. You can expect to be shown how to carry out some or all (or more) of the following exercises:

Palming: Most people, Bates claimed, obtain some benefit simply by closing the eyes and relaxing. "But some light comes through the closed eyelids, and a still greater degree of relaxation can be obtained, in all but a few exceptional cases, by excluding it". The way to do this is to cover your eyes with the palms of your hands. Palming can be carried out two or three times a day, for about 10 minutes at a time.

Shifting and swinging: "One of the best methods of improving the sight, we now find, is to imitate consciously the unconscious shifting of normal vision" – the shifting, that is, which your eyes are continually doing as you read these words. This does not mean that you should make an effort to "swing" – Bates insisted there must be no strain. The aim of this exercise is to relax the eyes and help to mobilize them.

> ❛ *Whether I used my mind and bespectacled eyes well or badly, and what might be the effect upon my vision of improper use, were . . . to practically all other orthodox ophthalmologists, matters of perfect indifference. To Dr Bates, on the contrary, these things were not matters of indifference; and because they were not, he worked out, through long years of experiment and clinical practice, his peculiar method of visual education. That this method was essentially sound is proved by its efficacy.* ❜
>
> Aldous Huxley
> *The Art of Seeing*

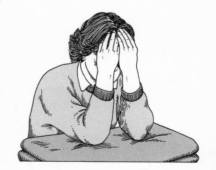

Palming
Close your eyes and cover them with your palms, making sure they do not touch the eyes. Think of something pleasant or listen to music – don't daydream. If the mind is blank, the eyes will not be relaxed.

Blinking: The purpose of blinking is to lubricate the eyes. People with defective vision, particularly those who are accustomed to wearing glasses, are apt to stare more, as if straining to see. "Learn to blink once or twice every 10 seconds", Harry Benjamin advised, "but without effort, no matter what you may be doing at the time, and especially when reading".

Splashing: The eyes should be splashed with water at least 20 times, morning and evening.

Near and far focusing: This involves holding pencils or other objects at a certain distance from your face and focusing with both eyes, first on one and then the other, blinking each time you change focus. This exercise can be repeated at odd intervals throughout the day whenever the opportunity arises, and it will help to rest the eyes.

Remembering and imagining: Bates laid great emphasis on the importance of the memory and the imagination as aids to better vision. Remembering colours while palming, he found, enabled people to see them better in actuality. The eyesight of one of his patients was "corrected by the memory of a yellow buttercup", and imagining a beautiful sunset could have a similar effect.

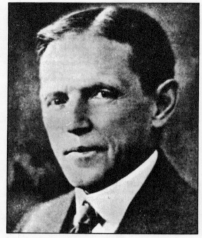

Dr William H. Bates
Dr Bates (1881–1931) became perturbed by the fact that although his patients were apparently responding to treatment, many continued to complain of headaches and eyestrain.

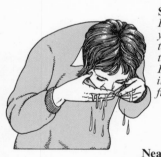

Splashing
In the morning, splash your closed eyes 20 times with warm water, then 20 times with cold. Repeat this in the evening but use cold water first, then warm.

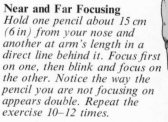

Near and Far Focusing
Hold one pencil about 15 cm (6 in) from your nose and another at arm's length in a direct line behind it. Focus first on one, then blink and focus on the other. Notice the way the pencil you are not focusing on appears double. Repeat the exercise 10–12 times.

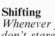

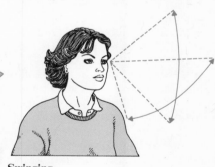

Swinging
With feet apart, stand in front of a window and sway gently from side to side 100 times. Blinking at left and right, look at something outside; notice how the window seems to move in the opposite direction to you yourself.

Shifting
Whenever you look at an object, don't stare but keep your gaze constantly shifting up and down and from one side of it to the other. The smaller the shift, the more the eye muscles will be exercised.

Bates was convinced that "presbyopia" – ageing sight – could be fought off with these methods, if they were used with determination. And he cited a case which Oliver Wendell Holmes had described in *The Autocrat at the Breakfast Table*, of an old gentleman living in New York State "who, perceiving his eyesight to fail, immediately took to exercising it on the finest print, and in this way fairly bullied Nature out of her foolish habit of taking liberties at five-and-forty, or thereabout" – so much so that his eyes became like "a pair of microscopes".

Suitable cases

Bates' exercises are suitable for people whose eyesight is failing so long as it is failing from what are ordinarily considered to be "natural" causes.

In other words, if there is any doubt in your mind that your eyes are basically healthy, it is important that you have them checked to ensure that there is not something organically wrong with them, such as glaucoma.

Self-help

While it is obviously preferable to be taught the method by a qualified Bates practitioner, if this is not practical (and they are few and far between) you can study Bates' book, *Better Eyesight Without Glasses* or Aldous Huxley's book on the subject, *The Art of Seeing*, as well, and work from them. But Bates' book is rather confusing in parts, and indeed, some practitioners these days have modified his technique. The techniques mentioned here only give you a guide as to how your vision can be improved without recourse to mechanical aids.

If you do take a course of Bates lessons, however, it will always be useful to practise the exercises between sessions so that your eyes are constantly being used and exercised in the correct way. Simply learning to blink regularly and consciously avoiding bad habits such as staring, which come with the wearing of glasses, the eyes will benefit.

Tissue salts therapy

The idea behind tissue salts therapy is that in today's society our bodies tend to lack certain essential and naturally occuring inorganic minerals or "tissue salts" which need to be replaced. Research has shown that particular disorders can be traced to deficiencies in specific salts.

Schüssler's twelve tissue salts

Biochemic name	Chemical name	Common name	Function	Indication
Calc. Fluor.	Calcarea fluorica	Fluoride of lime	Gives elasticity to connective tissues	Relaxed conditions (e.g. strained muscles, haemorrhoids, ruptures, etc)
Calc. Phos.	Calcarea phosphorica	Phosphate of lime	Helps build new cells for blood; promotes growth in children; good for bones and teeth	Wasting diseases; poor circulation; restorative in convalescence; skin eruptions
Calc. Sulph.	Calcarea sulphurica	Sulphate of lime (plaster of Paris)	Purifies the blood	Skin eruptions
Ferr. Phos.	Ferrum phosphoricum	Phosphate of iron	Contained in red blood corpuscles	Inflammations; minor injuries; early stages colds; sore throats; bronchitis; rheumatism
Kali. Mur.	Kali muriaticum	Chloride of potash	Aids metabolic processes	Congested conditions
Kali. Phos.	Kali phosphoricum	Phosphate potash	Nutrient in structure of nerve and brain tissues, muscles and blood cells	Nervous conditions; insomnia
Kali. Sulph.	Kali sulphuricum	Sulphate of potash	Aids formation of healthy skin cells, in destruction worn-out cells and in carrying oxygen to tissues	Asthma; rheumatism; rheumatic fever; catarrhal conditions; headaches; indigestion
Mag. Phos.	Magnesia phosphorica	Phosphate magnesia	Nutrient of blood, bones, teeth, brain, nerves, muscles	Relief of shooting pains, cramp, spasms; neuralgia; itching
Nat. Mur.	Natrum muriaticum	Chloride of soda	Aids regulation of moisture content in body	Wherever there are imbalances of salt in the system
Nat. Phos.	Natrum phosphoricum	Phosphate of soda	Regulates acid level in cells	Imbalances of bile, uric acid; indigestion; nausea; heartburn
Nat. Sulph.	Natrum sulphuricum	Sulphate of soda	Stimulates natural secretions	Liver conditions; headaches; asthma; nausea
Silicea (silica)	Silicea (silica)	Silicea (silica)	Promotes suppuration; essential constituent of connective tissues	General debility; toxic conditions, foul discharges

Origins

The need for salt replacement was first expounded by a German homeopathic physician, Dr Schüssler, in the 1870s. It was the basis of a new therapy which he called "biochemistry" – an unfortunate choice, as biochemistry was soon to blossom into an academic discipline with a far wider range of activities. All disorders, Schüssler believed, could be traced to deficiency in one or more of the elements which are essential if our systems are to function properly. He nominated 12 basic tissue salts.

Research

Orthodox biochemical research has since confirmed and amplified many of Schüssler's findings, as Eric F.W. Powell has shown in his handbook *Biochemistry*. "For example, a deficiency of calcium will tend to disorders of nutrition and of the skeleton; a lack of sodium leads to digestive troubles, acidity, rheumatism and associated disorders", and shortages of magnesium, iron and other tissue builders all create problems.

Dr W.H. Schüssler
Schüssler (1821–1898), believed that all diseases result from a lack or imbalance of one or more of the 12 basic tissue salts.

Procedure

Tissue salts are prescribed by many naturopaths, herbalists, homeopaths and other natural therapists. The practitioner will be concentrating on trying to find from an examination of you and your symptoms, which tissue salt, or salts, may be lacking. Powell emphasizes, however, that the psychological aspect has to be taken into consideration, because "it frequently happens that the correction of a mental condition is followed by an immediate return to normal in the organism". In other words, it may be the mind which is disrupting the body's chemical manufacturing system to create the deficiency, in which case replacement with remedies should not be necessary if the mind's problems are dealt with. Where replacement therapy *is* necessary, the tissue salts are prescribed in homeopathic potencies, according to the practitioner's estimate of the patient's requirements.

Self-help

Any disorder *may* be due to tissue salt deficiency. This therapy is normally tried when other forms of treatment have failed, or where you have found that you are deficient in some respect.

You can buy the tissue salts individually or as "combination remedies" made for specific disorders from health stores and some chemists. The salts are safe and can be taken without fear of side effects. While they are non-toxic and non-habit forming, care should always be taken to read the instructions regarding dosage.

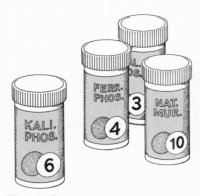

Tissue salts
Schüssler's tissue salts can be found in many health shops and homeopathic chemists.

HERBAL MEDICINE

As it is most widely practised, herbal medicine involves the preparation of the roots, leaves, stems and seeds of plants, either for consumption, in the form of medicine, or for use on the skin, as ointment. But as the many meanings of the term "balm" indicate, plants can be used in various ways. In aromatherapy, for example, they are often rubbed into the skin, usually through massage, and Bach remedies, made from flowers, are designed to have an effect on mood as well as on the body.

Attempts have been made to introduce a term which would embrace all the varieties of therapy which are based on the use of plants: "phytotherapy"; "botanotherapy"; "vegotherapy" are just a few. None of them except herbalism, however, has established itself in common use.

Herbalism

In a number of ways, herbal medicine lies a little outside the general run of alternative therapies. Herbs are available for anybody to pick, and they are in constant use in the kitchen; there is no clear line to be drawn between their culinary and their clinical use. They are in fact used extensively without reference to any medical herbalist's advice, either made up from plants or bought over the counter. And although there is a mass of information available about herbs from folklore and from the experience of individual herbalists, the range of agreement over what remedies to use for particular disorders is surprisingly small. Nevertheless, the use of remedies made from herbs (as distinct from medicine using only the "active ingredient" or synthetic versions), which had seemed to die out, is staging a recovery.

Origins

The question has often been asked: how did primitive people know which herbs were beneficial, and which were poisonous? The answer is simple: our early ancestors knew by instinct, as all species of wild animals (and to a lesser but still considerable extent, domestic animals) know instinctively, what they can and what they cannot eat and drink. More than that, animals even instinctively realize when, for some reason, their diet lacks certain vitamins or trace elements and they will migrate to new feeding grounds to find them (see page 16). Our forebears, presumably, had the same ability.

When instinct lost its powers, memory took over. For a time, however, memory and instinct worked in tandem. Tribal herbalists, investigators have found, combine traditional lore, handed

Free courses in phytotherapy (healing through plants) are being offered to members of the French medical profession by the privately financed Institut d'Enseignement de Phytothérapie (IEP).

In the last three years, the demand in France for herbal cures has increased enormously. The Institute was only started last May, and its courses have attracted more than 300 people a time, including dentists, pharmacists, biologists, veterinary surgeons and medical students.

Dr Moatti, IEP president, hopes the Institue will soon be recognized officially . . ."

*Times Health Supplement
25 December 1981*

down through generations, with intuition when prescribing and even when looking for herbs. The belief has lingered on in some folklore. In the west of Ireland, the tradition is that the right herb to treat an illness will not be found if it is searched for, but only if the seeker allows himself to be guided by the fairies – in other words, by clairvoyance.

Herbal medicine and astrology

In many early civilizations the medicinal plants came to be used in their own right, though often with an astrological element attached. Herbals came into standard use recommending specific plants for the treatment of specific symptoms, many of which are still in use today. In the Middle Ages, however, English physicians began to favour drugs compounded from a number of herbs, along with other substances such as ground animal horn. Druggists came into being, whose job it was to make up the physicians' prescriptions. Herbalists lost caste, but they did not go out of business altogether, for physicians were few in number, and mostly concentrated in London and a few other cities.

Culpeper's *Herbal*

Herbal remedies continued in use throughout the country. Two seventeenth-century herbals give a good idea of the medicinal plants then in use, and of how they were employed. One, compiled in the 1630s by John Parkinson, listed some 3,000 plants. The other, better known herbal was by Nicholas Culpeper.

Although he trained as an apothecary – the forerunner of the general practitioner of today – Culpeper believed in astrology, and in its importance in relation to plant life as well as to human life (such beliefs were not, at the time, considered eccentric: his contemporary Robert Boyle was fascinated by alchemy, as indeed was Isaac Newton, in the next generation). Nevertheless Culpeper's belief in astrology did upset those members of his profession who were beginning to try to make medicine a more exact science, separating it from what they were coming to regard as a superstition.

Still less did his contemporaries approve of Culpeper's decision to publish a translation of the then current *Pharmacopeia* from Latin into English. It was consequently Culpeper's book on herbal remedies, rather than other works, which was to establish itself as *the* English herbal, running through edition after edition, and making his name synonymous with the craft, as indeed to many people it still is today.

Plant extracts

Although remedies continued to be the mainstay of medical treatment, all the time the use of "simples", (single herbs prescribed for specific complaints) was being eroded. This was

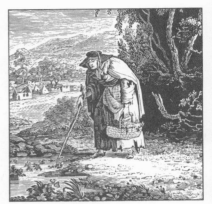

The herb gatherer
An antique woodcut by John Bewick (1753–1828) depicts an old woman collecting wild herbs. Today an increasing number of people are harvesting and drying their own herbs, normally for use as infusions.

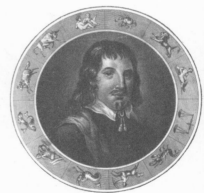

Nicholas Culpeper
Shown here, Culpeper (1616–1654), is famous for his Herbal, *which combines astrology with herbalism, hence this representation of him surrounded by the signs of the zodiac.*

partly a result of the physicians' passion for polypharmacy, (ever-weirder compounds of substances were being prescribed as drugs), and partly because of the discovery that it was possible to extract what was understood to be the medicinal component of the plant.

This enabled the medical profession to appropriate effective herbal remedies, and claim the credit. Thus when in the 1780s an English country doctor, William Withering, gave up all hope for one of his patients, a dropsical old woman, only to see her later, recovered, because she had taken a herbal tea made from dried, powdered foxglove leaves, he undertook experiments which led to its curative action being attributed to the ingredient digitoxin, rather than to the plant itself. Following this Withering was the first to see the connection between cardiac disorders and dropsy.

The development of synthetic drugs

Early in the nineteenth century, morphine was derived from the juice of the opium poppy, eventually supplanting the herbalist's remedy, laudanum, which consisted of tincture of opium in alcohol. Later still, heroin came from the same source, along with cocaine, originally used as a pain-killer, from the coca plant. In due course synthetic drugs arrived; these were imitations of the plant drugs but, it was claimed, as effective and more reliable.

By the beginning of the present century, the march of science on the one hand and of commerce, with its "patent medicines" on the other, meant that herbalists were being squeezed out of the high street into some hole-and-corner establishment, if indeed they survived at all. Ironically, two of the greatest names in the history of proprietary medicines (Thomas Beecham, who got to know his herbs while working as a shepherd boy, and went on to make a fortune from his pills and powders, and Jesse Boot, whose chain of chemists shops did much to make the proprietary medicines generally available) began their careers as herbalists.

Chemists replace the herbalists

A few individuals fought to keep herbal remedies before the public. Notable among them was Hilda Leyel who, between the wars, founded the Society of Herbalists, initiated and organized the Culpeper shops, and wrote a number of books about herbs, both medicinal and culinary. Leyel was also largely responsible for rousing opposition to a Pharmacy and Medicines Bill, (which, as originally drafted, would have made it difficult for herbalists to continue to practise in Britain) and for securing modifications.

Restoring herbalism to public acceptance

In 1947, Mrs Leyel gave an address to the King's College Biological Society which, in retrospect, can be seen as the start of the campaign to restore herbalism to public acceptance on the grounds that, successful though the new products of the pharmaceutical industry were, to place too much reliance on them was going to be dangerous.

One of the great objections to herbal medicines was that they were not standardized. But "it is the very fact that herbal medicines are *not* standardized that makes them of value", Leyel countered. "They are organic medicines instead of inorganic ones". It was strange, she thought, that at the very time when medical scientists had been discovering the importance of vitamins and enzymes, "modern practice is devoting so much ingenuity to devitalizing foods and medicines, depleting them of their vitality for the sake of standardizing them".

The drawbacks of the new drugs

In the same speech at King's College, Hilda Leyel drew attention to a feature of the new drugs which people then were hardly aware of. Herbalists, she pointed out, do not like to use poisonous remedies. "Some of the new synthetic drugs like penicillin are very poisonous. The modern problem when a new drug or compound is discovered is that the substance which is supposed to kill the germs of the disease is equally competent to kill the patient" – a warning she was to reiterate three years later in connection with the introduction of cortisone when she pointed out the link between cortisone and the plant from which African natives extract poison for the tips of their arrows.

Mrs Leyel died in 1957, when the wonder-drug era was still in its prime, before the revelations of the Kefauver enquiry and the thalidomide scandal. Events since have justified her arguments. Herbalism now enjoys the renaissance for which she laboured.

One of the reasons has been that "straight" plant remedies have been found necessary where modern drugs either create allergies, or breed resistant strains of bacteria. In his *Adventures in Healing*, published shortly after Mrs Leyel's death, Dr Heinz Graupner drew attention to the value of some of the contents of "nature's medicine chest", such as the birthwort plant, long used to clear up ulcers and infected wounds, and invaluable in cases where the patient cannot take penicillin without serious adverse reactions.

The revival of plant remedies

The most striking example of the value of natural remedies in recent times has been a report from a London hospital of the successful treatment of a patient suffering from an infected wound following a kidney transplant operation. When antibiotics proved of no avail, a member of the surgical team recalled that he had seen African tribal healers cure similar infections by placing thin strips of papaya fruit in the wound, "like cement in a crack". Somebody went out to buy a papaya and within a week, the wound had healed.

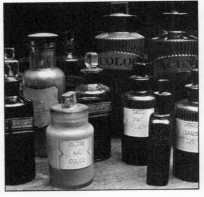

Herbal remedies
Herbalists concoct their remedies from plants or extracts, each treatment being specifically blended for the individual patient. They aim not only for relief of the patient's symptoms, but also for an improvement in his general standard of health.

Isolating active ingredients

At the same time, with faith in synthetic drugs being shaken by the depressingly high failure rate in the production of new types, more attention has been given to the investigation of herbal remedies, some of which have been in use for millennia. The manufacturers hope, of course, to be able to isolate the pharmacologically active substance, refine it, and market it. Ordinarily this would bring no benefit to the herbalist. But one of the consequences of the renewed interest in plants as the source of drugs has been the discovery that it can be the whole plant, not the supposed active ingredient, which has the beneficial action.

This has been emphasized by Dr William A.R. Thomson, for many years editor of *The Practitioner*, and Chairman of the British Academy of Forensic Science. In his *Herbs that Heal*, he has described how the realization has begun to dawn that the "active principle" sometimes mysteriously ceases to be active when isolated. Worse, it may become active in unwanted ways, producing side-effects.

A possible explanation is that nature endows plants with a balance which is somehow lost if the whole plant is not used. As an illustration, Thomson cites the risks to patients who are prescribed "glycosides", the active principle of the foxglove leaf. In one American hospital where patients were treated for heart conditions with glycosides, one in four suffered severe side-effects, and some of them died as a consequence.

This point has since been taken up by Malcolm Stuart, originally a researcher into viruses, whose work in Africa convinced him that plant drugs, which he had originally thought were simply quack cures prescribed by superstitious witch doctors, really were effective. The fact that digitoxin from foxglove leaves is as effective as, and safer than, the active glycoside ingredient, strikes him as important. "I have a theory that the whole plant contains secondary effect-enhancing substances", he has explained, adding that more research was needed into "the buffering effect, the synergistic effect" in such cases.

Herbal remedies have also been given a boost by the World Health Organization, which has been supporting efforts in the undeveloped countries to extend the use of plant drugs, to enable them to spend a lower proportion of their limited resources on proprietary drugs. The ecological movement, too, and the spread of health food shops have helped to make herbal preparations more widely available.

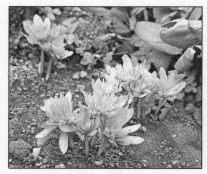

Autumn crocus
The autumn crocus is a member of the lily family. The flower grows in autumn on a stem bare of leaves, giving it its common name "Naked boys". The seeds are sometimes used in the treatment of gout.

Procedure

There are trained herbalists who take patients and examine them, take a case history, and follow the usual course before prescribing their remedies. But the majority of people who use herbal remedies do so on the advice of friends, or with knowledge gained from reading articles or books. To a great extent, therefore, herbal medicine is a matter of self-medication, and often far removed from herbalism proper.

However, you may find that there is a practitioner of herbal medicine in your vicinity as distinct from somebody simply selling herbs. If so, it will probably be under some title such as "medical herbal consultant", and it will be necessary to make an appointment. The consultation is likely then to follow the same course as it would with a naturopath. Moreover, the herbalist may also be a naturopath, for many nature cure practitioners now recommend herbal remedies.

Consulting a medical herbalist

At your first consultation, the medical herbalist takes a complete case history, recording all previous illnesses, inoculations, allergies (if any), genetic tendencies, trips abroad, and reactions to drug therapy or other forms of medical treatment. Your diet, and any stress factors at home or at work are considered and a physical examination is given.

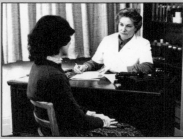

1 *The herbalist starts by taking a full medical history, concentrating especially on your present symptoms. This patient has a rash on her forehead.*

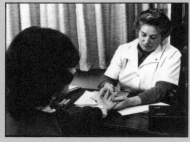

2 *She examines the patient's hands to check whether there are any lesions on the skin or nails.*

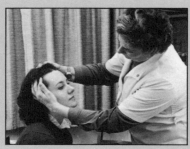

3 *The patient's rash near the hairline and the patch of dry skin between her eyebrows is observed.*

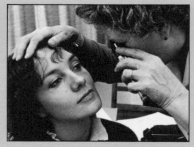

4 *The herbalist concludes the examination by inspecting the eyes for clarity; looking particularly at the retina.*

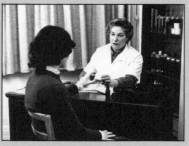

5 *Having reached a diagnosis, the herbalist prescribes plant remedies. These will be given to the patient before leaving but they may be adjusted later as the patient progresses.*

Struggle for the soul of herbalism

At this point a problem arises. The great majority of people who take up herbal medicine, whether or not they go to a herbalist, take it up for the treatment (or prevention) of symptoms. "What irks experienced users of herbal remedies, professional and lay, is how far this view differs from reality and how severely it misconstrues the real advantages of the therapy", Simon Mills, Director of Research at Britain's National Institute of Medical Herbalists, has complained. "As symptomatic remedies, frankly, herbs are rather pathetic: do we need to go back a century to fight again their miserable fight against the really successful symptomatic remedies of modern man?"

What Mills is saying, and many thoughtful supporters of herbal remedies agree with him, is not that herbs are entirely useless as symptom-removers (they have a role there, too, and a growing one, now that the symptom-bashing remedies of modern man are all too often proving less successful, or causing adverse reactions). But herbs ought to be regarded as a contribution to the holistic health movement, and not as just another method of getting rid of the outward and visible signs of inward and invisible disease processes.

This struggle for the soul of herbalism is not something which we can deal with here. Anybody who wishes to become familiar with the background should read Barbara Griggs' *Green Pharmacy: A History of Herbal Medicine*, a carefully researched and well-written survey which sets the struggle in its historical perspective. For our present purposes, it is sufficient to make the point that medical herbalism should not be regarded as just a matter of trying out herbal remedies to find whether any of them relieve your headache or your asthma.

Most people, however, who contemplate trying herbal remedies for the first time, are likely to do so in the hope of curing or warding off some unwelcome disorder. And they can expect to be advised on this by the practitioner, though he or she may also (and is now increasingly likely to) encourage you to think in terms of removing the cause of your symptoms, rather than simply of removing the symptoms themselves.

We do not propose to go into the way herbal remedies are selected and prepared, as anybody who wants to try them without first taking a herbal practitioner's advice would be wise to obtain them from a specialist shop, and use them strictly according to the instructions on the packet or bottle. Selection is very much a matter of trial and error, as the herbals, past and present, offer a variety of possible remedies for almost every symptom in the book. At least you have one consolation, however, and that is that even if some herbal remedies do not work for you, they are very unlikely to be attended by unwelcome side-effects.

Research

One of the criticisms constantly levelled against herbal medicine is that its remedies have not been properly tested. This is only partly true. In *Green Pharmacy* Barbara Griggs describes what happened in connection with one research project, set up to test "Bio-Strath Elixir", a herbal product marketed by a Swiss business man, Fred Pestalozzi.

The Bio-Strath story

A Zurich trial with mice showed that if mice were subjected to X-rays, Bio-Strath protected their fertility, they had more and larger litters. In a controlled trial, in the Netherlands, with 123 mentally retarded children, those who had been taking Bio-Strath showed a significant improvement in their powers of concentration and self-expression. In another trial in Switzerland, in which 60 doctors were asked to test Bio-Strath on patients, "the overwhelming majority were so impressed by the improvement produced that they said they would prescribe it again".

Accordingly, Pestalozzi and his British agent, the naturopath Michael van Straten, applied for a licence to market Bio-Strath in Britain. The Committee on Safety of Medicines refused it on the ground that the tests had not proved it to be safe, so Pestalozzi organized laboratory tests to prove that it had no toxic effects. In the meantime, a further trial in Switzerland on cancer patients recuperating after surgery showed "dramatic improvements in appetite, physical activity and general condition; the patients taking it gained on average around seven pounds more than the control patients". Yet even then, the Committee rejected three out of the nine preparations which a licence had been applied for, in spite of the fact that all of the ingredients in the three rejected preparations were available over the counter in Britain.

At the same time, the research effort was suddenly blocked. The doctors who had seen Bio-Strath's remarkable results with cancer patients were asked to continue the trials, at Pestalozzi's expense. But, "after originally agreeing, they changed their minds a month later and stopped the trials without explanation. Neither Pestalozzi nor van Straten has been able to persuade a single hospital to run similar trials".

Campaigns against medical herbalism

There can be little doubt about the reasons for the unwillingness of orthodox medical researchers to investigate herbal remedies – rank prejudice, coupled with the fact that there is rarely any money in it. In the United States, the position is even worse, as the Food and Drug Administration (FDA) has run a relentless campaign against medical herbalism, even to the point of confiscating a consignment of honey on the ground that it was wrongly claimed to be nutritionally valuable. A claim that a herbal product has medicinal properties, or advice on how it should be used medicinally, removes a herbal product from the "culinary" category and transfers it to the "drug" category – where it is at once required to satisfy FDA requirements. These entail setting up research projects on a scale, and at a cost far beyond the herb industry's resources, even when there is no serious doubt about the safety of the remedy.

The plain fact, Professor Norman Farnsworth, a leading US expert on plant drugs, has complained, is that the FDA "don't want to know, don't want to get involved and are unresponsive to suggestions". Congress has not allocated the FDA funds with which to regulate the herb industry, and, "from my experience with the FDA their current personnel have little understanding of the inherent toxicological and technical aspects of herbs. They are primarily interested in interpreting current laws in a way that will cause them the fewest problems".

Ginseng – a much maligned drug

Nevertheless, there are signs that the prejudice is being broken down – among them, the progress of research into ginseng, a root which has been used as a mild stimulant for millennia in the Far East, but has only recently become popular in that capacity in the West. "Ginseng is another old, much-maligned drug that is being reexamined and proving most interesting", Professor E.J. Shellard of London University observed in his inaugural lecture in 1974. "It has anti-infective and anti-fatigue properties and there is accumulating evidence of its anti-stress activity".

The maligning had been due to the fact that what were thought to be ridiculously exaggerated claims for the drug were made in the Chinese *Pharmacopeia* where it was described as preventing, among other things, headache, exhaustion and depression, as well as being a useful adjunct in the treatment of diseases of the circulation, the kidneys, and the nervous system. But three years later, Dr Stephen Fulder, a lecturer in human biology at the same college, described how he had found a "surprisingly extensive literature on the pharmacological effects of ginseng", chiefly from the Soviet Union and the Far East and, he said, "even after discarding poor-quality papers, I was left with a bewildering array of positive results".

As with all the psychoactive drugs, the effects of ginseng have proved hard to quantify in trials because so much depends not just on the individuals taking it, but on their mood at the time. Still, Fulder has found a general pattern emerging from experiments: "the stress response, whether behavioral (such as fear) or homeostatic (such as temperature regulation) is exaggerated, but then returns to normal more quickly. Therefore in the long term adrenal capacity is maintained and even increased". Ginseng, in

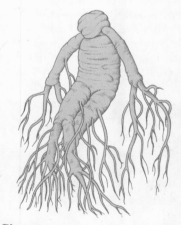

Ginseng
Ginseng, an Asian plant, is notable for its calming and restorative properties, particularly when dealing with stress, although many other wider claims are made for its powers. The root of the plant is used and readily available in tablet form.

other words, does not do the homeostatic system's work for it, as some drugs do, thereby weakening it; it is one of a class of drugs for which he proposes the name "adaptogens", which are normally harmless but can help to restore body processes to normal "when faced with stress or damage".

Evening primrose oil

There are other signs of the prejudice against herbal remedies breaking down. Last year, in an article in *World Medicine*, Geoff Watts, the BBC's Health commentator, asked what links schizophrenia, Parkinsonism, eczema, dry eyes, alcoholism, obesity, rheumatoid arthritis, cardiovascular disease, breast disease, brittle nails and the premenstrual syndrome? "What links the maladies in this apparently random collection is that all respond to, or might in theory respond to, treatment with an oil extracted from the seeds of the evening primrose plant".

This kind of assertion, Watts admitted, was not likely to win medical friends and influence scientific people; "but evening primrose *is* winning some medical friends, *is* influencing some scientific people" – among them the well-known medical researcher Dr David Horrobin, who has been exploring the effects of cis-linoleic acid and gammalinolenic acid which the seeds are rich in. Although results have been mixed, they have been promising in connection with some of the disorders Watts listed, and with multiple sclerosis. But as the evening primrose grows

At a herbal shop
Many plant remedies are available over the counter in herbal shops. It is generally best to take advantage of the herbalist's experience and seek advice on the most suitable herbs for your specific complaint than to try to decide for yourself.

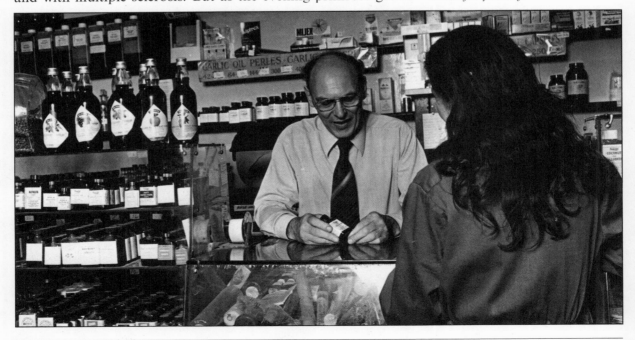

wild, its oil cannot be patented, so there has been little interest from the major drug companies, except in the possibility of producing a synthetic version, should the trials produce more evidence in the oil's favour.

Worldwide research into herbalism

Although research into herbal medicines has been taken much further in the Far East, particularly in China where it has been extensively and carefully conducted, the findings are not yet taken seriously in the West. Research in the developing countries, though it is now being conducted on an ever-increasing scale, has rarely fulfilled the West's protocol requirements.

One reason is the difficulty of holding controlled trials of the kind that orthodox medicine now relies upon to test drugs, as an article in the *New Scientist* by Joseph Hanlon has indicated. Research into medicinal plants in Ghana has "a high priority", he explains; the researchers use "sophisticated analytical chemistry techniques, collaborate with laboratories all over the world and publish in prestige western journals". The results demonstrate beyond all question that many medicinal plants have therapeutic properties: "analysis shows they contain many compounds already familiar to pharmaceutical chemists and do have the antibiotic and other properties claimed for them". Some even work for ailments "which cannot be effectively treated by modern 'scientific' drugs".

But to demonstrate the effectiveness of plant drugs in formal controlled trials in Ghana would present formidable problems. For a start, they are ordinarily prescribed by local medicine men, who would be unlikely to be fitted easily into the rigorous protocol of a modern investigation. Nor can plant drugs be tested in the same way as synthetic drugs, because they display wide variations according to where and when they are collected.

"Plants vary widely according to soil and the time of the year (and sometimes the time of day) when they are picked", Hanlon points out. This should come as no surprise, in view of the striking differences in the quality of wine, according to the location of the vineyard and the weather. Plants do not necessarily keep their potency when stored, which should also come as no surprise, considering the difference between vegetables straight from the garden, and vegetables bought in shops. And their manner of preparation can also make a difference.

Reviving Culpeper's ideas

Paradoxically, the realization of the importance of some of these variables – notably the influence of the time of day the plant is picked – is doing something to rescue Culpeper from the disfavour into which he had fallen in the eyes of modern, "scientific" herbalists.

"The quasi-herbalist Nicholas Culpeper attempted to take herbalism back into the world of astrology and the occult", as Frederick Hyde, Chairman of the British Herbal Pharmacopeia Committee, has put it, explaining that such views are no longer taken seriously. "Their ideas are not consistent with those generally accepted by herbalists, and give the false impression that herbal medicine is atavistic and archaic. Nothing could be further from the truth". But the recent investigations of lunar cycles on plant growth, along with research into biorhythms and paranormal phenomena, suggest that some of the occult notions of the old herablists may not have been so crazy, after all.

Until recently, scientists felt there was no more to be said about occult beliefs. But "a growing body of perfectly respectable scientific opinion suggests that there may, after all, be plenty more to be said", Barbara Griggs observed, "and that we are only at the beginning of a new knowledge of what plants and men and life

Making herbal remedies

Mixing the tinctures
Many medical herbalists have their own dispensaries in which they prepare tinctures and make up remedies according to the needs of their patients.

To make such tinctures, the roots, leaves and/or flowers of herbs may be used. In the course of a fortnight dried herbs are macerated in a variety of liquids, usually alcohol and water, and then the mixture is placed in a special press to obtain the actual tincture. After filtering, the tincture is ready for use.

Mixing Remedies
In herbal medicine it is usual to administer more than one herb at a time, so that the herbalist dispenses a mixture of tinctures. The first step is to measure out each of the tinctures precisely.

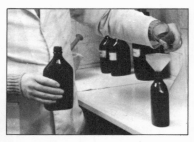

The tinctures are poured into a medicine bottle and mixed together. A reaction may occur between the various medicines, making further pharmaceutical adjustment necessary.

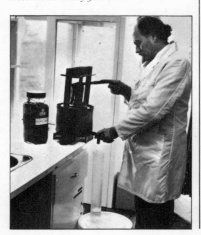

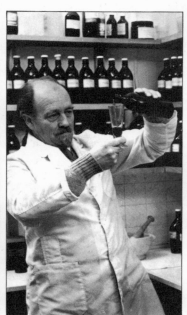

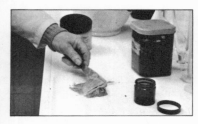

The herbalist also uses creams, ointments and cerates made from organic materials such as beeswax, lanolin, alcohol and/or oils, to administer herbs to the patient. These need careful blending.

itself are about, and how intricately man and plant interrelate". One suggestion is that plants, "in common with all living beings, have a non-physical energy field which may react directly on the 'energy field' of people they may be used to treat". This would help to account for such phenomena as the "green fingers" of some gardeners, and the evidence for plant sensitivity provided by John Whitman in *The Psychic Power of Plants*, and Peter Tomkins and Christopher Bird in *The Secret Life of Plants*.

Suitable cases

The chief value of herbal remedies for most people who use them for self-medication, is in the treatment of everyday disorders. Deciding which remedy to use is largely a matter of trial and error, because "placebology" plays so large a part in determining how effective they are going to be.

Over-the-counter herbal remedies are commonly used as palliatives designed to soothe away the pain, the irritation, or whatever the disturbance may be. Their justification in this role is that they are cheaper, safer, and can be more effective than many of the suppressors which are mass-marketed.

The role of herbs in preventive medicine

Herbal remedies are also widely used in preventive medicine – for example, in place of tea or coffee by people who want to cut down their intake of caffeine, and as an addition to the bath water to keep the skin in good condition.

According to Maurice Mességué of Provence, the best-known contemporary herbalist (his patients have included King Farouk, Ali Khan and Pope John XXIII), herbal remedies can be of help in almost every known disease. In his influential book *Health Secrets of Plants and Herbs*, Mességué lists herbs which can be used in treating well over 100 disorders. One snag is that he offers so wide a choice for some complaints – as many as 20 or 30 possible remedies. As with *Homeopathy* (see pages 66 to 73), this is inevitable if the herbalist is prescribing for a type of patient, not just for a type of disease.

It is particular patients, too, rather than particular disorders, that are regarded as most likely to benefit from herbal remedies. But some symptoms feature on all lists – catarrh, colds, coughs, tonsillitis, headaches and other pains; rheumatic and arthritic pains; diffuse aches; non-specific urethritis and thrush; earache; toothache; loss of appetite; insomnia; skin troubles, such as acne and dandruff; digestive disorders such as dyspepsia, nausea, constipation and diarrhea; and minor accidents and injuries – burns, scalds, cuts, bruises, insect bites and so on. It is commonly emphasized that herbal remedies, internal or external, are of value as adjuncts to other forms of treatment.

Self-help

Although Simon Mills of the National Institute of Medical Herbalists disapproves of what he describes as "the growing fashion to use simple herbs for many of the common prescriptions dispensed for everyday ailments", because the information about them is so often "confused and contradictory", he is all for the exploration by individuals of herbal remedies: "there is something very appealing about choosing a remedy from the garden, field or hedgerow rather than relying on an unfamiliar, isolated chemical". He suggests starting with 10 common herbs, to see what effect they have, and lists burdock, dandelion, horseradish, parsley, garlic, chamomile, ribwort, comfrey, wild oat and meadowsweet, which cover most of the everyday non-serious disorders. No two herbalists would have the same list, nor do the standard herbals agree what each plant should be used *for*. But a look through a few herbals will give you an idea of which herbs are most commonly recommended for your problem.

Preparing a herbal infusion

There is one simple standard method of preparation: a pint of boiling water poured over an ounce of dried herb or ground-up root (or 30g to half a litre) left to steep in a covered vessel for 5 to 15 minutes, and taken by the cupful 1 to 3 times a day according to instructions. The aim, Mills reiterates, should be to use herbs which you personally find improve your general health.

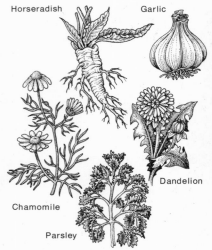

Herbs and their remedial properties
Clockwise from top right: *garlic is an antiseptic and can be used as a wound dressing; dandelion treats the liver, gall-bladder and urinary organs; parsley is a gentle laxative and diuretic; chamomile is an appetite stimulant and general tonic as well as being a pain-reliever; and horseradish can be applied directly to stings and bites.*

Aromatherapy

The term aromatherapy implies the use of our sense of smell in the prevention and treatment of disorders, and it is still occasionally used in this sense – for example in Benjamin Walker's *Encyclopedia of Metaphysical Medicine*. Walker describes it as one of the techniques of breathing used to promote health: a branch of "ophresiology" (from the Greek *ophresis*, meaning smell), the study of the effects of different smells from flowers, herbs, spices etc. The belief was that "the natural fragrance from living plants as well as the aromas from compounded ingredients, are equally efficacious in aromatherapy, but each kind of odour has its own particular virtue . . ."

Nowadays, however, "aromatherapy" is most commonly used to describe a particular type of treatment in which essential oils or "aromatic essences" are rubbed into the skin, or used as inhalants, or in baths and footbaths, and, less often, ingested.

> *Physicians might, . . . make greater use of scents than they do, for I have often noticed that they cause changes in me, and act on my spirits . . . which makes me agree with the theory that the introduction of incense and perfume into the churches . . . was for the purpose of raising our spirits, and of exciting and purifying our senses, the better to fit us for contemplation.*

Montaigne
Essay on Smells c. 1580

Origins

Essential oils were used in medicine in China as far back as the records there go. They were in common use in all ancient civilizations. They even feature in the *Bible* in one of the most familiar of all Jesus' parables, about the man who fell among thieves, who left him half dead. After the priest and the Levite had passed him by on the other side, the good Samaritan had compassion on him and "bound up his wounds, pouring in oil and wine".

Synthetic drugs replace essential oils

Oils continued in common use for a variety of purposes until they were gradually squeezed out by the discovery of the chemical constitution of plants and by more easily mass-produced chemical substances. Eventually preparations such as morphine and later heroin, cocaine and many more in which the essential oil of a

An aromatherapy factory
At Charabot and Co. in France, essential oils are distilled from plants to be used in aromatherapy. The essences can be found in the roots, flowers, leaves, bark or resin, depending on the plant. In all cases, though, they are found in minimal quantities and this makes them very expensive.

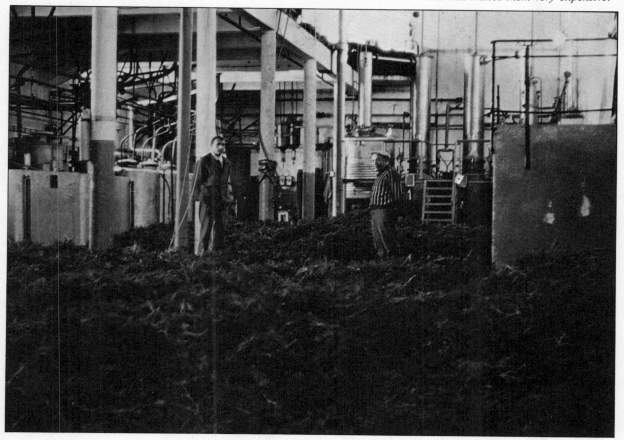

plant was displaced, therapeutically, by its alkali, which came to be regarded as the vital ingredient. The antiseptics, too, began to replace oil in the treatment of wounds.

During the First World War, however, the limitations of carbolic acid and other antiseptics became apparent, and the French chemist Professor René Gattefossé began to try out oils once again (after having accidentally burned his hand, he put it into a jug containing lavender essence, and found that it prevented blisters from forming). His work was followed up by Marguerite Maury and others in France, though it is only in the last decade that it has begun to make progress in Britain, largely through the efforts of Robert Tisserand, himself the author of several books on aromatherapy and the proprietor of a company producing essential oils.

Aromatic essences, according to Dr Jean Valnet in *The Practice of Aromatherapy* "are volatile, oily, fragrant substances which can be obtained from plants in a variety of ways; sometimes by *pressing* (e.g., cloves), sometimes by *tapping* (laurel, camphor), sometimes by *separation* using heat (turpentine) in some cases by *solvents*, or by *enfleurage* (absorption of the perfume by a greasy substance from which it is afterwards separated)". But they may have to be distilled, a process which requires considerable quantities of the plant.

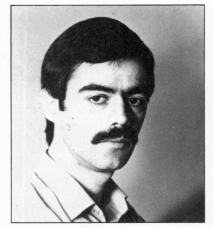

Robert Tisserand
Research by Tisserand has shown that natural essences have a mysterious influence on mood and emotions. Essence of Jasmine, for example, is uplifting, while essence of Linden Blossom has relaxing properties.

Procedure

Essential oils are most commonly applied during massage. The patient benefits both through the oil penetrating the skin and, at the same time, through inhaling it. Oils can also be applied as creams (usually in beauty treatments), ointments, lotions, or potions – though controversy continues over whether they should be taken internally. In his *Aromatherapy* Dr W.E. Arnould-Taylor states bluntly that the practice is to be deprecated, citing Marguerite Maury, who found that the mucous membrane of the digestive tract was too sensitive to essential oils, and adding that the oils can be dangerous when taken with other forms of medication. But Dr Valnet, probably the most experienced medical practitioner of aromatherapy in the world, does prescribe internal applications.

Distinguishing aromatherapy and herbalism

In some treatments, the normally clear-cut distinction between herbalism and aromatherapy becomes blurred. Aromatherapists, however, tend to try to distance themselves from the herbalists, so that they can be looked upon as therapists in their own right, rather than simply as a spin-off group. In Britain, the training of herbalists has been formalized into recognized schools and an institute, but this has not happened with aromatherapists.

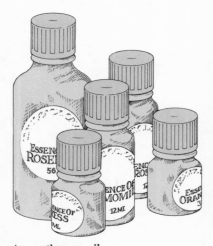

Aromatherapy oils
Essential oils used in aromatherapy are extracted from a variety of herbs, spices, flowers, woods and resins. The oils are highly concentrated and need to be kept in dark bottles to protect them from light.

As far as the raw materials are concerned, "in herbalism, usually a large quantity of the distillation needs to be taken because of its comparative weakness", Arnould-Taylor claims. "In essential oils, the quantities used are very small because of the high concentration". He adds that the quantity and quality of the product is easier to control in essential oils.

Consulting an aromatherapist

Aromatherapy is used to treat the whole range of disorders but it is especially effective with psychosocial complaints. The way the oils are applied varies according to the nature of the disorder – urogenital disorders, for example, may be treated orally or with hip baths, whilst respiratory problems are normally treated with inhalation or back massage. Your preferences with regard to methods of treatment will always be taken into consideration.

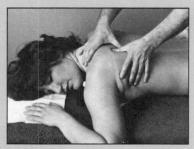

1 *The therapist establishes the patient's symptom picture and the background to her problem. Then he selects the appropriate spectrum of oils for this condition from a stock of about 40 different ones.*

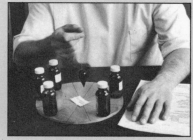

2 *Placing a "tally" from the patient in the centre of a dowsing disc – a lock of hair or a handwriting sample – the therapist will dowse to find the most suitable oil and then the best method of treatment.*

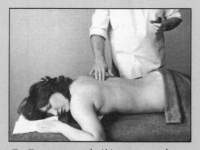

3 *Concentrated oil is massaged into the spinal reflex. Spinal massage is effective for many disorders – the specific complaint determines the exact point on the spine that will be treated.*

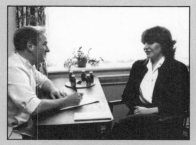

4 *The therapist massages a large area of skin in the affected region of the body with diluted oil. This patient was suffering from a respiratory complaint.*

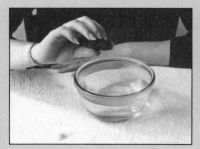

5 *Inhalation is also commonly used as a method of treatment. The patient sprinkles a few drops of concentrated oil into a small bowl of boiling water.*

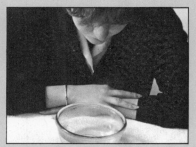

6 *Then she hangs her head over the bowl and breathes deeply. Inhalation is most frequently prescribed for disorders originating in the lungs or head.*

Robert Tisserand gives another reason. He claims that the basic difference between herbs and essences is due to "the ethereal nature of the oils", which are highly volatile, giving them "a profound effect on the mental/emotional level, an effect comparable to the Bach Flower Remedies". As this effect can be even more powerful than their action on the body, "aromatherapy lends itself to a holistic mind/body approach which goes beyond normal practice".

Varying effects of the same herb

To judge from one of the case histories Tisserand has provided in a recent issue of the *Aromatic Oil Company Bulletin*, the mind/body effect can indeed be startling. An aromatherapist decided to try out clary sage on a patient suffering from depression; "during the treatment he was convinced he was floating in the air and kept opening his eyes, fearing he would bang his head on the ceiling". The therapist reported that he had barely finished the massage "when I had to crawl off to the nearest empty floor space where I 'passed out'". All had ended well, with the patient leaving on a "high", but the therapist had not cared to try clary sage again. Experiences with the same ingredients differ widely, however, because patients are unique, and each one will probably have a slightly different reaction to the same herbs. For example, Donald Stevens, another English aromatherapist, also dealing with a long-term depressive (this patient had been treated conventionally, homeopathically and with acupuncture before coming to him for help) reported that "these previous treatments had given minimal benefit and created too great a reaction. But clary sage made her feel both mentally and physically lighter, and a course of five treatments changed the situation dramatically".

Although the term aromatherapy is only occasionally used to refer to treatment or prevention of disorders simply with the help of the sense of smell, it is by no means improbable that this method, too, will make a comeback. (The ancient tradition that certain herbs could provide protection from the plague lingers on in the posy which is carried before a judge on his way to an assize.) Although swooning is no longer fashionable, the role of smelling salts in prompting recovery is still remembered. Herbal pillows, too, are on the market, to offer protection from a variety of ailments, and to aid sleep.

Research

According to Tisserand, research in Italy has shown that essential oils sprayed from an aerosol can be used in the treatment of patients suffering from anxiety or depression: "The effect of odours on the emotions has been known for centuries, but it is only in the last 30 years or so that we have begun to realize the healing potential of this deep, inherent response to fragrance". The actual perception of fragrance by the patient, he believes, is an important factor.

Suitable cases

Arnould-Taylor's case histories in his book *Aromatherapy* suggest that almost any disorder in the psychosomatic or stress-induced range may be treated with satisfactory results. The combination with massage extends its scope. Valnet gives a list of disorders which, he claims, have responded well to aromatherapy – among them shingles, skin disorders (including the effects of burns or wounds), and rheumatism.

Bach flower remedies

These consist of 38 specially prepared remedies derived from the flowers of plants. Based on the method invented by Dr Edward Bach, these remedies are prescribed as treatment for what Bach believed to be the underlying cause of any physical disorder – a negative emotional state. Dr Bach's theory was that if you work on a patient's anxiety, depression, bitterness or resentment the physical symptoms associated with the problem will disappear.

Origins

Bach originally trained as a pathologist and bacteriologist, qualifying in London shortly before the First World War. On becoming dissatisfied with orthodox medicine, he switched to *Homeopathy* (see pages 66 to 73), experimented with homeopathic remedies, and in the course of his work he came to the conclusion that the homeopathic belief in the importance of the patient, as distinct from the nature of the patient's symptoms, could be utilized more effectively by prescribing remedies on the basis of the patient's emotional condition. This could be linked, Bach believed, to the appropriate remedy, partly by rule of thumb (some remedies were particularly effective in cases of, say, depression), partly by intuition.

"Throughout his years of medical practice, he had been seeking for scientific proofs, using his intellect", Bach's colleague, Nora Weeks has recalled. "A change now came about. He became extremely sensitive to his intuitive faculty, for he found that by holding his hand over a flowering plant he would experience in himself the properties of the plant". In other words, if he were

> *Disease is in essence the result of conflict between soul and mind – so long as our souls and personalities are in harmony all is joy and peace, happiness and health. It is when our personalities are led astray from the path laid down by the soul, either by our own worldly desires or by the persuasion of others, that a conflict arises.*
>
> Dr Edward Bach

worried, holding his hand over plants enabled him to find which one would be appropriate to treat worry and its symptoms.

Eventually Bach isolated 38 wild flowers from which he prepared remedies which could be used in this way. But he insisted that they must be prepared by the method he had evolved. This meant "placing the flower heads on the surface of water, in a plain glass bowl, in full sunlight, for three hours", before bottling.

The problem Bach left to those who have continued to use his method is that by the end of his career (he died in 1936) he was explaining and justifying his intuitions with mystical arguments. His remedies worked, he claimed, not because of their chemical composition, but because they had "the power to elevate our vibrations, and thus draw down spiritual power, which cleanses mind and body, and heals". Had he worked with the radiesthetists, who were exploring along similar lines, they might together have provided a firmer foundation on which to build – and a few radiesthetists and radionics practitioners do, in fact, use Bach remedies, as part of their treatment (see *Radionics and radiesthesia*, pages 257 to 264).

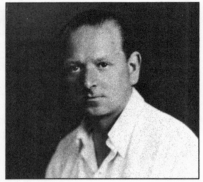

Dr Edward Bach
Dr Bach (1880–1936) gave his name to a process whereby personality disorders were healed by the use of water "impregnated" by the powers of flowers.

Procedure

Anybody can follow Bach's instructions and use any of his remedies. As they are "absolutely benign in their action, they can never produce an unpleasant reaction under any condition", claims the *Handbook of Bach Flower Remedies*, "therefore they can be safely prescribed and used by anyone, and this was Dr Bach's intention; that man could bring about his own healing".

These days Bach practitioners are almost extinct but the Remedies themselves are readily available from health centres and other such outlets, and direct from the Bach Centre at Wallingford, near Oxford. They are intended "not directly for the physical complaint", the introduction to the latest edition of the handbook explains, "but rather according to the sufferer's state of mind, according to his moods of fear, worry, anger or depression. An inharmonious state of mind will not only hinder the recovery of health and retard convalescence, but it is the primary cause of sickness and disease." Not merely did Bach differentiate between the various negative states of mind – fear, loneliness, despondency, and so on but he also further differentiated, for prescribing purposes, between the various types of fear. Under that heading "there are five Remedies for five different kinds of fear such as: terror, fear of a known cause, fear of an unknown cause, fear of the mind losing control, and fear of other people". One of the most popular is the *Rescue* remedy for emergency first aid. This is a combination of five remedies and can be used in all cases of "panic, sorrow, shock, terror, sudden bad news and accidents".

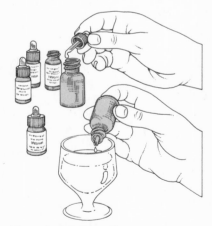

Preparing the remedies
Two or three drops of the concentrated remedy (or each remedy if you are taking more than one) are placed in a special "treatment" bottle which is then filled with pure water (not tap water). Take the remedy as necessary by placing two or three drops of this solution in a glass of water or fruit juice

Suitable cases

Because these remedies are not prescribed for any physical complaint, (their aim being to deal with causative factors), they are recommended for people with underlying emotional problems which may be found to relate to physical symptoms.

Bach's flower remedies

Dr Bach divided his 38 remedies into seven groups to cover all the known negative states of mind. Each flower is used to treat a different state of mind as listed below.

Group name and remedy	Negative aspect treated	Group name and remedy	Negative aspect treated
FEAR		Oak	Despondency through lack of progress, plodding and struggling against all odds
Rock rose	Terror, extreme fear or panic		
Mimulus	Fear of known things, shyness	Crab apple	Feeling unclean in mind and body, self-dislike
Cherry plum	Fear of mental collapse and uncontrolled temper		
Aspen	Fear of the unknown, anxiety and apprehension	**OVER-CARE FOR THE WELFARE OF OTHERS**	
		Chicory	Possessiveness, self-pity, craving attention
Red chestnut	Excessive fear or anxiety for others	Vervain	Over-enthusiasm causing strain and tension, stress, being highly strung and incensed by injustices
UNCERTAINTY			
Cerato	Self-distrust, foolishness, repeated seeking of advice		
Scleranthus	Indecision, procrastination and imbalance	Vine	Feeling of domination, being inflexible, ruthlessness and craving power
Gentian	Depression from a known cause, doubt and pessimism	Beech	Intolerance, arrogance and being critical of others
Gorse	Hopelessness and despair	Rock water	Self-denial, self-repression and martyrdom in pursuit of an ideal
Hornbeam	Doubt of own strength to cope, tiredness and the ''monday morning feeling''	Olive	Exhaustion following stress and suffering mental fatigue
		White chestnut	Persistant, unwanted worrying thoughts, mental arguments
Wild oat	Dissatisfaction and lack of direction	Mustard	Deep depression, gloom and melancholia all for no apparent reason
LACK OF INTEREST IN THE PRESENT			
Clematis	Daydreaming and indifference, inattention and escapism	Chestnut bud	Being slow to learn life's lessons, continually repeating same mistakes
Honeysuckle	Living in the past and holding on to it, homesickness	**LONELINESS**	
		Water violet	Pride, reservedness, enjoying being alone, feeling superior or aloof
Wild rose	Resignation and apathy	Impatiens	Impatience and irritability
DESPONDENCY AND DESPAIR		Heather	Feeling too concerned for yourself, dislike of being alone, being a poor listener
Larch	Lack of confidence, anticipation and fear of failure preventing action, inferiority		
		OVER-SENSITIVITY	
Pine	Feelings of guilt, self-reproachfulness, feeling unworthy, taking the blame for other people's mistakes	Agrimony	Anxiety and mental torment hidden behind a brave face
		Centaury	Weak will, overanxious to please, 'doormat' tendency, easily exploited
Elm	Temporary feeling of being overwhelmed by responsibility	Walnut	Major changes in life (for example, puberty and menopause) over-sensitivity to strong outside influences
Sweet chestnut	Extreme anguish and desolation (not suicidal)		
Star of Bethlehem	All forms of shock and sorrow — physical, mental and emotional		
Willow	Resentment and bitterness	Holly	Jealousy, hatred and suspicion

SYSTEMS OF MEDICINE

This section includes two systems of medicine: Homeopathy, based on the principles of Samuel Hahnemann; and Anthroposophical medicine, based on the teachings of Rudolf Steiner, but derived partly from homeopathy. Most homeopathic and anthroposophical practitioners are in a different category from other natural therapists as traditionally they have first completed a training in orthodox medicine. Homeopathy, however, is coming to be used more and more by therapists who have not been to medical school.

Homeopathy

Most people, when they fall ill, think of their symptoms as the result of an attack by a germ, virus, toxin or other assailant. Homeopathy is based on the principle that symptoms are often the consequence of the body's resistance mechanism working to repel an attack, and that far from seeking a way to suppress symptoms, it may be desirable to take some form of treatment calculated to help the resistance.

Although most homeopathic remedies are derived from herbs and minerals which have been used therapeutically for centuries, they are used for different purposes. Where a doctor would prescribe a drug that lowers temperature for a feverish patient, a homeopath would prescribe a drug which, given to healthy people, would raise their temperatures – the assumption being that fever is the body's way of fighting off the disorder.

At the same time, homeopaths believe that the effectiveness of a remedy cannot be gauged by its "strength", as measured conventionally. A remedy may actually be made more effective by what would appear to be dilution of its strength.

Origins

Some 200 years ago Samuel Hahnemann, a young doctor from Saxony, took up the study of biochemistry. In the course of his research he began to try out the effect of some of the drugs then in common use to treat illness, the difference being that he experimented with them to see what effect they would have on him when he was *not* ill.

The effect of quinine

Hahnemann was particularly impressed by quinine, which had long been successfully used by South American Indians to treat malaria, and had been introduced to Europe by Jesuit missionaries. What impressed Hahnemann was that when he took a

6 *Wherever she goes, the Queen takes a battered black box full of medicines many chemists have never heard of . . .*

The Queen, . . . uses arsenic for sneezing, or an upset stomach, onion for a runny nose, and anemone when someone is down in the dumps after an illness . . .

The Queen's interest in homeopathy – a system of "alternative" medicine developed at the end of the eighteenth century – stems from childhood. Her father, the late King George VI, used to treat both his daughters this way. 9

James Whitaker
London *Daily Star*
1 February 1980

dose of quinine it made him feverish; it gave him, in fact, the symptoms he would have expected, had he been suffering from a bout of malaria.

The explanation, he surmised, must be that the symptoms of malaria are not the symptoms of the disease, but of the body's resistance to the disease. Could this be true of other types of illness? By trying the notion out with other drugs, both on himself and on volunteers, he found that it was. A drug which produced certain symptoms in healthy subjects was the drug of choice to treat those symptoms when patients fell ill with them.

"Like cures like"

The homeopathic principle, as Hahnemann elaborated it, was that "like cures like". This was far from being a new idea. It had been observed by anthropologists in tribal medicine, though usually in a rather different form: symptoms were sometimes treated with herbs which resembled the suffering organ, so that a plant with ear-like leaves would be prescribed for earache. That like could cure like in Hahnemann's sense, however, had been known to the Hippocratic physicians, and it had been one of the principles expounded by Paracelsus, at the time of the Renaissance. Thomas Sydenham, the father of British medicine, had also emphasized, in the seventeenth century, that symptoms ought to be regarded as indications of the fight the body was putting up against illness. They were signs, he claimed, that whatever was causing the disorder was being thrown off, enabling the patient to recover.

Orthodoxy, however, continued to think of symptoms along the allopathic lines Galen had laid down under the Emperor Marcus Aurelius in the second century. Fevers, for example, were invariably treated with drugs to lower the patient's temperature. Only one homeopathic practice had won limited recognition: the inoculation of young children against smallpox, with small amounts of pus taken from a mild case of the disease – a method which, if it did not kill the children there and then, had been found to give them some protection against smallpox later.

Hahnemann's "potencies"

By chance, while Hahnemann was conducting his research in Germany, Dr Edward Jenner in Britain was taking the principle a step further. Investigating the old wives' tale that a mild attack of cowpox gave immunity from smallpox, he was able to provide evidence which convinced his colleagues that inoculation with a vaccine made from cowpox pus would also protect those who had been vaccinated from smallpox epidemics.

Had Hahnemann concentrated on presenting the case for homeopathic treatment and immunization in its simplest, like-cures-like terms, he might well be revered today as one of the

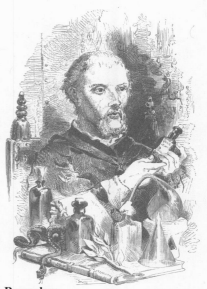

Paracelsus
Theophrastus Bombastus von Hohenheim (1493–1541), a Swiss chemist commonly known as Paracelsus, *revolutionized "hide-bound" medical methods by experimenting with new chemical compounds.*

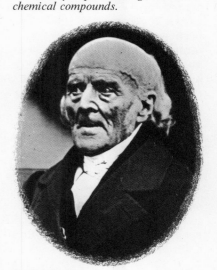

Samuel Hahnemann
The founder of homeopathic medicine, Hahnemann (1755–1843) was photographed towards the end of his life in Paris on 30 September 1841 by Foucault.

greatest of innovators in the history of medical science. But in the course of his research he made another discovery: that the *potency* of a homeopathic remedy was not related to its *strength*, as conventionally measured. If a drug were diluted in one hundred times its volume of distilled water, his "provings" of drugs appeared to show, it actually became *more* effective.

Hahnemann did not stop at dilutions ("potencies" as he thought of them) of one in a hundred; he would take a drop of the diluted mixture and "potentize" it again and again, until, on accepted scientific principles, there would not be so much as a molecule of the original drug left. Yet it was then, he claimed, that the remedy would be at its most effective.

This "potentizing" principle appeared so contrary to common sense that it was rejected by the great majority of physicians. Inevitably, too, it aroused the antagonism of the drug manufacturers and the pharmacists, who realized their livelihoods would be in danger if the heresy spread. From 1810, when Hahnemann published his *Organon of Rational Healing*, to the present day, orthodox medicine has rejected homeopathy, often making open war upon it.

Homeopathy in Britain

In one respect, however, homeopathy stands apart from other natural therapies – it is not so segregated from the medical profession. This happened largely by accident. During the great cholera epidemics of the last century the rumour got around that homeopathic remedies were effective, adding to the growing number of people who, dissatisfied with the bleedings and purgings and repulsive drugs of that era, were turning to homeopathy. In 1854, when the figures were collected for the mortality rates in London hospitals, the record of the homeopathic hospital was so much better than that of all the others that at first the Board of Health, dominated by orthodox doctors, tried to suppress the figures by leaving them out of the published record. They were only prevented from doing so by the intervention of a young member of Parliament, sympathetic to the homeopathic cause.

Two years later, the same man, by then in the House of Lords and a friend of Dr Quin, first president of the British Homeopathic Society was instrumental in persuading parliament to strike out a clause in the bill setting up the medical profession. As drafted, this would have given the General Medical Council the right to erase from the Medical Register the name of any doctor who practised homeopathy. (Some medical schools had actually been refusing to grant degrees to students who had qualified, unless they pledged themselves not to practise homeopathy.) As a result, would-be homeopaths could continue to practise; but they had first to qualify as doctors in the usual way, before taking a further qualification in a homeopathic hospital.

This system worked satisfactorily enough while medical students' training was short. But when it was lengthened to five years and more, prospective homeopaths found themselves subjected to ever-increasing amounts of orthodox specialist instruction with which, as homeopaths, they disagreed. At the same time they were subjected to conditioning of a kind calculated to make them accept that the basic homeopathic principle of potentizing through dilution was unscientific, and indeed ludicrous. Not surprisingly, the number of students who survived this brain-washing process at their medical schools and went on to qualify as homeopaths began to dwindle.

The pharmaceutical revolution of the 1940s and 1950s, associated with sulpha drugs, penicillin and the antibiotics, appeared to be the last straw for homeopathy. Here were orthodox remedies which really worked, and could work consistently well – better, as homeopaths had to admit, than their own remedies. Although by this time they had the advantage of recognition within the National Health Service as well as a certain social cachet (Queen Mary had been a devotee of homeopathy, and her children, and some of her grandchildren, had homeopathic treatment for minor ailments), the number of practising homeopathic physicians continued to decline. As a result, when the "wonder drug" image became tarnished and the public began to look around for alternative therapies, homeopathic treatment was hard to come by.

Opposition from the medical establishment

In Britain the medical fraternity has also been doing its best to make the homeopath's lot even harder. When a recent NHS reorganization in Liverpool necessitated the transfer of a homeopathic clinic to the new Royal Liverpool Hospital, the doctors there rebelled on the grounds that medical students "should not be exposed to any unorthodox medicine before qualification" and that the clinic's presence would "cause alarm to many doctors and patients", among other objections. As Tom Ellis, MP for Wrexham, put it, it would be hard to find a better example of the professions' "sheer blind prejudice and bigotry".

As the current shortage of medically qualified homeopaths cannot be quickly remedied, the availability of homeopathy through public health services is certain to remain restricted in the immediate future. Increasingly, however, practitioners of other forms of natural medicine have been taking courses in homeopathy. Its links are particularly strong with radionics, where there is a half-century old tradition of practitioners using their gadgetry not just to diagnose disorders but to select the appropriate homeopathic remedy and broadcast it to their patients (see *Radionics and radiesthesia*, pages 257 to 264).

Procedure

The initial visit to a homeopath differs little from a visit to a doctor, except in one important respect: the case history taking is lengthier, and puts much more emphasis on you as an individual, rather than on the disease you may be suffering from.

Diagnosis is made not so much on the basis of objective tests of the kind that allopathic physicians use to decide what illness a patient has, as on the evaluation of what the homeopath sees, feels and hears. The course the homeopath will take in deciding upon treatment is little changed from Hahnemann's time.

A very special approach

A few years ago the Homeopathic Trust for Research and Education asked the medical correspondent of a national daily, himself a doctor, to write an objective reporter's-eye-view of homeopathy, which has been published as a brochure, *Medicine in the Round*. Perhaps the most striking feature, he found in the course of his enquiry, was "the doctor's attitude towards the patient". As in orthodox medicine, the first step with a new patient is history-taking, "but history-taking with a difference. Not only are the diagnostic symptoms considered, but also the patient's personality and constitution – physiological and psychological – as manifested in temperament and disposition". Even his or her likes and dislikes are taken into consideration; "the patient is upset by the cold, will not touch fat, wants to be alone when ill – all such information is noted and collated to form the basis of a decision as to how he should be treated".

The second step is for the homeopath to decide upon a remedy. The procedure of choosing a remedy has been described in *Homeopathic Prescribing* by Adolf Voegeli. Even for the common cold, the choice of remedy is based not just on the type of cold and the stage the symptoms have reached, but also on the lifestyle and the personality of the individual who has the cold. Thus, *Nux vomica* is most often indicated at the start of a cold and "is particularly effective for the type that corresponds to this remedy – the choleric and irritable stay-at-home, the person who lives under extreme pressure of business and who can't stand cold"; *Arsenicum album* is "especially suitable for thin people who feel chilly and lack energy. It is one of the few remedies where a head cold improves in a warm room"; and *Pulsatilla* "often indicated at the end of a head cold", acts best "on people of a delicate temperament, who are sensitive to remarks and even have tears in their eyes as soon as anyone offers them the slightest reproach".

Preparing the remedies

The next step consists of the preparation of the remedy. If the remedy is a solid, it is pounded in a mortar along with some

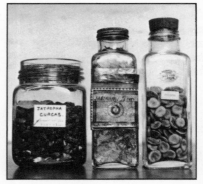

The raw materials
These are the main ingredients for three plant-based homeopathic remedies – Jatropha, Jaborandi, and Nux Vomica. To make a "mother tincture", each will be left in alcohol and distilled water for a month, then pressed and filtered.

therapeutically inert substance; if it is a liquid, it is diluted in distilled water and "succussed" – rapidly shaken up on a machine – until infusion is complete. Remedies are prepared to whatever degree of "potency" the homeopath decides is required.

An issue upon which homeopaths diverge is the lengths to which the potentizing process need be carried. A single potency, in the proportion of one part of the remedy to 99 of dilutent, is described as "1 C", but the process may be continued to "10 C", or even "2,000 C". For obvious reasons, then, it is unwise for people who have not been to a homeopathic practitioner to shop around for homeopathic remedies – though these are now becoming more widely available. There are books which list the remedies for symptoms ranging from abscesses to yellow fever, but they are designed primarily to assist the prescriber.

Homeopathic remedies need to be protected from contamination. They should be kept in airtight containers and exposed to the air only for as long as it takes to extract the pills, and consume them. They should not be taken in conjunction with other medical drugs (though this has been the subject of debate). Some homeopaths have a more extensive list of "don'ts", including coffee, sweets and other stimulants.

Homeopathic remedies come in different styles: pills, powders, granules, tinctures and ointment. The potency of the remedy and the frequency with which it is taken are a matter for the judgement of the homeopath in the first place, and for the experience and common sense of the patient thereafter.

Preparing homeopathic pills
Once the "mother tincture" has been diluted to the required potency and "succussed" (shaken up), a few drops are introduced into a small bottle of unmedicated pills, made from lactose and sucrose.

Research

The arguments chiefly used by the medical establishment to discredit homeopathy have been that it is inherently unscientific, and that homeopathic "provings" of drugs in fact prove only that the drug produces symptoms in healthy people similar to those of the disease the homeopaths treat with it – which is not the same as saying that it is effective. Why should homeopaths not accept the discipline of controlled trials of their remedies, of the kind all prescription-only drugs are put through before they are allowed on the market?

The "inherently unscientific" argument is usually derived from the commonsense belief that dilution *cannot* really increase potency. On the contrary, surely, it must remove all trace of remedy? But a quarter of a century ago, a Glasgow doctor published the results of trials which demonstrated that this is incorrect. A remedy which had been diluted to the point where, in theory, nothing at all could be left of it was nevertheless found to be capable of affecting enzyme levels. And in the late 1970s, other doctors from the Glasgow homeopathic hospital accepted the challenge, and submitted their therapy to controlled trials.

The main problem earlier (apart from the unwillingness of the medical profession to sanction trials of homeopathic remedies and a chronic shortage of funds to support such research) had been that homeopaths disliked the principle on which orthodox trials had come to be run; the patients were divided at random into two groups, and then treated "double-blind", so that neither doctors nor patients knew who was getting the drug, and who was getting the placebo. As the homeopath chooses remedies according to the patient, rather than according to the type of disease, such randomized double-blind trials could not be expected to give fair results.

Clinical trials

It was not until the late 1970s that a compromise was reached so that a trial could be held in Glasgow. Doctors from the city's Homeopathic Hospital, the Centre for Rheumatic Diseases, the University's Department of Medicine, and the Royal Infirmary collaborated. The patients had all been diagnosed as suffering from rheumatoid arthritis, and had been treated for it by orthodox methods for periods varying from four months to 10 years. They were divided into two groups and 54 were given homeopathic treatment, 41 treated with aspirin (still the standard orthodox treatment, though periodically new varieties of anti-rheumatic drug enjoy a brief vogue).

By the end of the trial period 24 of those who had been treated homeopathically were better; only six were better after the aspirin treatment. The failure, or drop-out, rate was 33 percent for the homeopathic patients, 85 percent for the aspirin patients. Of the drop-outs in the homeopathic group, none were due to adverse side-effects; in the aspirin group, 39 percent quit for that reason.

Made bold by this success, the homeopaths decided to risk accepting a modified double-blind trial. They saw 50 patients and chose whatever homeopathic remedy they considered appropriate. But half of these patients were given a placebo instead of the remedy and nobody knew which patients had received the remedy. This trial was also unusual, in that patients continued to take whatever orthodox remedies they had been taking before – otherwise their doctors would not have let them participate.

If orthodox assumptions had been correct, patients taking the homeopathic remedies would have fared no better than those on the placebo. But after three months, when the code which showed which patients were on the placebo were revealed, it was found that they had continued to deteriorate, whereas those on the homeopathic remedies had significantly improved. To be on the safe side, the two groups of patients were then switched, and the trial continued. Again, after three months those on homeopathic remedies were faring significantly better.

In view of these results it is difficult any longer to dismiss homeopathy on the ground that there is no scientific evidence for its effectiveness. Even the *Lancet* has given cautious approval. If the improvements are confirmed in further trials, an editorial has conceded, "then homeopathy would provide a yardstick against which workers with more toxic agents could measure their effects" – a reminder, incidentally, that homeopathic treatment should be assessed not simply in terms of the effectiveness of its remedies, but also in terms of the freedom of the remedies from unwanted side-effects.

Suitable cases

Homeopathy is regarded by its practitioners as offering alternative remedies to almost all those of conventional medicine – and remedies that are, in general, better and safer. Most homeopaths would admit that in cases when disease is a danger to life, as in virulent infections, a powerful allopathic remedy such as an antibiotic, where a suitable one is available, can still be the drug of choice. But patients who entrust themselves to a homeopath ordinarily do so with the expectation that any kind of illness can be diagnosed and treated.

Self-help

"First-aid kits" are available containing 10 or more standard homeopathic remedies, along with instructions on how they can be used to treat most minor disorders – cold, indigestion, seasickness, and so on. Homeopaths do not disapprove of this, but they urge you not to go in for first aid of this kind until you have learned something about homeopathy in general and about your own needs in particular, as some of the standard remedies may not be right in your case.

Some of the standard remedies have names that sound alarming, *Nux vomica* or *Arsenicum* for example, and they could be lethal if they were given "neat" derived as they are from poisonous plants such as the deadly nightshade or from toxic minerals. But in homeopathic doses they are safe. At the stage which orthodox medicine has reached in relying on powerful drugs which all too often have unwanted side-effects, homeopathy's great strength is that the only adverse reaction you can experience is one which homeopaths, along with naturopaths and other practitioners of natural therapy, all warn about. When the human body is encouraged to throw off toxic materials, it may do so violently, for a time, with vomiting or diarrhea and perhaps other symptoms such as rashes and itching. These are not side-effects, however, they are merely an indication that the treatment is working.

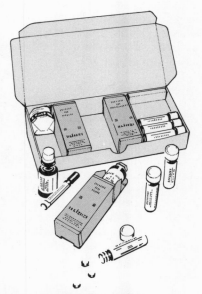

A homeopathic first-aid kit
Such a first-aid kit contains medicines, in the form of tablets, ointments and tinctures. Their combined cures range from pre-examination nerves to boils.

Anthroposophical medicine

Not so much a therapy as an alternative attitude to health and illness, anthroposophical medicine is based on the wider teachings of Rudolf Steiner. It is practised only by medically qualified doctors who have also undergone special training.

Origins

Steiner's beliefs, which are essentially Christian in outlook, were originally similar to those of the theosophists. When theosophy came into being a little more than a century ago, its followers accepted the eastern tradition of *prana*, or life-energy, as the mainspring of good health. The basic aim of medicine, they believed, is to liberate the mind and body from anything which obstructs the force's flow. They did not reject the tenets of orthodox medicine, but they insisted that instead of relying on drugs and other forms of treatment, doctors should encourage patients to look to their own lifestyles to find out why they have fallen ill. "All healing is self-healing", they advised.

More than that, patients must realize that the life they are currently living is only one of their lives. Their health is related to what they have brought with them from past lives, as well as what they are doing with their present ones – the "karma" principle. This "load" carried from the past, however, must not be regarded as something they can do nothing about in the present. Their aim should be to make the most of their lives with the ultimate objective of Nirvana, or salvation, in mind, and with good health as a by-product.

Steiner's own beliefs

The Austrian thinker and scientist Rudolf Steiner joined the theosophists towards the end of the century, but split with them in 1909 to form the Anthroposophical Society. Steiner's preferred term, anthroposophy, was based on the Greek words *anthropos*, meaning man, and *sophia*, wisdom. He said anthroposophy should be understood to mean "awareness" of one's humanity. Steiner also began to take a more positive interest in the problems of prevention and treatment of illness. At this stage, his movement had some affinities with what F. Matthias Alexander had begun to preach: the fundamental unity of the human organism; the inter-relationship of mind and body; and the need consciously to recognize and eliminate bad habits, notably of posture (see also *The Alexander principle*, pages 104 to 108). "With certain things we do, no matter whether or not they are of enduring importance, it is good practice to look carefully at what is being done", Steiner recommended in a lecture in 1912. We should learn to watch how we stand, and walk, and gesture, with a view to establishing a greater measure of control by the higher centres of the personality over the lower.

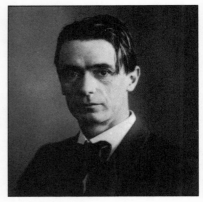

Rudolf Steiner
The teachings of Steiner (1861–1925), founder of anthroposophy, embrace the fields of education, science, religion, and medicine.

Steiner schools

Steiner went on to develop new ways of training people, based upon what came to be defined as his fourfold picture of humanity: "To the concept of man as a physical body, he adds the concept of man as a living organism possessing a body of formative forces (termed the 'etheric' body); man as a sentient being experiencing an inner life of emotions and drives (and so possessing what Steiner called an 'astral' body); and man as being conscious of himself (and so possessing an ego or 'I')".

He established schools where his ideas could be applied to the education of children. These were later adapted for use with the mentally handicapped. Through meetings and discussions with a small group of doctors interested in applying his principles to the care of the sick came the development in the 1920s of anthroposophical medicine.

It stands quite close to *Homeopathy* (see pages 66 to 73), with which it has many links (although it is not restricted to one therapeutic procedure, such as the giving of medicines). Steiner, for example, agreed with the homeopaths that the practitioners of anthroposophical medicine should first qualify as doctors, and only then begin to apply his principles in their practice. He died in 1925, without realizing just how difficult it was for those principles to be maintained in the face of orthodoxy's strongly materialist trend.

This has meant that anthroposophical practitioners are closer in their ideas and attitudes to natural therapists than they are to most of their fellow doctors. Only among the medical homeopaths have they found fellow-feeling and sympathy.

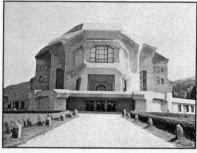

The Goetheanum
Rudolf Steiner designed and built his first Goetheanum in Dornach near Basle in Switzerland. It was to be the headquarters of the Anthroposophical Society but in 1923, it was destroyed by fire and replaced with this version, built from 1924–8.

Practising anthroposophical medicine

Like the homeopaths, they found the "wonder drug" era hard to survive. "Until a few years ago, the prospects for any future at all for anthroposophical medical work in England seemed very slim", Dr James Dyson wrote in a paper on anthroposophical medical training in 1978. The prospects now look brighter, but as with homeopathy, the problem remains that the orthodox training which practitioners are still required to go through is now so far removed from anthroposophical principles that it is difficult to reconcile the two.

Doctors who wish to practice anthroposophical medicine must attend a postgraduate course run by members of the medical section of the School of Spiritual Science in Switzerland. Steiner Schools, curative homes, and clinics are to be found in many parts of the world, though it is in fact interesting to note that anthroposophical medicine is much more firmly established in the rest of Europe than in Britain. In Europe, anthroposophical doctors run into the hundreds, and there are two general and eight specialized hospitals.

Procedure

What you should expect depends very much on the practitioner. Anthroposophical doctors may use some orthodox medicines, but more commonly, they prescribe homeopathic or herbal remedies or specially prepared anthroposophical medicines. Curative eurhythmy (a system of promoting self-expression through music), and special massage, hydrotherapy, art therapy, music and speech therapy may also be provided by therapists trained in Steiner's methods.

Suitable cases

Everyone, theoretically, is a suitable case. But a better way of looking at it, if you are dissatisfied with conventional medical care (and like Steiner's notions) is to find out whether there is a practitioner of anthroposophical medicine in the vicinity (they are few and far between), and if so, to ask for an appointment, and see whether you establish rapport. The well-established Steiner system will take things on from there.

Eurhythmy dancing
Steiner advocated the use of eurhythmy, in which movement is linked to the sounds of speech. Certain kinds of movement represent the vowel sounds, others the consonants. Besides being used for a variety of physical and mental disorders, eurhythmy is very beneficial for children, developing their suppleness and sense of rhythm.

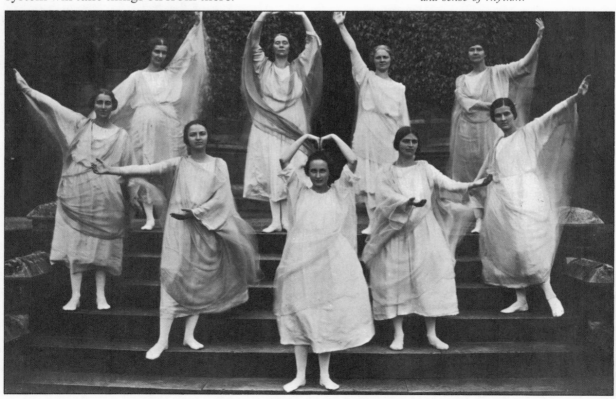

MANIPULATIVE THERAPIES

In all civilizations people have existed whose role it was to look after the workings of the musculoskeletal system – from undertaking running repairs, as when a bone is broken and has to be reset, or when a joint is dislocated and "reduction" is employed to get the part back into its proper place, to toning up muscles with the help of massage. But few physicians have felt it necessary to learn these skills and as a result, they have usually been carried out by auxiliaries.

The importance of touch in primitive societies

Over the years, various researchers have come to realize the significant role that touch has played in primitive societies. The great American ethnologist Daniel Brinton found that some American Indians used a technique of light stroking, sometimes with no apparent physical contact. Edward Evans Pritchard, Professor of Anthropology at Oxford University, described how the Azande tribe of central Africa had individuals who were much admired for their skill in reducing fractures, but who also gave light massage. In Samoa, according to the missionary J.B. Stair, the verb "to doctor" was synonymous with "to rub", the process involving anything from the gentlest of finger-tip pressure to energetic kneading. The natives of Tonga, the eighteenth-century traveller William Mariner reported, also used rubbing, along with more violent measures: small children were employed to trample upon patients.

In such practices it is easy to discern the early origins of manipulative and postural therapies. But touch was also esteemed for its own sake. Often there was an element of magic in it. In the Solomon Islands, the English anthropologist, William Halse Rivers watched a therapist using techniques of a kind "which so closely resemble those of our own massage that, if simply observed, and not made the subject of special inquiry, they would undoubtedly be regarded as the equivalent of this remedy as practised by ourselves". But when he did make them the subject of special inquiry, he found that the aim was "to act upon an imaginary octopus, which was supposed to have taken up its abode in the body of a patient; while in other cases the object was to extract from the body the immaterial object or principle, which was held to be the cause of fever or other form of disease".

Three key factors for treatment

Three elements, in other words, need to be taken into consideration when it comes to treatment: the actual physical consequences, the psychological impact, and the possibility that there is an as yet, unexplained healing force. No clear-cut line can be drawn between manipulative therapies which are basically physical and those which have a strong psychological component; we deal with both in this section. Those which, like hand healing and

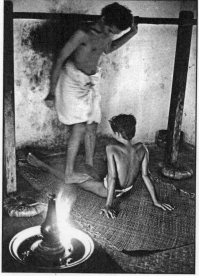

Kathakali training
Manipulative therapies are very common in primitive societies. This Indian Kathakali dancer is using his feet to massage his pupil's legs, thus releasing the boy's muscles.

therapeutic touch, are derived from the assumption that some psychic force is at work, will be found in the section on *Paranormal therapies* (see pages 223 to 271).

Bonesetters versus doctors

That manipulative therapies are practised largely outside the medical profession (even physiotherapists make little use of manipulation, though it looks as if this may be changing) is largely due to the fact that when in 1858 the medical profession was set up in the form we know it today, and given extensive monopoly powers, "bonesetters" (as they were then commonly known) were left outside. As a result; any doctor who referred a patient to a bonesetter risked the penalty of having his name erased from the Medical Register. In the circumstances, the leading medical figure of the Victorian era in Britain, Sir James Paget, concluded, members of the medical profession must themselves learn the craft, or they might find that a bonesetter could become a serious rival: "If he can cure a case which you have failed to cure, his fortune may be made and yours marred", he warned. His forebodings were soon to be justified. The bonesetter Herbert Barker began to make a big reputation towards the end of the century. In spite of professional hostility he won national acclaim and in 1922 was awarded a knighthood for his services to society.

By this time, however, the old-style bonesetter was gradually ceasing to be a serious threat to the profession's monopolistic powers. The introduction of X-rays had given orthopedic physicians and surgeons the advantage which had enabled them to undertake "reductions" without the need to open up the body to see what they were doing. And the art of manipulation was being taken over by practitioners who, though they were also outside the medical profession, had qualifications. Unlike the bonesetters, they had gone through training courses to qualify as osteopaths and chiropractors.

Since that time, massage, which used once to be practised by physiotherapists, has now become predominantly an alternative therapy. And a number of other techniques have been introduced in the present century which also come (though some of them only partially) in this general category: the Alexander principle, rolfing (and postural integration), polarity therapy, reflexology, applied kinesiology (and touch for health).

Vertebral manipulation

Before we go on to survey the alternative manipulative therapies, however, it is worth having a look at what has been loosely called vertebral manipulation. This technique of manipulating the spine does not owe allegiance to any school, as osteopathy and chiropractic do. And as it has mainly been practised by some physiotherapists and a few doctors, it is not, strictly speaking, in the alternative camp. Yet it has never really been accepted in the orthopedic world either, and the results of research into this technique have implications for manipulation in general.

The best-known form in Britain was developed by Dr James Cyriax, who was once a consultant at St Thomas's Hospital, and after his retirement in charge of an institute of orthopedic medicine. Cyriax did his best to persuade his colleagues, ortho-pedic surgeons and physicians, that they should learn manipu-lation, but with little success.

Cyriax disagreed with both osteopaths and chiropractors on the cause of back pain, as he did not believe that misalignment of the vertebrae was responsible. He also disagreed with the conventional orthopedic view that the responsibility commonly lay with a "slipped" disc. His assumption was that the guilt lies with a displaced fragment of disc, which manipulation can often shift to a point where it will cause no further trouble.

Unable to persuade the medical profession to introduce manipulation as a part of the medical student's training, Cyriax, anxious to prevent it from being monopolized by osteopaths and other medically-unqualified practitioners, has taught his method chiefly to physiotherapists. Many physiotherapists have also learned a technique popularized in Australia by G.D. Maitland.

Whichever method is applied, however, the consensus is that the rapport between therapist and patient plays a decisive part in the treatment. The type of manipulation, therefore, may be much less important than the ability of the manipulator to achieve the necessary relationship with his patients.

The difficulties of setting up trials

It is this fact which brings up an important point in connection with research. Insofar as the results of treatment depend upon the rapport between manipulator and patient, for a variety of reasons (the most obvious being that the success of the manipulation may depend on the degree of the patient's relaxation) it becomes very difficult to set up a controlled trial of a particular type of manipulation. And this is not the only problem – as some of the contributors to the US Department of Health's recent symposium on the subject have recognized – that has yet to be solved.

One of medical science's cherished research postulates is that in any trial patients should be "randomized" to prevent the practitioner selecting those which he or she thinks are most likely to be treated successfully. This goes against the equally cherished belief of the manipulators that half the battle, in their job, is selecting the appropriate patients for treatment.

It would also be extremely difficult to set up a fully controlled trial with one group of patients having manipulative therapy, and the other group getting only "pretend" manipulative therapy.

Patients would have to be very ignorant not to guess, or suspect, which they were getting.

And unlike a trial of a drug, where it can be arranged that all the patients are getting precisely the same dose, a trial employing more than one manipulator may mean that patients will be receiving different levels of treatment according to the manipulator's skill. Even if only a single manipulator is used, their treatment may vary according to circumstances. Early in the day, for example, the therapist is fresh, while later on in the afternoon he or she will undoubtedly have become tired.

It follows that any attempt which is made to assess the value of manipulative therapies of any kind will need to be more flexible in its protocol than is customary in controlled trials, allowing for the often highly subjective elements involved.

And how best this can be done is a problem which has as yet eluded solution – not that there have been many attempts to solve it, because of the unwillingness of the medical profession to investigate unorthodox forms of treatment, and the lack of funds for research projects of all kinds.

Osteopathy

In his *Manual of Osteopathic Technique* Dr Alan Stoddard describes osteopathy as "concerned with the establishment and maintenance of the normal structural integrity of the body". This is done primarily through manipulation of joints, in order to restore them to their normal positions and mobility, thereby relieving abnormal tension in muscles and ligaments. The greater part of an osteopath's work relates to the spinal column, not merely because its integrity is basic to the whole bone and muscle system, but also because it houses the spinal cord, through which the autonomic nervous system exercises its authority.

Origins

The founder of osteopathy, Andrew Taylor Still, was, in fact, a practising doctor who worked on the Union side in the American Civil War, before he became disillusioned with the orthodox medical principles and methods of the time. From personal experience and from treating patients he became convinced that good health is dependent upon the integrity of the spinal column. When the vertebrae slip out of alignment we fall ill.

Animals realize this instinctively. A dog or a cat, rousing itself after sleep, splays its limbs fore and aft and stretches until its backbone is concave, at the same time yawning and generally

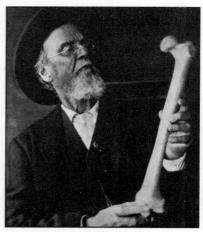

Andrew Taylor Still
Dr Still (1828–1912) the founder of osteopathy, believed that in order to function properly the structure of the body must be sound.

establishing that its range of muscular capability is in working order. Men, women, and especially children often instinctively go through the same routine. But we do not always carry it out, if it might make us late for school or for the office. During the day we slump in car seats or sit hunched over our work, often putting a strain on the spine without taking the exercise necessary to keep it, and its associated ligaments and muscles, in working order.

If Dr Still had contented himself with impressing upon his patients the fact that they must look after their spines or they would suffer backache and rheumatic disorders, his orthodox colleagues might well have accepted him and his disciples. But he went further. The spinal cord, he argued, regulates what is happening throughout the body, through its link-up with the nervous system. Even the circulation of the blood can be affected by the condition of the spine.

Many symptoms which we take to be the results of some local disturbance – skin disorders, stomachache, headache and so on – are in reality, Still asserted, the consequence of the spinal vertebrae being slightly out of position. Find the spot, realign the vertebrae, and the body's homeostat, its self-regulating system, can take over again, causing the skin blemish, the stomachache or the headache to disappear.

Osteopathic lesions

The concept of "the osteopathic lesion", as it came to be called, is still central to osteopathy. A pamphlet *Osteopathy: an explanation*, published by the British Society of Osteopaths, claims that it has "contributed to medicine an understanding of an important – but not generally recognized – type of lesion".

The lesions are of two kinds. Where a lesion occurs in the spine, "it represents an imbalance of normal tensions to the extent that the information reaching the spinal cord from the deep muscles of the spine becomes confused and contradictory" – perhaps because they have become unduly stretched or are in spasm. Or it may be that "the nerves from this part of the spinal cord become over-sensitive", passing on their irritability to joints, ligaments, and muscles, "this irritability affecting the arterial and venous circulation to organs and tissues whose nerve supplies originate in the segments of the spinal cord concerned". These days osteopaths increasingly also use the term "segmental dysfunctions" which includes an awareness of the structures associated with joints – that is the nerves, muscles and ligaments as well as the bones themselves.

No actual vertebral displacement is necessarily implied by the term "lesion" and this has given the medical establishment the chance to insist that the lesions are a myth. But the establishment's real objection has been to the idea that manipulation can be used to treat a wide range of symptoms – those

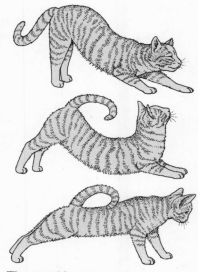

The stretching cat
All animals stretch after sleep, arching and then hollowing out their spinal columns so that the vertebrae are given the opportunity to "mesh" into the right alignment.

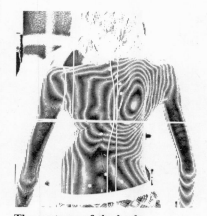

The contours of the back
This moiré topographic photograph shows the back of a 13-year-old boy with pronounced congenital scoliosis. The positions of the vertebrae are marked by the white dots. Osteopathy prevented the spinal curve from deteriorating further.

arising from the "irritability" effect. It was this that led to a protracted campaign against osteopathy in the United States and, later, in Britain, when osteopaths began to practise here.

The campaign for recognition
In the USA osteopaths have recently managed to establish themselves as doctors in their own right, recognized as such even by the medical profession. But in Britain they have not yet won formal recognition. Some doctors have taken courses in osteopathy and practise it, but ordinarily when people talk about going to an osteopath, they are referring to somebody who has no formal medical qualifications, but who has trained at one of the osteopathic teaching institutions.

Consulting an osteopath

Before treatment you will be examined for areas of muscle tension and joint strain, both while standing and while performing a range of spinal movements. The actual techniques used in treatment are adapted according to your age and the amount of pain you are in.

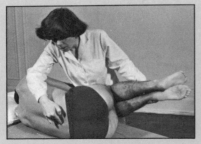

1 *This osteopath begins her examination by obtaining an overall impression of the patient's state of health, his posture, and the amount of discomfort standing gives him.*

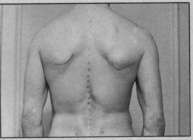

2 *She then focuses attention on areas of the body that may be contributing to his complaint. This patient's shoulders, shoulder-blades and hands are at different levels and his spine curves slightly.*

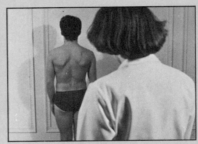

6 *Osteopaths spend much of their time examining the lumbar spine for signs of poor joint movement, muscle spasm, pain, bone disease or degeneration, while the patient lies completely passively.*

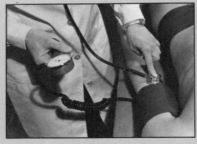

7 *Here the osteopath is checking the function of the middle thoracic ribs and vertebrae before deciding what treatment is needed. The patient's arms are crossed in front of his chest for convenience.*

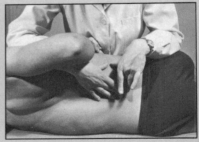

8 *To check the patient's health thoroughly, the osteopath may measure the blood pressure, listen to the heart and lungs, take blood or urine samples, and examine the eyes for clarity.*

Orthopedic surgeons used to have a supply of horror stories about patients who had gone to an osteopath for manipulation, only to find out, too late, that what was the matter with them was spinal tuberculosis. Occasionally such tales can still be heard, but when the medical journal *General Practitioner* combed through the records, no single case could be discovered where osteopaths had been sued for malpractice, as they surely would have been had such tales had any foundation.

Procedure

An appointment with an osteopath initially follows the same course as an appointment with a doctor. (However, as Dr David

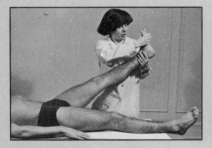

3 The straight leg raising test stretches the sciatic nerve. If the patient has intervertebral disc damage or muscle spasm anywhere along the nerve's length, raising the leg will be painful.

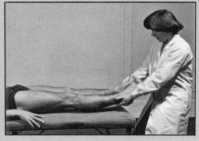

4 The osteopath asks the patient to relax his muscles while she compares the lengths of his legs. Lateral curves in the spine or asymmetry in the pelvic bones may result from any discrepancy.

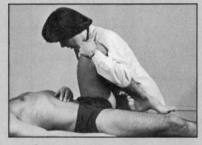

5 By flexing and pushing down on the patient's knee, the osteopath assesses the amount and quality of movement of the sacroiliac joint and discovers whether it is causing the pain.

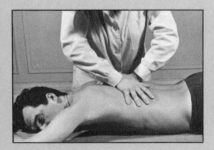

9 Manipulating one of the joints of the lumbar spine, the osteopath executes a short, sharp rotational movement which slightly separates the surfaces of the joint and results in a small "click".

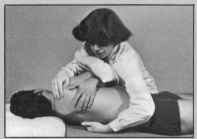

10 "Soft tissue" work involves stretching and relaxing muscles and connective tissue. Massaging tissues that are hypercontracted decreases tension and improves blood supply to the tissue.

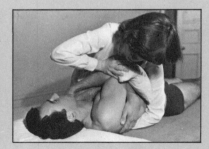

11 To manipulate the mid-dorsal spine, she places a flat hand under the patient's spine, then applies rapid downward pressure on his arms which is transmitted through his chest.

Delvin noted in an article in *World Medicine*, when he decided to try *his* local osteopath, he found the man booked up 12 days ahead, and "even the busiest of busy general practices can't compete with that".)

Visual clues to diagnosis

On your first visit a general case history will be taken, but whereas all too many GPs simply listen to the patient's replies to questions, jotting down the answers, an osteopath will watch you come in to the room, observing how you stand, how you walk, how you sit down, how you sit in a chair (upright or slumped), and so on. He or she will be looking for connections between the information you provide and how you hold yourself. Increasingly, these days, the osteopath will also be paying attention to how you express yourself, because of the growing recognition that the symptoms which prompt people to come for treatment are frequently related to stress.

Deciding on treatment

The clues picked up from patients in this way decide what osteopaths do next. They may decline to treat you if they realize, say, that you require surgery, or that there are psychiatric undertones to your disorder which lie outside their competence. In such cases they would suggest you see another practitioner.

If you have come with what you believe to be a back problem, the next step is ordinarily to look at your spine – or, in a sense, to look *through* your spine – to try to make the connection between your symptoms and your vertebrae. It may be that some fault will immediately be found which can be set right by a simple twist, using your arms or legs for leverage. The majority of patients who go to an osteopath are backache cases. Many of them have simply "ricked" their backs, and it can be a relatively simple matter, with training and experience, to put the spine right. But in other cases the manipulation needed is going to be more complicated, because it may not just be the vertebrae, but other bones and muscles, which need attention.

Lately, the emphasis has increasingly shifted away from the simple search for a spinal lesion to a wider outlook, as reflected in a recent article called "The Holistic Approach of Osteopathy" by Harold Klug in the *Journal of the Society of Osteopaths*. "As the nervous system is clearly designed to operate as a unit, any aberration of function, in whatever body system it may be expressed, must be viewed as a reduction in the efficiency of the homeostatic and integrative functions of the nervous system", he explains. "Thus the osteopathic physician's concern is to re-integrate the nervous system by relieving those disturbed reflexes, wherever they may occur, and thus permitting the homeostatic mechanism to reassert itself".

The high-velocity thrust

The kind of manipulation you may expect is consequently impossible to describe in general terms and not even easy to show in pictures, though Stoddard in his manuals gives a good idea of what is entailed. It really needs film to illustrate the techniques, but even this is inadequate, because the amount of leverage which the osteopath decides to exercise depends on his or her "feel" for the resistance to the movement. Although "one of the most frequently used manipulative approaches is the high-velocity thrust which releases the joint" the Society of Osteopath's publication *Osteopathy: an Explanation* remarks, "many patients require extremely gentle treatment or find the thrust techniques a little overwhelming. For them, a system called 'functional technique' can be used gently to coax the tissues".

The value of pain

The high-velocity thrust, the pamphlet insists, is "normally painless, and most effective in removing pain quickly". And although where adhesions need to be broken down, a short, sharp wrench may be painful, it will be less painful in the long run than more gradual methods. There is fairly general agreement among osteopaths that anesthetics should be used sparingly, if at all, because they disguise the pain, depriving the manipulator of a useful source of information.

Osteopaths also realize that the pain can be a reflection of a state of mind and the patient ought, if possible, to be made aware that it cannot be removed simply by some manipulative manoevre. Pain can sometimes "habituate" itself to certain actions, like bending down. In certain circumstances, hypnosis may enable a patient to bend down painlessly. In such cases, the patient may be more in need of some psychological therapy than of manipulation, or perhaps both may be required.

Research

Only one serious attempt has been made to mount a controlled trial of osteopathy, and unluckily it was poorly designed. Four hundred and fifty patients with backache were put at random into four groups. One group was treated by an osteopath, one by physiotherapy, one had the standard orthodox prescription of rest and painkillers, and the fourth group were given corsets to wear. Representatives of the British Association of Manipulative Medicine, which consists of doctors who practise manipulation, declined to cooperate when they found that the patients were to be distributed at random beween the groups: a manipulator, they argued, must be able to select those patients he or she thinks will benefit, and reject the rest. However, an osteopath took on the allotted group, and the trials went ahead.

As reported in the *British Medical Journal* in 1975, the results of the trials appeared to show that patients treated by the osteopath did only marginally better than those in the other three groups. But a closer look at the report revealed that the effects of treatment on 70 of the patients had not been included, because they had not completed the trial. Of these, 40 had been treated by the osteopath, and 26 of them had stopped attending because they felt so much better that they could not see the point of continuing. Had they been included in the results, the osteopath's group would have had a far higher rating than the rest.

Suitable cases

In most countries the great majority of an osteopath's patients have been, and still are, backache sufferers. Usually they have lower back pain or what used to be called lumbago. Osteopaths' experience in putting right "ricked" backs – the kind that come suddenly, when you are digging in the garden or stooping to pick something up – makes them a natural first choice in such circumstances.

But quite often in the course of treatment patients find that other disorders from which they have been suffering are relieved or removed altogether: *Respiratory disorders, Digestive disorders, Circulatory disorders* (see *Disorders*, pages 300 to 339). While it is still unusual for anybody to go to an osteopath for the first time with, say, asthma or high blood pressure, it is becoming increasingly common for patients who have initially been to an osteopath for backache, or some associated disorder such as sciatica, arthritis, or "tennis elbow", to go back for treatment for other types of disorder when conventional treatment fails.

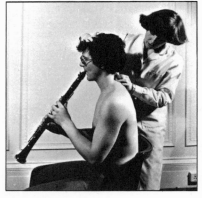

Treating a musician
To assess why a musician suffers from pain, the osteopath first observes him playing, then feels for the amount of muscular effort and joint strain present in the neck. One of the aims of treatment will be to instruct him in, and help him maintain, a comfortable posture while playing.

Cranial osteopathy

This is a spin-off from standard osteopathy in which the "osteopathic lesions" are traced and treated principally by palpation of the skull and the pelvic area. Few practitioners specialize in this technique alone, but many use it as an adjunct to straightforward osteopathic treatment.

Origins

The term cranial osteopathy is a little misleading, in that this technique bears little resemblance to straight osteopathy. This version is an approach to the treatment of the whole body, as well as the head, by using the rhythmical pulse of the cerebro-spinal fluid as an aid to diagnosis and treatment. It was originally developed by an osteopath, William Sutherland, who shortly before the end of the nineteenth century, convinced himself by experiment that it was possible to diagnose and treat disorders simply by using his hand to explore his patients' skulls.

Procedure

Cranial osteopathy is generally used as part of treatment, and is so gentle that patients are hardly aware of it. The therapists explain that they are "feeling" the cerebro-spinal fluid by palpation, similar to the way a GP feels the pulse of a patient, but intuition as well as basic knowledge are used here. The pulse can be felt anywhere on the body, but is particularly clear on the skull and in the pelvic area. Feeling the pulse not only enables osteopaths to make a diagnosis, but it also prompts them to make slight changes of pressure which can lead to significant changes in the patient.

Suitable cases

Cranial osteopaths take on much the same kind of patients as osteopaths. They claim some success in treating conditions which have resisted other forms of treatment, such as epilepsy, deafness and migraine, and also find it useful in the treatment of autistic children and new-born babies, particularly those who have had a difficult birth.

Cranial osteopathy techniques

Cranial osteopathy is an extremely subtle form of diagnosis and treatment in which the therapist feels for the "involuntary mechanism" – very slight rhythmical expansion and contraction movements which constitute the pulse of the cerebrospinal fluid. The quality and symmetry of this pulse give useful information about the general state of health of the tissues.

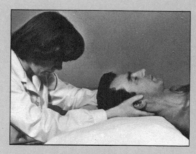

1 *With the weight of the patient's cranium in her hands, the osteopath can detect quite complex "strain patterns" in the cranial tissues.*

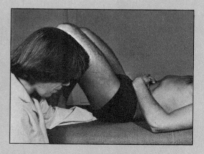

2 *Working on the base of the spine, the osteopath affects the relationship of the pelvic bones to one another, as well as the muscle tone of the pelvis and lower spine.*

Chiropractic

Chiropractic has been defined by the British Chiropractors' Association as "an independent branch of medicine which specializes in the diagnosis and treatment of mechanical disorders of the joints, particularly those of the spine, and their effects on the nervous system". The term is taken from the Greek, and means "manual practice", or "treatment by manipulation"; the practice is said to have originated with Hippocrates.

Origins

Chiropractic is derived from similar roots as *Osteopathy* (pages 80 to 86). It was founded in 1895 by David Daniel Palmer of Iowa. "Displacement of any part of the skeletal frame", his belief was, "may press against nerves, which are the channels of communication, intensifying or decreasing their carrying capacity, creating either too much or not enough functioning, an aberration known as disease". Slight displacements of the spinal vertebrae ("subluxations", as his disciples began to call them) might be reflected in a great range of symptoms, not just backache, but headache, indigestion, asthma and psoriasis. Unlike orthodox medicine, the aim of chiropractic was not to concentrate upon dealing with the symptoms, but to find the subluxation and correct it manually; as a result of this the symptoms would disappear.

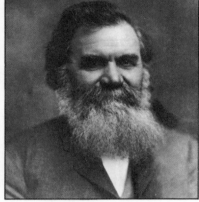

David Daniel Palmer
Palmer (1845–1913), the founder of modern chiropractic, a therapy which seeks to cure spinal and nervous disorders by manipulation.

The main differences between chiropractic and osteopathy

Ian Hutchinson of the British Chiropractors' Association explains: "The differences in the theories behind these treatments are mostly historical. The early osteopaths believed that the effect of their treatment was via the blood circulation, whereas chiropractors emphasized the role of the nervous system. Recent surveys have shown that there are great similarities between the two groups. The major differences were that chiropractors used X-rays about five times more frequently than osteopaths and were more likely to perform orthopaedic tests and neurological or physical examinations on their patients.

In treatment, osteopaths make more use of mobilization of joints and use more soft tissue techniques. Traditionally, the difference between chiropractic and osteopathic manipulative techniques has been that osteopaths use greater leverage while chiropractors employ less leverage and more direct technique. Using osteopathic leverage techniques, contact is still often made some distance from the joint being manipulated, whereas in chiropractic techniques, leverage is often used but contact is made directly over the vertebra being adjusted. Chiropractors will usually adjust a joint in a specific direction to free it in this direction, whereas osteopaths are less concerned with the direction of their manipulation".

Developments in modern chiropractic

Although in theory chiropractors today still owe allegiance to this principle, in practice they have moved away from it, albeit in different directions, according to the nationality. In the United States, largely owing to the way in which members of the medical profession have increasingly tended to specialize, chiropractors have been taking over primary care in many parts of the country, where general practitioners are scarce. This has meant that they have been placing less reliance on manipulation. In Britain, where there are far fewer chiropractors in proportion to the population and where almost everyone has free access to GPs, chiropractors have tended to become specialists in the use of manipulation in the treatment of back pain and related disorders.

A survey of British chiropractic published in the journal *Rheumatology and Rehabilitation* in 1977 showed that more than half the patients came with pain in the lower back, and a further one in five with neck pain. To the question "Do you find that patients sometimes seek your help because of a reluctance to take drugs?", no less than 98 percent answered "yes", and a majority added that the patients were usually reluctant to inform their doctor that they were going to try chiropractic.

Procedure

As described by a working chiropractor, Stephen North, the procedure involves first, the taking of a case history. As patients are not, as a rule, referred from their GP, a chiropractor, unlike a physiotherapist, has to take a very full medical history. Then there will be a physical examination "to assess the general

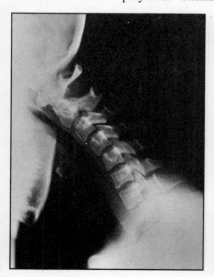 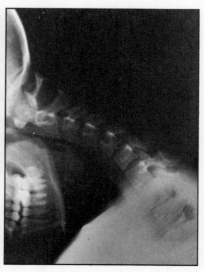

Chiropractic treatment for migraine
This patient had been suffering from migraine headaches, with associated vertigo, nausea, and vomiting. An X-ray taken before treatment (see left) shows reduced movement of the lower neck probably caused by a minor whiplash as a child. After six weeks of chiropractic treatment (see right), normal movement has been restored.

condition of the patient and to shed light on disorders relating to the condition complained of". Third, an X-ray and fourth, in some cases, the taking of blood and urine specimens for analysis in a laboratory.

Treatment, North explains, "is based on the combined assessment of all levels of examination and is specifically designed for the individual. Its aim is to achieve and maintain a state of mechanical equilibrium in the back consistent with freedom from pain and disability".

The long-term aims

Although the immediate approach is usually towards spinal adjustment (specific manipulation), the prevention of recurrences

Consulting a chiropractor

Chiropractic treatment is based on the principle that mechanical dysfunction is best corrected by mechanical means. The main method used in treatment is "adjustment" – specific manipulation of a fixed joint using a high-velocity, low-amplitude thrust, applied directly to a vertebra; this varies according to the area being treated.

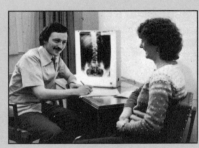

1 *The chiropractor takes a full case history, followed by orthopaedic tests, a neurological and physical examination, and often an X-ray, to exclude other conditions that might be causing the symptoms.*

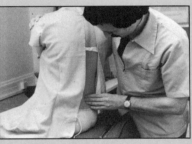

2 *With the body twisted, each of the lumbar spinal joints is palpated, to reveal which show 'fixation" – lack of movement – or hypermobility – excessive movement.*

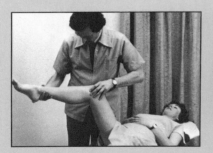

6 *The chiropractor tests the rotation of the hip joint, with the leg raised and bent at the knee.*

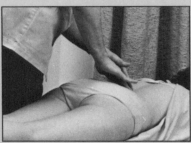

7 *During the examination the chiropractor also feels for any increases in muscle tone and other tissue changes around joints.*

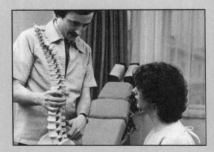

8 *Using a model of the spine and pelvis, the chiropractor explains what he has discovered during the examination before proceeding with the treatment.*

requires cooperation between patient and chiropractor. The patient's critical interest is encouraged by attention to mobility, strength, posture, gait, obesity and occupational stress. Sometimes patients are encouraged to become active in "self-help" areas such as relaxation classes, *Yoga* or *T'ai chi* (see pages 138 to 146). Until recently, chiropractors used a recognizably different technique from osteopathy. Instead of exerting leverage through arms and legs, they relied on a thrust to restore the displaced vertebrae to their correct alignment. They also tended to concentrate most of their attention upon the cervical vertebrae, where the head joins the body. But over the years, the difference between the two therapies has dwindled, and many chiropractors now use some osteopathic techniques, and vice versa.

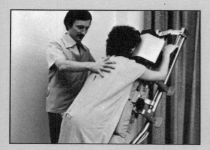

3 *A patient who is in too much pain to lie down can be lowered from a standing position on a specially designed chiropractic couch.*

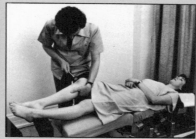

4 *Using a hammer, the chiropractor checks the patient's reflexes – in this case, he is checking the quadriceps reflex.*

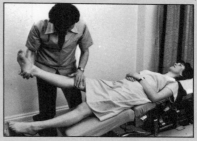

5 *One of the orthopaedic tests involves stretching the sciatic nerve – if there is any pressure on the nerve, raising the leg straight up will be painful.*

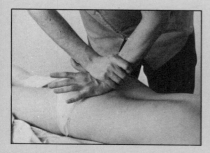

9 *To adjust one of the sacro-iliac joints – the joint between the spine and the pelvis – the left hand is in contact with the pelvis and equal pressure is exerted through the right and left arms.*

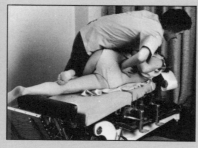

10 *With the patient lying on her side, one of the lumbar spinal joints is adjusted.*

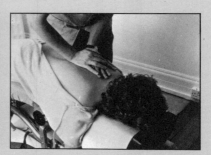

11 *The chiropractor uses both hands to adjust one of the joints in the thoracic spine.*

Research

How effective is chiropractic? Indirect evidence of its effectiveness has been provided by statistics about the use of manipulation in the treatment of industrial back injuries in the United States, through workmen's compensation records.

A study in Florida in 1960 of nearly 20,000 cases revealed that the average cost per case was 60 dollars, compared with 102 dollars for medical treatment and that the average work time lost was only three days for cases treated by chiropractic, compared to nine days for medically treated cases.

Similar studies from other states of the Union have shown a similar pattern. And a recent report from a government commission set up to investigate chiropractic in New Zealand, whose members collected, sifted and assessed evidence from the United States, Canada, Britain, Australia and other countries, came to the conclusion that manual therapy of the kind chiropractors provide "can be effective in relieving musculoskeletal symptoms such as back pain, and other symptoms known to respond to such therapy, such as migraine".

The safety factor

As with osteopathy, the allegation has often been made that a chiropractor has missed some simple diagnosis, and used manipulation in circumstances where it can do no good and may do harm – for example, if there is a bone tumour. But the chiropractors' use of X-rays makes this sort of occurrence unlikely, and in any case, in Britain at least, the great majority of their patients come to them after diagnosis by a member of the medical profession has disclosed that there appears to be nothing organically the matter with them (though chiropractors sometimes find there is).

In the hands of a trained, registered chiropractor, the New Zealand commission reported, "spinal manipulative therapy is safe"; they are sufficiently well-trained "to determine why there are contra-indications to spinal manual therapy in a particular case, and whether the patient should have medical care instead of, or as well as, chiropractic care".

Impressive statistics back up safety claims

Striking evidence for the relative safety of chiropractic, as compared to orthodox medical treatment, has come from the United States. In the early 1970s, a check on the insurance premiums paid by orthopedic specialists in cities such as New York and Los Angeles as protection from malpractice suits was around $5,000; by the mid 1970s it had increased in New York to $25,000, and in Los Angeles to $50,000. The equivalent premiums for chiropractors worked out at about one fiftieth of these figures.

Gradually it has begun to dawn in orthodox medical circles

that chiropractic can no longer be derided and dismissed. "What is to be done about chiropractors?", the *New England Journal of Medicine* asked in a recent editorial. "Efforts by organized medicine to eliminate them have been unsuccessful. The label 'quack' has not stuck. Despite the most strenuous opposition, they have attained licensure in every state in the United States and in Canada and many foreign countries. Over 23,000 chiropractors treat some eight million Americans for a wide variety of conditions. Reimbursement for their services has been authorized by Medicare, Medicaid, Workmen's Compensation plans, and by many Blue Shield plans and other private insurance carriers. Chiropractors received more than 30,000 dollars worth of Medicare funds in 1978. Over 2,000 new chiropractors will be graduated this year, more than 70 percent of them from colleges federally recognized as accredited. Chiropractors appear to be winning their struggle to survive".

Ten years ago, the editors of *The New England Journal of Medicine* would not have even considered printing such subversive stuff. Twenty years ago, if they *had* printed it, they would have been either sacked or certified insane. But now, chiropractic has broken through in North America to the point where the medical profession can no longer block its progress to recognition.

Establishment objections to chiropractic

In Britain, the medical profession has felt less threatened by chiropractors, partly because there are so few of them (there are currently only about 150), partly because so much of their time is spent on backache, which doctors have to admit is not an ailment they can deal with effectively. Nevertheless, when the Chiropractors' Association decided in 1975 to apply for registration under the Professions Supplementary to Medicine Act, the doctor-dominated PSM Council turned the application down. Although the Council declined to give its reasons, the chiropractors were unofficially informed that they could not be considered as "supplementary" so long as their method was based on a different *principle* from orthodox medicine.

The fundamental objection is not to chiropractors treating backs – if they stuck to that, the general impression is, they would be acceptable. What irritates the medical establishment is their presumption that chiropractic manipulation of the spine can be effective in treating other types of disorder. This is an attitude which found expression in a recent editorial in the *British Medical Journal* (*BMJ*).

Some alternative systems of medicine, it observed, have begun to seriously compete with orthodoxy – in spite of the fact that "for treating conditions other than bone and joint abnormalities chiropractic, for example, ought to be as distinct as divination of the future by examination of a bird's entrails".

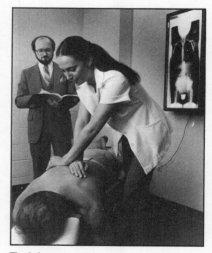

Training as a chiropractor
Chiropractors use X-rays both to diagnose their patient and to monitor them during treatment. Here, observed by her teacher, a student performs a high-velocity, low-amplitude thrust to free an immobile joint.

The same *BMJ* editorial went on to make the point that there is no evidence of a kind acceptable to medical science that chiropractic works. The profession was not simply being bloody-minded it believed. "No: what is wrong is the refusal by the critics and the fringe practitioners to accept the standards of proof that medical scientists have developed in the last hundred years; not for nothing has the concept of the randomised, double-blind control trial been described as one of Britain's most important contributions to medicine since the war. In the case of chiropractic, for example, the fact that many patients treated by chiropractitioners get better is seen as evidence enough of professional respectability. Yet what is the basis of some chiropractitioners readiness to treat diabetes or psoriasis by manipulation of the spine? The underlying theory has not been subjected to scientific testing – it is an article of faith, no more rational than the acupuncturist's belief in *yin* and *yang*".

The lack of controlled trials

To this there were, and still are, two answers. As we observed in the introduction to this section, "randomised, double-blind controlled trials" can be used to test drugs, but not to test chiropractic manipulation. It cannot be given "blind" because patients, unless they are singularly obtuse, will be able to guess whether the manipulation they are receiving is or is not genuine, and the chiropractors will know whether the manipulation they are giving is genuine. And randomizing patients would deprive the chiropractors of their chance to reject patients they feel will not respond to manipulation. Besides, as correspondents wrote in to the *BMJ* to point out, the success of chiropractors does not depend exclusively upon their technique. "The modern doctor tends to depend more and more on scientific medicine at the expense of viewing the patient as a whole person", one correspondent pointed out. "Chiropractors and the like go to the other extreme, setting themselves to understand how the patient feels and to explain what is wrong".

Even if full controls are not practicable, however, it is possible to set up trials which give some indication of whether or not manipulation works satisfactorily, and enable a rough comparison to be made with standard medical techniques. The New Zealand committee of enquiry took the trouble to collect, sift and assess the results of all the trials which have been reported where manipulative methods, not just chiropractic, have been used in western countries. The overall message, its conclusion was, "appears to be quite clear. It is that spinal manual therapy, even if performed by relatively unskilled and inexperienced practitioners, is more effective in providing quick relief of pain of musculoskeletal origin than are conservative methods. Furthermore, there was no evidence of any harm being done to patients.

Thus spinal manipulation, at least for a clearly defined type of condition, appears to be safe and effective".

Suitable cases

The British Chiropractors' Association lists low back pain (lumbago), disc lesions, sciatica and other leg pains, hip and knee problems, headaches, neck pain, shoulder and arm pain, and pins and needles or numbness sensations. Muscular aches, and joint pains such as those in the elbows, feet and ankles, can also be treated, it claims.

Massage

Massage is easier to demonstrate than to describe. As a technique, it lies between the laying on of hands and therapeutic touch, on the one hand, and shiatsu, acupressure, physiotherapy and rolfing on the other. It is primarily concerned with the soft tissues, the chief aim being to promote relaxation – paradoxically, though, it can act as a stimulant – perhaps because by relaxing muscles and removing tension, massage frees previously contained energies.

Origins

Massage is as old as history and can be found in every culture in the world, in one form or another. In the East, children learn to massage at a very early age. It's as normal in most parts of the world, and as familiar, as taking a bath.

The mystery is why it should so largely have drifted out of fashion in the West. Presumably, the advances in scientific medicine during the nineteenth century led to the belief that massage would no longer be required as a form of therapy. For a time, however, it continued to be provided by medical auxiliaries, and was extensively used in the First World War to rehabilitate wounded soldiers. Later, however, it went out of fashion, as physiotherapists became attracted to other, more "modern" forms of treatment and began using a variety of mechanical gadgets.

Recently, massage has been coming back into its own. It is not, strictly speaking, a therapy, as many of those who seek it do so simply because they enjoy it. But many people do find it therapeutic, either because they feel that it sets them up for what they are doing – professional footballers, for example – or because they find that the relaxation is beneficial for mind and body alike.

❛ Giving a massage is something everybody ought to be able to do. It isn't a mystique – it's a natural thing, and very easy. I'm not talking about the hour-long professional body massage, but about easing somebody's shoulders in the office, or massaging your husband or wife when they get in tired from work. ❜

Clare Maxwell-Hudson
Masseuse

Procedure

Sometimes the therapist will come to the patient's own home –
this is often the case with elderly or bed-ridden people, or those
who cannot get about easily – more often than not, however, you
go to them for the treatment.

Many masseuses (women now predominate in this field) like to
use a special massage table; others prefer to work on the floor

Massage techniques

*All you need for a body massage is some oil,
several towels to keep the person warm while
you work on exposed areas, and a firm*
*surface. Don't talk too much during the
massage and try to keep your hands in contact with the body all the time.*

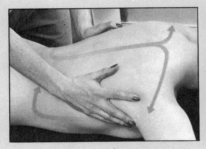

1 *Make sure your hands are well
oiled. Stroke both hands firmly
up either side of the spine, continue
out across the shoulders and glide
your hands gently down the sides
and in at the waist; "stroking" is
used to link movements.*

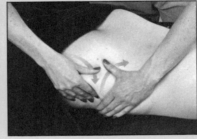

2 *Kneading is particularly good
for fatty areas like thighs and
buttocks. Imagine you are kneading
dough: grasp and release the flesh
first with one hand and then the
other, working in flowing, circular
movements.*

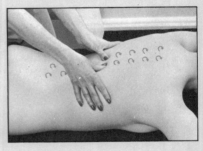

3 *To relax tense back and neck
muscles, make small, firm, circular movements up either side of
the spine with your thumbs; push
the muscle up and out, gliding your
hands gently from one point to the
next.*

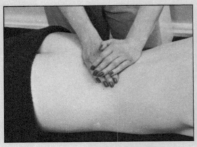

7 *Finish off the back massage by
creating heat in the small of the
back. Cup both hands together for
a minute or two to build up heat,
then very slowly, lift them off the
skin.*

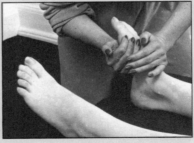

8 *Working on the front of the
body, begin by stroking the
whole leg and then work down to
the feet. Using both hands, firmly
stroke the instep, arch and toes.
This is very soothing and relaxing.*

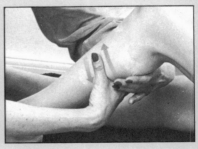

9 *Working from the ankle to
knee, cross-cross the hands
around the calf without losing contact with the skin. This is particularly effective for loosening up
tight calf muscles.*

(most beds are impractical because they are too soft). The room will be warm enough for the person being massaged to remain comfortable, lying undressed (or nearly) prone on a blanket, or towel, on a table or on the floor.

The techniques of massage

The course which the massage takes will vary according to the predilections of the therapist. One of the clearest accounts of

In the following photographs several different techniques are demonstrated but you can give a relaxing massage by simply using "stroking". *The movements should be rhythmical and firm on the upward stroke and gentle on the return.*

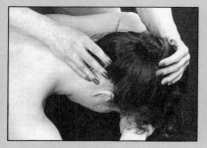

4 *To relieve tension in the neck, continue with the same movement using the thumb and forefinger of one hand. Work up the neck and support the head with your other hand. Pressure should be firm but not painful.*

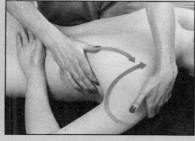

5 *Stroke around the shoulder working in a clockwise direction to relax the muscles. One hand should make a full circle and the other a half circle making one continuous movement.*

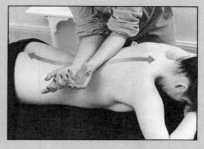

6 *Stroking the back is very pleasant. Centre the forearms on the middle of the back and push them apart working down towards the buttocks and up to the hairline, gliding gently over the neck. Hold for a second and repeat.*

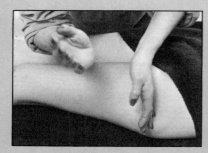

10 *Stimulate areas like the buttocks and thighs with fast hacking movements. These should not hurt, so use only the sides of the hands, making "bouncy", upward movements.*

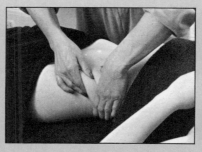

11 *After stroking the centre of the stomach in a clockwise motion, knead (see step 2) the area around the waist by grasping and releasing the flesh with alternate hands.*

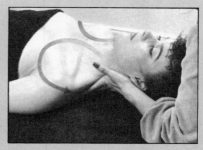

12 *Work the chest by sliding both hands together down the breastbone and out across the shoulders. Mould the hands around the shoulders and behind the neck.*

what to expect of massage was provided by Clare Maxwell-Hudson in *Your Health and Beauty Book*. She is writing from her own experiences as a masseuse, and while other practitioners may not agree with her on details, they would be in broad agreement on her general description.

Treatment almost always begins with *effleurage* – stroking movements, which also spread oil over the surface of the back. The oil is not essential, but it makes things easier for the therapist, and pleasanter for the person being massaged. Vegetable, mineral or baby oils are commonly used and they are mixed with essential oils; talc is sometimes used as a substitute, but this is less effective, and it feels less pleasant.

As well as stroking, you can expect a number of other techniques: friction, energetic rubbing, of the kind which you would expect to use to warm somebody up; *pétrissage*, a kneading process, which is used on the fleshy areas of the body. "It is used on the underlying muscles and fatty areas; it stretches shortened muscles and tissue, and helps to relax hard, contracted muscles", says Clare Maxwell-Hudson. There may also be circular movements up either side of the spine and neck, alternating pressure and then relaxation. There are many other variations on the massage theme: gentle slapping; "hacking" with the sides of the hands; clapping with slightly cupped hands; pummelling and "piano playing" (the fingers drumming on the fleshy area at the base of the neck).

Pain can be good

Most people, contemplating taking massage for the first time, are likely to ask whether it hurts or not. This depends on the therapist. Some feel that no pain should be felt and that there is something wrong if it *is* felt. Others, a minority, incline to the "rolfian" view – that pain can be integral to the success of the treatment (see pages 101 to 104). A middle-of-the-road attitude which is increasingly encountered is that pain can give a useful indication of an area of tension, and although there may be a painful moment, a split-second later the relief from the easing of the tension makes it almost pleasurable in retrospect.

How frequently massage is carried out depends on your inclinations and your income. If you like being massaged, and are rich enough to afford it, you may enjoy it daily – as do some sports people and athletes. Many people have a regular weekly massage; some go only when they feel they need it. Most people who enjoy massage would say they would have it more frequently if time or money would allow. Only the very tense or the very inhibited would prefer to take a tranquillizer than be massaged, if the choice were left to them.

A problem faces anybody who wants to try massage, but has no idea who to go to. Qualifications, such as they are, mean little.

Skill depends partly on innate knack, partly on experience, partly on the ability to achieve a kind of psycho-physiological rapport with the recipient so that, in some way not as yet understood, the hands of the therapist move in harmony with the muscles on which they are working.

"Massage should be pleasurable"

Even if you know little or nothing about the techniques of massage, you can often tell within minutes whether a practitioner is any good. Much can depend simply on mutual liking between client and therapist. An hour in the company of somebody who is irritating is unlikely to be very beneficial, however proficient the operator. "I am constantly surprised", Clare Maxwell-Hudson observes, "that today's massage training lays all the emphasis on technique. The consequence is that the massage is clinical and soulless, which neither the giver nor the recipient enjoy. Massage should be pleasurable".

Because it should be pleasurable, the hour must not be boring, and this means a readiness on the part of both people involved either to talk, or not to talk, as the mood takes them. During massage, Clare Maxwell-Hudson feels talk is to be avoided. The therapist, she argues, should concentrate on what he or she is doing; and there is no doubt that massage given properly is physically taxing on the therapist.

Suitable cases

Deciding who is likely to benefit most from massage presents a problem, for the obvious reason that response to massage depends largely on the subjective reaction of the patient – or client, the term some practitioners prefer. People who come to them, they point out, are not patients; they could more accurately be described as people who want to *avoid* becoming patients at a later stage.

As massage is primarily a technique of relaxation, it is most commonly sought by tense people and those who suffer from stress symptoms such as headaches. But its practitioners emphasize that it adapts itself to individual needs, in particular, those of athletes, dancers, musicians, and other people who regularly use certain sets of muscles which can become strained, fatigued or injured.

When rapport is established, massage can be used either as a stimulant, or as a soporific. You don't therefore need to be ill to have massage or seek it and there should be no *unsuitable* cases for treatment. But the therapist ordinarily will wish to know if you have any serious disorder such as thrombosis and he or she may advise you to have it checked by another practitioner before continuing with massage.

Self-help

Almost anybody can learn to give massage, even if not everybody can learn to give it professionally; and this is useful in the case of large families, or groups living together. It takes time and practice to develop a good technique, but remember that there's a good chance that if you picture what you like having done to you, that it will feel good to someone else. If you are simply suffering from sore feet, for example, spend a few minutes stroking them.

Face massage

Nothing short of plastic surgery can get rid of lines and wrinkles, once they have formed. But massage can help prevent new tension lines from appearing for not only does it help relax the muscles but it also stimulates the blood vessels under the skin.

Begin by cleansing your face thoroughly and then follow the procedure illustrated here, using the basic movements – stroking, pinching and stimulating.

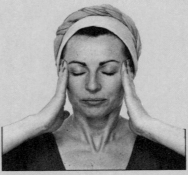

1 Start by stroking the whole face. Use both hands and work up the neck, out across the cheeks, then glide gently inwards, work up and out over the forehead. Finish by applying gentle pressure to the temples.

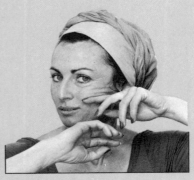

2 Stimulate the skin by using the back of your hands and loosely rolling your fingers up the cheek. This can also be used on the neck and under the chin.

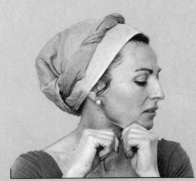

3 With your thumb and fore-finger, gently pinch the skin along the jawbone and under the chin. This is very stimulating and helps prevent a double chin.

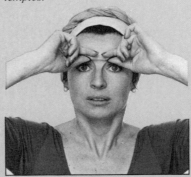

4 To release tension around the eyes, firmly squeeze the eyebrows with your thumb and fore-finger. Always work from the bridge of the nose towards the temples.

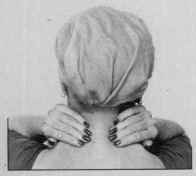

5 For tension in the neck and shoulders make firm circular movements working up either side of the neck then out across the shoulders.

Rolfing

Rolfing or Structural Integration is a particular technique of connective tissue manipulation which seeks to liberate the physical structures of the body, so that they are able to realign and integrate themselves "properly with respect to gravity".

Origins

Manipulative therapy in general tends to regard the spine as having the key role – like a tent-pole upon which the body relies to maintain its posture integration. Dr Ida Rolf, who gained her doctorate in 1920 in biological chemistry and then went on to work in organic chemistry at the Rockefeller Institute, began (for reasons which those quizzing her always found her reluctant to talk about) to question this assumption. A tent-pole, she pointed out, is of little use unless it is securely supported all the way round by pegs and guy ropes, and the body works on the same principle. So in the 1940s she initiated a method of working on those pegs and guy ropes – the connective tissue and muscle – by the application of manual pressure.

Rolf's "pile of bricks"

Another way she had of viewing the human body was in terms of a child's tower of bricks – so long as the body is correctly aligned, all is well, but if any part is out of alignment, as can happen as the result of an injury, an emotional trauma, or just bad postural habits, then the structure becomes unstable. Instead of the muscles performing their natural function of coming into action when, and only when, required, some of them have to spend their whole time shoring the structure up. Eventually they lose their elasticity, adhesions develop in the connective tissue (which also hardens) and energy is lost as the body adjusts to coping with supporting itself in its new, out-of-kilter arrangement. Gravity, instead of reinforcing balance and integration of the body, is now the cause of stress.

To correct this, Rolf decided, what is needed is a form of manipulation that will use gravity as a tool, to stretch and shift the connective tissue back into a state of symmetry, when the body will be free to take its natural – and therefore correct – posture, which in turn restores the entire nervous system to efficient working order. "Man has become aware of himself as a more patterned structure: he feels himself revitalized".

Relating emotions to posture

Rolfing, however, is not simply a matter of restoring physical equilibrium. Rolf came to believe that feelings create postural change (as when we speak of somebody being bowed with grief, or tense with rage), so that working to rebalance the physical body will often involve the release of emotional pain, and memories

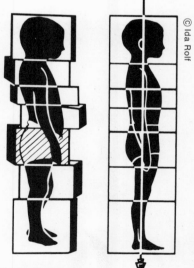

© Ida Rolf

The Rolfing bricks
This diagram of a child with whom Ida Rolf worked has become the symbol of rolfing. Each brick relates to a part of the body and the aim of rolfing is to make the "tower of bricks" perpendicular, as in the second diagram.

may even be recalled of traumatic episodes in a person's life as specific parts of the body are rolfed. The technique, then, offers the possibility of changes in behaviour and attitudes – and also of "enhanced abilities".

It was not until the mid-60s – after around 35 years of work with her technique – when Dr Rolf had moved to Esalen, on the west coast of California, that the 10-session course which is now the accepted practice first became established. Rolf began official classes for training students at this time and it was not until the 1970s that the Rolf Institute – still the only training centre for prospective therapists – was established.

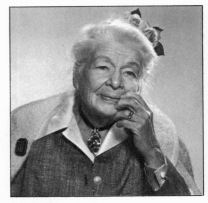

Ida Rolf
Ida Rolf is the founder of rolfing, a deep-massage technique which frees the mind and emotions as well as the body from their conditioning.

Procedure

The sessions usually take place once a week, and last about an hour. After your case history has been taken you will be photographed from the front, back and both sides – in order to compare yourself before and after the course – and then asked to lie down, usually on a massage couch, though the floor will do.

The therapist works with the connective tissue around the chest and neck, using knuckles and fingers to stretch and to separate out the layers of tissue. He or she will then proceed to work on the feet and ankles, the sides, legs, abdomen, diaphragm, ribcage, the pelvis – in a systematic way covering everything from head to foot, including even the inside of the mouth. Then the "after" photographs will be taken – often after each session – and you can see as well as feel for yourself all the changes that have taken place in your body.

There are any number of opinions on what the experience of being rolfed is like. According to the account of one journalist, Lisa Connolly, the sessions range "from the pleasure of firm massage to intensely, but momentarily searing pain". But the degree of both the pleasure and the pain "depends on the emotional and/or physical experience present in the particular part of the body being rolfed, and the inner willingness and participation of the rolfee to be rolfed. . . . It is vital in this most intimate experience of physical contact that the rolfer and rolfee share mutual trust and affinity".

Research

In a project sponsored recently by the Rolf Institute of Structural Integration, 48 subjects were divided into two groups (that were as far as possible matched), and one of the groups was rolfed. Measurements and tests were made in a variety of ways ranging from electroencephalogram (EEG) recordings to *Kirlian photography* (pages 273 to 275). The report claimed striking benefits: "Rolfing makes consistent and progressive changes during each

Rolfing techniques

A course of rolfing typically consists of 10 one-hourly sessions. During the first seven sessions, the rolfer will concentrate on manipulating individual parts of your body, and during the final three sessions reintegrate and realign the whole body. Rolfers emphasize that you should make a conscious effort to relax during sessions, in this way you will help to release tension.

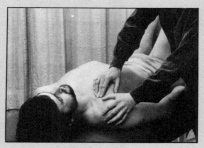

1 The rolfer photographs each client from the back, front, and each side before the course starts and again at the end of each session.

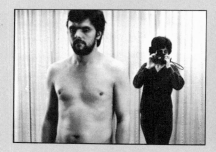

2 While the client lies on a flat couch, the rolfer uses her fingertips, knuckles, and, occasionally, her elbows to free shortened connective tissue.

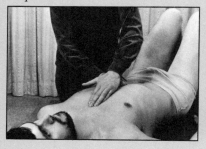

3 This work will be continued down the center of the rib cage around the breastbone.

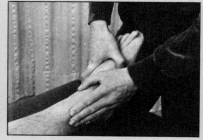

4 In one of the early sessions the rolfer will concentrate her work on the legs and feet to help improve the client's balance enabling him to feel more "centred".

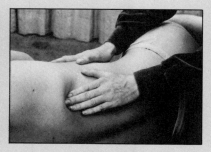

5 To promote easier breathing, the rolfer works on expanding the sides of the rib cage.

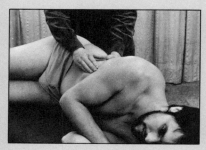

6 The rolfer will work on both sides of the rib cage to ensure even expansion.

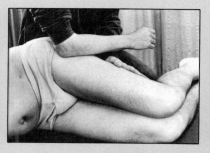

7 Elbows may be used to stretch the connective tissue along the side of the upper thigh.

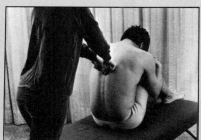

8 Each session ends with the rolfer working on the client's back and the neck.

session, and based upon the areas of the body processed", it concludes "the widespread implications for psychophysical health are profound".

How profound the implications are will have to await further research, monitored by independent assessors. What is clear, however, is that rolfing has a striking effect on many of those who elect to try it – from physical changes, that from photographs it can be seen are maintained over a year after the treatment sessions, to psychological changes that it might be expected could only take place through some form of psychotherapy.

Suitable cases

Looking around a roomful of people, Ida Rolf would often cheerfully claim that everybody present would be all the better for a course. Rolfing, though, is not designed for treatment of any disorder – although it may be of help with certain types of headaches or backache – but is aimed rather at prevention. The assumption is that re-establishing structural integration will help liberate the body's homeostatic mechanism to perform its functions unimpeded, and so reduce the risk of illness of any kind. But for many clients, it primarily represents a way towards personal growth.

The Alexander principle

The Alexander principle is not easily described. It is a type of therapy which aims to treat, and prevent, a range of disorders by what is essentially a system of postural changes.

Origins

Towards the end of the nineteenth century, an Australian, F. Matthias Alexander, found that his career as an actor and reciter, which had hitherto been successful, was in jeopardy because he kept inexplicably losing his voice during performances. "Having the true scientific spirit and industry", Bernard Shaw was to recall, Alexander "set himself to discover what it was that he was really doing to disable himself in this fashion. In the end he found this out and a great deal more as well". He discovered that the immediate cause of his loss of voice was that he was pulling his head backwards and downwards during his performances. "The great deal more" that he found was to be the basis of the therapy that has become known as the Alexander principle.

Alexander agreed with Still and Palmer (the founders of

It is now possible to conceive of a totally new type of education, affecting the entire range of human activity . . . which would preserve children and adults from most of the diseases and evils that now affect them.

Aldous Huxley
Ends and Means

Oestopathy and *Chiropractic*, see pages 80 to 100) about the importance of the integrity of the spinal column, but he differed from them in two significant respects. If the vertebrae were out of alignment, he believed, the reason was generally *misuse*. We can get into bad habits, standing or sitting, walking or talking. By adopting postures for which our bodies are not designed, we subject them to strains for which they are unfitted. Habit, he asserted, influences the use we make of our bodies, and the use we make of them influences the way in which they function.

Secondly, Alexander believed, "our manner of use is a constant influence for good or ill upon our *general* functioning". Alexander was not thinking exclusively in physiological terms. We must, he asserted, "appreciate the part played by an improving manner of use in the restoration and maintenance of psycho-physical efficiency and conditions of well-being". Mind and body, to him, were interrelated.

Alexander's basic premise was that we must stop doing what comes naturally, because that is often the product of years of misuse and bad habits: slouching, slumping, tensing up, and so on. Postural habits may have to be quite deliberately broken, so that they can be replaced with new and better habits. His method, he emphasized, did not consist of a series of set exercises, because what was needed would be different for each individual who took his course. He preferred to regard it as a system of reconditioning.

Procedure

Alexander admitted that his method could not be described for instructional purposes in a manual, defending himself from criticism by pointing out that neither can the game of golf. Teachers of his method and their pupils would agree. There has never been a good description of what to expect if you decide to take an Alexander course, nor is there likely to be. In general terms you can expect a series of lessons. But how many weeks, months, or even years they will take varies greatly from patient to patient. Some complete a course after, say, 12 visits, others, with more serious problems, may need much longer.

A patient's eye view

Perhaps the most revealing account was included in Dr Wilfred Barlow's *More Talk of Alexander*. This was the diary of an American woman who could not walk, and could stand only with the help of a stick, who had been persuaded while in London to take a course of lessons from Alexander, and kept a diary describing what happened.

Even these diary entries are tantalizingly short of descriptions of what Alexander actually did, apart from constantly reminding her to keep her joints moving and flexible. But his aim, clearly,

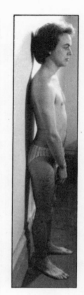

Demonstrating faults in posture
If a patient is asked to stand against a wall, as shown, certain common faults will be apparent. These may include the shoulders touching the wall before the buttocks, and an excessive hollow in the back.

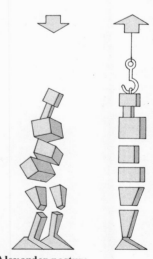

Alexander posture
F.M. Alexander taught that spinal energy should flow upwards so that all movement comes from the head. An imaginary hook pulls the spine up into the correct alignment, that of a gently curved vertical.

Learning the Alexander principle

Teachers of the Alexander principle all work in slightly different ways. Some work with you in a sitting position, others find that patients relax more easily if they lie down. As part of your course, you will be taught how to maintain the directions given during training.

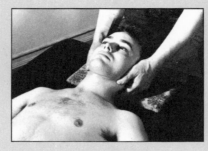

1 *The patient is told to concentrate his total attention on the words "Neck free, head forward and out", while the teacher lets him experience what the correct position feels like.*

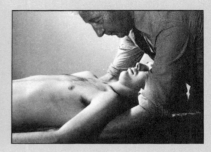

2 *The patient focuses on the words "Back, lengthen and widen", while the teacher slides his hands under the patient's back and moves it into the correct position thereby releasing the tension.*

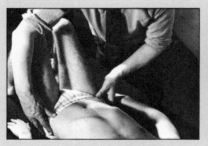

3 *If, like most people, the patient arches his lower back, he is instructed to think of the words "Back, back", while the teacher flexes his pelvis.*

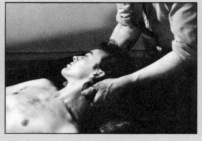

4 *To control tension, the patient must learn to check immediate responses to stimuli. For example, when told that his head will be moved, he must relax and think "Head forward and out", while his head is turned.*

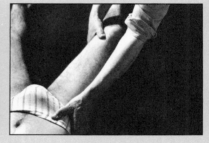

5 *While his leg is rotated and flexed, the patient is taught to keep still, inhibiting any movement, and to run through the verbal instructions for steps 1 and 2 (above), adding the words "Hip free, knee out".*

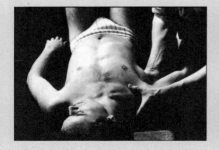

6 *People often hunch their shoulders up and forward. To correct this, the patient is told to concentrate on the words "Back, down and widen" while the teacher encourages the shoulders to go back on the couch.*

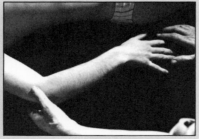

7 *All patients learn the above instructions before being taught to release other, more individual tensions. Here the patient concentrates on "Wrist in, elbow out", to regain the correct line for the forearm.*

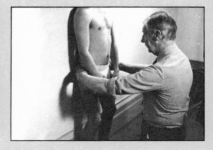

8 *After the work on the couch, the patient goes through the same instructions for head, neck and shoulders standing against a wall with feet apart, heels 5 cm (2 in) from the wall and knees slightly bent.*

was to make her visualize her posture as it would be if she was in full health and strength, so that she could consciously correct faults in the way she was actually standing. This meant that she continually had to do things with, say, her neck and head – things which felt all wrong. As she herself put it, "all the things which feel right for me to do are wrong. So I must not do the wrong thing – that is, the thing that to me feels right". By nagging at her to break habits of misuse, Alexander managed to liberate her joints and muscles – which was sometimes a painful process – until eventually she returned home able to walk again and having recovered her general health.

Research

The Alexander principle does not lend itself easily to controlled trials. Recently in England, however, Dr Barlow collaborated with Professor J.M. Tanner of the Institute of Child Health to put a group of 50 music students through the course and compare their posture over a period of nine months with a matched group of acting students who were given routine gymnastic training. Dr Barlow has since reported that: "the figures showed a marked postural improvement in the Alexander group and a deterioration in the (acting) group".

On an anecdotal level, the principle can claim enthusiastic testimonials from some eminent people. The great American educationalist, John Dewey, for example, had been clumsy all his life. While he had found this a nuisance and sometimes an embarrassment, he assumed there was nothing that could be done.

According to Edward Maisel in his introduction to *The Alexander Technique*, Dewey realized, from his work with Alexander, "that his own bodily activities were as appropriate a domain as any for the exercise of his highest abilities. He credited the technique therefore not only with having effected a marked improvement in his health, but also with having made him conscious of his total ignorance of a whole field of knowledge".

Aldous Huxley and Alexander

Sir Stafford Cripps thought that the course he took with Alexander was "one of the fortunate experiences of my life". Aldous Huxley, though he admitted that he could not explain *why* the Alexander method worked, said he was sure, "as a matter of personal experience and observation, that it gives us all the things we have been looking for in a system of physical education: relief from strain due to maladjustment, and consequent improvement in physical and mental health", along with a heightening of consciousness at all levels, and a way "to prevent the body from slipping back, under the influence of greedy 'end-gaining' into its old habits of mal-co-ordination".

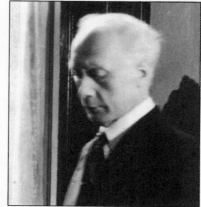

F. Matthias Alexander
Alexander (1869–1955) gave his name to the Principle which stressed the importance of re-educating the muscular system as a means to achieve physical and mental well-being.

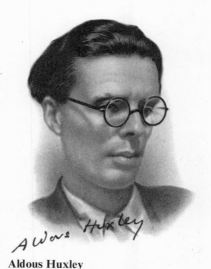

Aldous Huxley
One of the Alexander principle's many devotees, Huxley (1894–1963), said that, together with improved physical and mental health, he found that it brought about "a general heightening of consciousness on all levels".

Tinbergen's Nobel oration

More recently, the Nobel Prizewinner Nikolaas Tinbergen actually devoted his speech, on receipt of his award, to a eulogy of the Alexander principle as "an extremely sophisticated form of rehabilitation, or rather of redeployment, of the entire muscular equipment, and through that of many other organs, which made other forms of physiotherapy look crude in comparison".

Suitable cases

Practitioners of the Alexander principle commonly assert that almost everybody can benefit from a course, because most people have some postural defect or other. Their main source of patients, however, comes from people who feel, without knowing why, that they are not quite up to par – that they suffer too often from the syndrome of just being sick (see pages 303 to 304) or one of its concomitants (lassitude, headache, or whatever they may be), or from sporadic attacks of some bone or muscle disorder, including severe low back and sciatic pain. It has also been found useful in such varied conditions as high blood pressure, spastic colon, trigeminal neuralgia, osteoarthritis, asthma, and so on.

Sometimes, as with Alexander himself, it is a recognition by patients that they are not performing as well as they ought to be, which makes them feel that they are in need of what amounts to a kind of physico-psychological advisory service.

Self-help

Teachers of the Alexander principle will show you techniques which can be carried on at home. They are designed for the special needs of the individual, rather than for general use – because of Alexander's insistence that we should think in terms of working not on our bodies but ourselves.

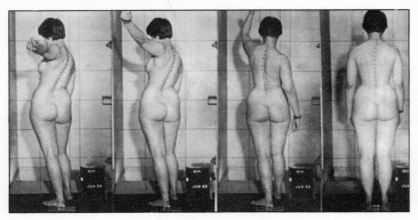

The effect of misuse
Any recurrent patterns of movements can lead to postural deformity. Here the repeated sequence of movements of a young left-handed javelin thrower has produced scoliosis, or a sideways curvature of the spine. A teacher of the Alexander principle will show you how you are misusing the body and re-educate you to a new pattern of use.

Feldenkrais technique

This system of body movement and retraining was designed by Dr Moshe Feldenkrais to improve posture and general health. It consists of two related but different techniques – "awareness through movement", which is grouped-based – and private, manipulative treatment called "functional integration".

Origins

Feldenkrais, a Russian-born Israeli, began his career as an engineer and physicist. Having received his science doctorate at the Sorbonne, he stayed in France and worked on the atomic programme with Frédéric Joliot-Curie. Following the German invasion of France in 1940 he escaped across the Channel to England and, for a time, worked for the British Admiralty. Feldenkrais was also accomplished at judo and a keen soccer player, and it was the flaring up of an old knee injury that first caused him to begin what has become a life-long study of the mechanics of human movement and how it relates to behaviour and learning.

Feldenkrais insists that he does not treat people but rather he "teaches principles"; he has only "pupils", never patients. He claims to be simply a teacher. His method is certainly difficult to explain quickly and easily. Using principles and exercises the aim is to programme the brain so that the whole mind-body system works efficiently. Yet when Thomas Hanna, ex-Director of the Humanistic Psychology Institute attended a course in Functional Integration, on the first day he heard Feldenkrais explain "The first principle of my work is that there isn't any principle".

The links between body and mind

From Hanna's description in his *The Body of Life*, and from Feldenkrais' own book, *Awareness through Movement*, it is possible to get an idea of what therapy on Feldenkrais' lines is like. The aim, as with the *Alexander principle* (pages 104 to 108) is to improve posture by self-awareness, in particular awareness of stance, gesture, and so on. "The bulk of stimuli arriving at the nervous system is from muscular activity constantly affected by gravity", Feldenkrais argues, so "posture is one of the best clues not only to evolution but also to the activity of the brain".

Not merely does the body continually reflect and express what is going on in the mind: "the qualities of unconscious movement in the human body are as individual as one's personality or character structure", as Hanna puts it, "*because these habitual patterns of acting are the somatic structure of what we call personality and character*"; but also, if the patterns are changed, it will affect the personality structure: "if the neuromuscular system of a widow is depressed, then if she is taught to change the pattern, she will no longer be depressed".

> ❝ *He's not just pushing muscles around. He's changing things in the brain itself, so that the patient can gradually adjust his whole muscular dysfunction to what we call a normal image. In the motor cortex, there's a photographic image which I call an image of achievement. And it's that image which Feldenkrais transmits. He knows how it ought to be. He transmits the image and you organize your brain to meet it.* ❞

Professor Karl Pribram
Head of the Neurophysiology Laboratories Stanford University, USA

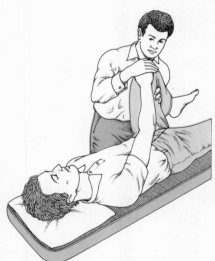

Correcting shoulder movement
Feldenkrais practitioners believe that it is often better to work on a problem area indirectly – attacking it directly may evoke the very patterns of movement that are causing pain. Here the shoulder is treated through the leg and pelvis.

Procedure

The debt to Alexander is obvious, and as with the Alexander principle, it is difficult, if not almost impossible, to describe the "therapy", except as an exploration of habits of posture and gesture, with a view to showing them *as* habits, often requiring to be un-learned.

"To begin with", Feldenkrais has explained", the lessons take place in the lying position, prone or supine, to facilitate the breakdown of muscular patterns" so that gravity does not exert the same pressures on the soles of the feet and the joints. A series of exercises follow, "done as slowly and as pleasantly as possible with no strain or pain whatever", designed to help the patient to come to terms with his body until by the end of the lessons, he "feels that his body is hanging lightly from his head, his feet do not stamp on the ground, his body glides when moving".

"Awareness through movement" is a series of simple exercises

Feldenkrais classes
Moshe Feldenkrais himself is depicted teaching his Awareness Through Movement technique to 235 pupils in a four-day-a-week, nine-week training course at Amherst, Massachusetts.

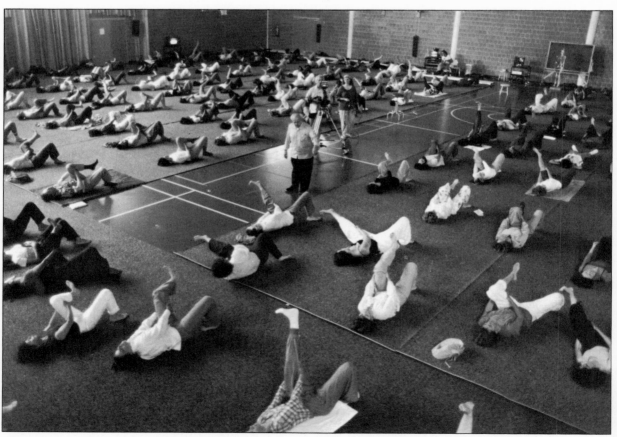

which can be taught to classes and workshops of up to 300 people in which the teacher verbally guides the class. The person-to-person technique, "functional integration" is indicated, according to Dr Carl Ginsburg, in a pamphlet on the method, "when a person needs added input to the nervous system beyond what can be achieved with self-exploration, and where there is pain or other disability"; it is an extremely gentle method – no force is ever used.

Suitable cases

Dr Ginsburg nominates people with neuromuscular difficulties, injuries and chronic pain, remarking that Feldenkrais has also taught "children with cerebral palsy or with learning disabilities, stroke victims and paraplegics". Actors, dancers, musicians, athletes and other professionals for whom physical fitness and versatility are important, may also benefit from learning Feldenkrais techniques.

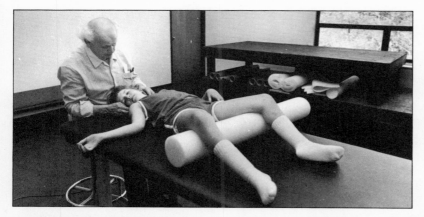

One-to-one sessions
Feldenkrais feels that "most of us use maybe five percent of our mind-body potential. In that sense we are all brain damaged". Left he is teaching a young girl who is suffering from cerebral palsy, an area in which he has an impressive reputation. Below he is working with an American basketball star Julius Erving, helping with an Achilles tendon problem.

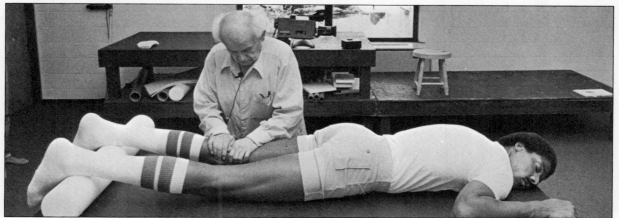

Reflexology

Both of these techniques are based on the proposition that the "life force" operates through channels as yet undiscovered by physiologists or neurologists. The discovery made by Dr W. Fitzgerald in the 1920s, that the body is divided into "zones" of energy which can be exploited in prevention and treatment, has since developed into what is commonly known as Reflexology. Some practitioners using what are essentially the same techniques, describe themselves as Zone Therapists.

The energy channels

For the reflexologist, there are 10 channels, beginning (or ending) in the toes and extending to the fingers and the top of the head. Each channel relates to a zone of the body, to the organs in that zone – the big toe relates to the head, for example. By feeling patients' feet in certain prescribed ways, reflexologists can detect which energy channels are blocked. By what is usually described as massage of the appropriate terminal on the foot, (using movements which range between of stroking and *Shiatsu*, see pages 133 to 137), they restore the energy flow to its correct balance.

In their *Reflexology: Techniques of Foot Massage for Health and Fitness* (a description of the technique, with photographs showing what to expect to see, though not what to expect to feel), Anna Kaye and Don C. Matchan claim that all the organs of the body are mirrored in the feet. This natural and drugless way of stimulating them "performs a set of functions, removing waste deposits, congestion and blockages in the energy pathways, improving blood circulation and gland function, and relaxing the whole system, including the mind".

Origins

References to a form of therapy in use in China five thousand years ago suggest that a form of reflexology must already have been in use there, and similar techniques have been observed in some tribal communities. Its use in western countries, however, is very recent, though a few naturopaths early in the present century were to adopt some of the techniques reflexologists now use.

Reflexology was established in the United States largely through the efforts of Eunice D. Ingham (Mrs Fred Stopfel) whose *Stories the Feet Can Tell* was first published in 1932.

Procedure

Following the preliminary case-history taking, you may be treated either sitting up in a chair, or lying down, according to which method is preferred by the practitioner and the patient. Your therapist will make a diagnosis and will not necessarily want to know your problems in advance.

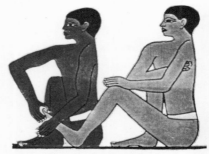

Reflexology in ancient Egypt
One of the only healing pictures from the Egyptian era, this drawing shows very early use of reflexology. It was found in the tomb of Ankhmahar at Saqqara – the Physician's Tomb – and dates from the early sixth dynasty, about 2,300 BC. An inscription above the figures reads: Don't hurt me I shall act in such a way as to obtain your favour.

Energy blocks

The initial stage is exploratory, the therapist working his or her way through the terminals of the energy channels on each foot, applying pressure (rotating toes, moving the foot up and down, rubbing the skin, and so on) to blocks of energy. These are commonly described by the therapists as minute lumps like crystalline deposits, under the skin. The object is to find them, and get rid of them, where possible, by specialized massage techniques. "Under a steady pressure, they are broken up" as Kaye and Matcham put it, "as a similar pressure would break up a sugar lump". Like those in a dissolving sugar lump, the theory is, these crystals are then easily absorbed in the body's waste disposal system, to be evacuated through sweat or in the urine, so that the energy will be free to flow freely again through the formerly blocked zone.

The massage may be gentle, like a form of stroking, or it may be more akin to shiatsu according to the nature and position of the obstacle which is to be removed. Where deep pressure is needed, pain, albeit momentary, can be severe. Patients "may be inclined to refer to it as a form of torture treatment" Ingham admitted. But, she adds, "strange to say, instinct seems to convince patients that the tenderness you have located indicates an abnormal condition", which satisfies them that the treatment is necessary for their ultimate well-being. Other practitioners fall back on the idea that there are two types of pain, one unnecessary and the other therapeutically desirable, and that patients can learn to live with, even enjoy, the desirable kind.

Reflexology chart
These diagrams show the individual massage points on the soles and sides of the feet and the parts of the body they govern, as used in reflexology.

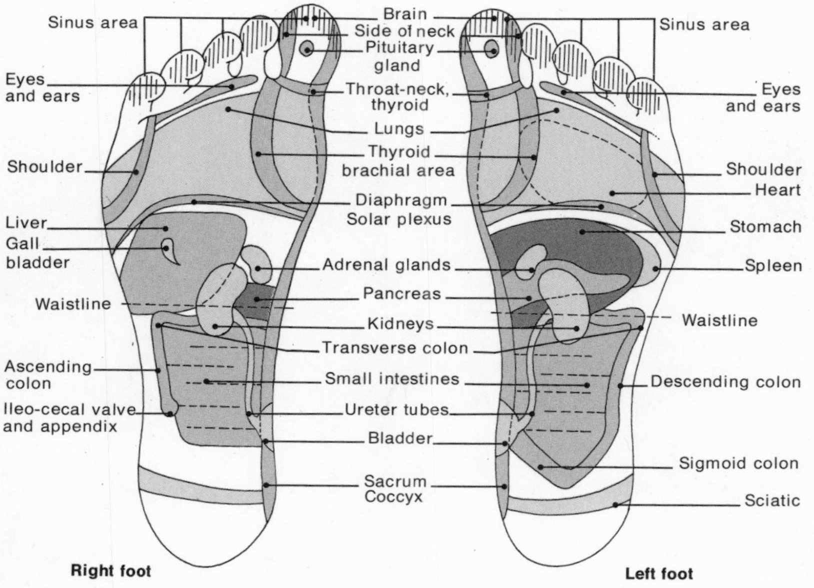

Sinus area
Brain
Side of neck
Pituitary gland
Sinus area
Eyes and ears
Throat-neck, thyroid
Eyes and ears
Lungs
Thyroid brachial area
Shoulder
Shoulder
Heart
Diaphragm Solar plexus
Liver
Gall bladder
Stomach
Adrenal glands
Spleen
Waistline
Pancreas
Kidneys
Waistline
Transverse colon
Ascending colon
Small intestines
Descending colon
Ileo-cecal valve and appendix
Ureter tubes
Bladder
Sigmoid colon
Sacrum Coccyx
Sciatic
Right foot
Left foot

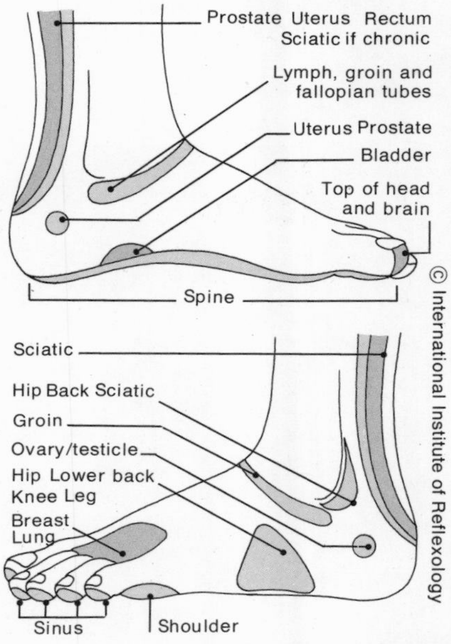

Prostate Uterus Rectum
Sciatic if chronic
Lymph, groin and fallopian tubes
Uterus Prostate
Bladder
Top of head and brain
Spine
Sciatic
Hip Back Sciatic
Groin
Ovary/testicle
Hip Lower back
Knee Leg
Breast
Lung
Sinus
Shoulder

© International Institute of Reflexology

Reflexology techniques

Reflexologists stress that the patient's body heals itself; the therapist is not responsible. He or she just acts as a mediator between you and your body's innate healing powers. You will be advised not to expect to obtain relief until you have had six weeks of treatment, but many people report feeling much better after only one session.

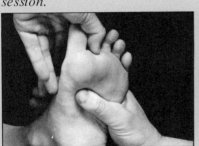

1 Before treatment, the therapist inspects the feet for callouses and corns as these can interfere with the nerve and blood supply to the parts of the body corresponding to their reflex zone (see charts, page 113).

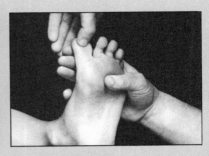

2 In the middle of each big toe lies the reflex to the pituitary gland, known as the master gland because it controls the other endocrine glands in the body.

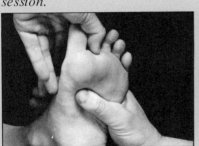

3 Here the therapist works the eye and ear reflex areas which are situated at the stem and base of the toes of both feet.

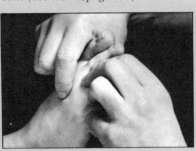

4 The therapist uses a "creeping" technique with his right index finger to work on the lung and breast reflexes which lie in between the metatarsal bones on both feet.

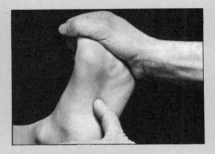

5 The thumb of the left hand massages the left kidney reflex – if this area is tender, it may mean that the patient is drinking too much alcohol, coffee or tea.

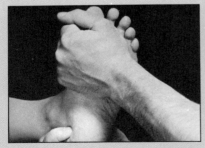

6 The middle finger of the right hand works on the reflex area corresponding to the uterus (or the prostate with a male patient) while the left hand rotates the foot.

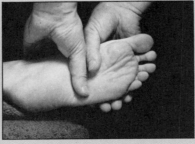

7 In the spinal twist, the therapist gently twists the bones in the foot. This is one of many relaxation techniques used both during and after treatment and is very soothing for the patient.

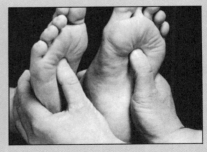

8 Another relaxation technique involves working on the diaphragm/ solar plexus reflexes of both feet at the same time while the patient breathes deeply. This is particularly effective for treatment of hypertension and stress.

Relaxation is important

All reflexologists emphasize the value, indeed, the necessity of relaxation in reducing pain and facilitating massage. Many begin their sessions with breathing exercises which help to relax their patients. They also point out that the reason for the blockage of the energy channels which they are trying to clear can often be tension. Ingham observed that worry is derived from the Saxon term for "choke", which fits in with her thesis that "one can choke off a portion of the normal blood supply to various parts of the body by refusing to stop needless worry". Needless worry, in other words, can be responsible for the crystallizing process, as also, she believed, anger can be.

The duration of a reflexology session depends upon many factors – including, as Kaye and Matcham have pointed out, the size of the patient's feet. Between 20 and 45 minutes is usual. The same principle applies in deciding how often treatments are required, whether once or twice a week, or whatever. How long they need to continue depends on their success, and that in its turn depends upon the severity of the patient's problems and the state of their vitality.

Suitable cases

Because reflexology, again like *Acupuncture* (see pages 120 to 133) is based on the proposition that if the balance of energy flow can be restored, symptoms of almost any kind can be banished, there are few disorders which practitioners feel they cannot help.

In an introductory pamphlet published by the Healing Research Trust, Wendy Stephenson claims that reflexology is "especially good for congestion; it will unblock sinuses, relieve migraine, assist the function of the pancreas and liven up a sluggish liver. It is very effective with constipation and in disorders of the kidneys". Ingham's list is more varied. Among the disorders for which she found reflexology valuable were apoplexy, arthritis, asthma, circulatory diseases, diabetes, epilepsy, glandular diseases, headache, hiccups, hypertension and kidney trouble. Most reflexologists report that many of their patients come simply because they find the treatment irresistible for dispelling symptoms of stress; they feel relaxed and calm after the session and go home to sleep like logs.

Reflexology has also had some success in the relief of pain; there is often a good response from people with back trouble. In cases of acute pain, such as that experienced by women in childbirth, or chronic pain, as in certain terminal illnesses, reflexologists report that their technique can be a particularly effective alternative to strong drug treatment. The advantage here, of course, is that, unlike with drugs, when the relief wears off, treatment can be repeated as often as required.

Applied kinesiology/touch for health

Practitioners of many different branches of natural medicine are becoming increasingly interested in the application of "touch", not as in manipulative and postural processes, for specific physical effect, but as a way of transmitting, or arousing, healing forces. Applied kinesiology, one such system, is based on special muscle-testing techniques through which weaknesses are identified and treated, thereby correcting imbalances in the body's energy systems. While applied kinesiology is practised by professionals, the aim of touch for health practitioners is to teach the skills of the professional kinesiologists to members of the lay public who are interested in preventative health care. In practical terms, kinesiology has affinities with therapies such as *Chiropractic* and *Massage*, while sharing the basic premises of *Acupuncture* and *Shiatsu* about energy flow (see pages 120 to 139).

A recent issue of the British Chiropractors' Association *Newsletter* had the headline "Applied kinesiology – the fastest growing healthcare approach in the States". The story suggested that it may be well on the way to becoming the fastest growing health-care approach in Britain, too, as nearly half the members of the Association recently attended seminars on the subject.

'We cannot believe that we were meant to have to learn to live with pain. Pain is the final alarm before some life-threatening malfunction takes place. Just prior to the pain and malfunction, there are signs and symptoms which can be recognized. One of these is a weakening of the muscles and a change in the posture. We must learn to listen and feel what is going on in our bodies and be able to correct the minor problems before they develop into serious illnesses.'

John Thie
Chiropractor

Origins

There is a sense in which all forms of manipulative and postural therapy, acupuncture and acupressure, and the laying on of hands can all be described as kinesiotherapies. But "applied kinesiology" most commonly refers to methods introduced by Dr George Goodheart, a chiropractor from Detroit, who stumbled across the new principles by accident. He discovered that some of the standard muscle tests he used provided clues to the workings of the entire body. Goodheart went on to teach his findings to other chiropractors, one of whom taught Brian Butler, who has introduced Touch for Health into Britain.

The assumption used to be that the main muscular trouble-makers in backache and associated disorders were muscles which were either in spasm, or too taut, thus affecting the spine. In the mid-1960s, however, Goodheart began to work on a different idea. It might not be muscle spasm or tautness that was responsible, he surmised, but rather (as Dr John F. Thie and Mary Marks put it in their book *Touch for Health*) that it was "weak muscles on the opposite side (of the body) which caused the normal muscles to seem to be or to become tight". Combining eastern ideas about energy flow with his own chiropractic techniques and other sources, Goodheart developed his new system. "This involves using muscle testing to determine the need for and effectiveness of treatment, and applying various techniques of kinesiology – the science of muscle activation – to restore muscle balance which is essential to good posture. . ."

Applied kinesiology techniques

Kinesiologists carry out a series of tests to determine your muscle responses. Each group of muscles is related to one of the meridians of acupuncture. Where energy is restricted or excessive, the muscle may be weak. Food allergies can also be discovered: foods to which the body is allergic make muscles weaker, while those that are beneficial strengthen them.

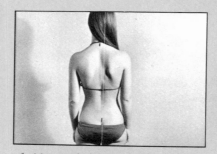

1 *Many imbalances are revealed by posture. This girl's right shoulder is higher than her left – a black line drawn at the crease of the buttocks and on the first thoracic vertebra deviates markedly from the plumbline.*

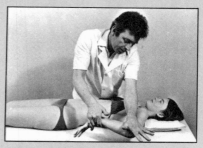

2 *Checking the strength of the subscapularis muscle involves rotating the humerus, using the elbow as the fulcrum.*

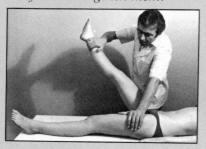

3 *Testing the psoas muscle provides valuable information, especially if the patient has low back pain, as this muscle is attached to all the lumbar vertebrae and affects spinal balance.*

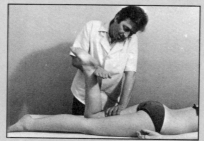

4 *The hamstrings are related to large intestine function and are vital for pelvic balance and stability. If weak, they can aggravate low back pain and cause tired legs. Strengthening them often brings immediate relief.*

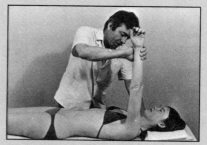

5 *The therapist tests the pectoralis major clavicular muscle. As it is strong, it can be used as an "indicator muscle" to check the body's response to various foods.*

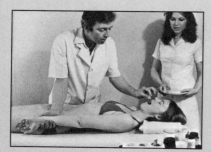

6 *The patient is offered a morsel of the food suspected of causing allergic reactions. After it has been chewed for a few seconds, the muscle is retested to see if its ability to function has changed.*

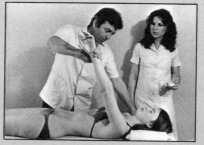

7 *In this case, the food has affected the functioning of the indicator muscle. The patient is far less able to resist the amount of pressure previously applied, and should avoid this food for some time.*

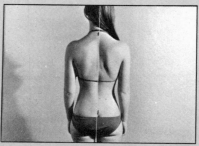

8 *Once the energies have been balanced and weak muscles strengthened, subtle improvements in posture can frequently be observed. The patient looks better and often experiences an immediate increase in well-being.*

Procedure

The distinguishing characteristic of applied kinesiology and touch for health, then, is the search for muscle imbalance, so that it can be corrected. Clues will be looked for in the taking of your case history; symptoms, kinesiologists find, are often related to muscle weakness – headache, for example, can be traced back to problems with the neck muscles. But the aim is not so much to correct individual weaknesses as to restore balance to the body. "A deviation in the normal posture can be the first stage of a problem or the result of years of compensation", Thie and Marks explain. "Recognizing the deviations or distortions is the first step in reversing them".

Practitioners of kinesiology vary considerably in their methods, some relying solely on techniques specific to it, others using it occasionally as an adjunct to, say, chiropractic. Muscle tests are likely to be carried out while you are lying down. The therapist usually works first on one side of the body, then on the other to detect the differences. Any imbalances of muscle tone will be corrected as they are found, using touch, or pressure, on the appropriate points.

Suitable cases

Applied kinesiology can be used for diagnosis in connection with other types of therapy, and for treatment when the diagnosis points to it. Kinesiologists claim that they do not rely on a knowledge of symptoms, in the usual clinical sense, since the patients' muscles provide them with all the information they need. They have achieved considerable success in allergy cases, particularly with food allergies (see *Allergy*, pages 309 to 310).

Self-help

Touch for health is designed specifically for lay people to learn kinesiology techniques so that they can detect and rectify muscle imbalances for themselves. The best way to learn touch for health is to take a short course. This does not enable people to practise as professional therapists, but it will provide a sound foundation for the safe domestic use of kinesiology techniques.

ORIENTAL THERAPIES

In this section we have included acupuncture, shiatsu and acupressure, therapies which share the fundamental belief that the energy which the life force transmits is distributed through the body along a system of invisible channels or meridians. In normal circumstances, in a healthy person, the life force, *chi*, flows evenly, maintaining a balance between the vigorous *yang* and the restraining *yin* elements (see below). But if either yang or yin becomes too dominant, the body's harmony is jeopardized and illness can result.

For treatment purposes, the nature of the imbalance has to be diagnosed and the meridians which need attention detected. With acupuncture, the balance is restored by the insertion of fine needles at specific points on the skin. These points are located on the appropriate meridian and selected to stimulate, or curb, energy flow, as required. Sometimes "moxibustion" may be used by the acupuncturist to stimulate the *chi* energy. With this technique, heat from a burning herb is applied to the acupuncture point. Imbalances can also be corrected without the use of needles by applying finger pressure to the acupuncture points, as found in shiatsu and acupressure.

In acupressure a finger, the ball of the thumb, or a knuckle is substituted for the needle. The points are the same as for acupuncture. but ordinarily only a few are used – those which the individual knows from experience are appropriate for his symptoms. Acupressure is sometimes encountered under different names: G-Jo – which roughly means "first aid" in Chinese – or Jin Shin Do.

The theory of yin and yang

The ancient Chinese believed that a life-force flows through all things; in ourselves along meridians or pathways which correspond to different organs of the body. The activating force behind *chi* is the constant movement of energy between two poles or extremes known as *yin* and *yang*; these correspond roughly to our ideas of positive and negative, or male and female, forces. In order to remain healthy the yin and yang forces must be perfectly balanced.

Within our bodies, the yin organs are those which are hollow and involved in absorption and discharge such as the stomach and bladder; the yang organs are the dense, blood-filled organs, such as the heart and lungs, which regulate the body. There is constant interaction between yin and yang forces and, if the yin/yang balance between the organs is interrupted, the flow of *chi* through the body will be affected and we will fall ill. Practitioners of oriental therapies aim to correct any imbalances and encourage *chi* to flow freely again.

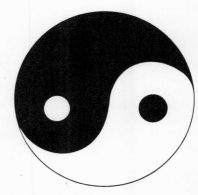

Yin/yang symbol
This symbol represents the perfect balance and constant interaction between the forces of yin and yang in every healthy organism.

Acupuncture

The term acupuncture derives from the Latin word *acus* (needle) and *punctura* (to prick). It is used to describe a technique in which needles are used to puncture the skin at certain defined points in order to restore the balance of *chi* energy, which, acupuncturists believe, is essential to good health.

Origins

Acupuncture's origins are lost in the mists of time, as writers on the subject have often remarked. Unlike nearly all forms of natural medicine, it has not been found in tribal use. The likelihood is, however, that it had its origins in a practice which has been common enough in tribal communities, that is, "scarifying" the skin, a therapeutic process presumably derived from the relief obtained by scratching when there's an itch. There are also travellers' tales of fine needles materializing at the behest of a witch doctor, as if to do the scarifying job for him by magic.

Acupuncture in ancient China

Whatever the explanation, the use of acupuncture in China has been traced back five thousand years, and sixth century BC Chinese medical textbooks dealing with it are still in existence. So cut off was China from the western world, however, that acupuncture was not introduced to Europeans until missionaries returned with information about it in the seventeenth century; though even then, it was regarded as little more than a curiosity.

When the term came into use here, it was for a type of treatment which may have originated in a similar way, but which was markedly different from the Chinese version. In the first issue of the *Lancet*, published in 1823, a Norfolk doctor described how he inserted needles into patients with dropsy to release the fluid, a procedure which he described as acupuncture. The term was also used to describe a form of treatment which came into quite common use to ease the pain of arthritis – this involved plunging a needle into the affected part. When it began to be better understood in Europe (largely thanks to a few Frenchmen, who had been impressed by its beneficial results while they were colonists in Indo China), Chinese-style acupuncture was found to be of an altogether more sophisticated kind, as was made clear in the first major treatise on the subject by the French diplomat Soulie de Morant in 1939.

Introducing "needle treatment" to the West

Although a handful of Chinese acupuncturists had been practising for years in British seaports (chiefly on their own countrymen from visiting ships), the general public remained largely unaware of their existence until the late 1950s. The story began to get around of the way that "the needle treatment" could work

❛ What is Acupuncture? It's concerned for the mental-emotional states of people; very much concerned with nutrition. It uses in its therapeutics not only needles, but finger pressure. It uses heat in the form of moxibustion. Nowadays, they are using things like laser beams and ultrasonics, and some people inject homeopathic remedies into acupuncture points. So there are all sorts of ways of dealing with the energy – Chi energy. ❜

Joe Goodman
Ex-President of the British
Acupuncture Association

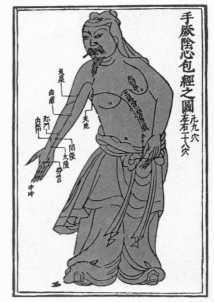

Early use of acupuncture
Acupuncture is a therapy which reaches back to the Stone Age. This Chinese acupuncture chart from "T'Ongen Tschen Kieou King" dates from 1031.

wonders for people with rheumatism, and a few other afflictions for which orthodox medicine had no satisfactory remedies. When a woman's magazine ran articles on the subject, it was inundated with letters from correspondents begging for more information and, in particular, for the names and addresses of acupuncturists. Some practitioners of other forms of natural medicine saw their opportunity – they took short courses on the subject (from books, if they could not find a teacher) and began to practise. Some, also, began to teach. By the early 1960s, acupuncture had begun to establish itself as the growth area in natural medicine.

The sceptics in orthodox medicine

The attitude of the medical profession was at that time less one of hostility than of derision. One British doctor, Felix Mann, took the trouble to study acupuncture in France in the late 1950s, and began to teach it to small groups of doctors. But his efforts to show that it should be taken seriously were greeted with amused contempt by most of his colleagues. How could sticking needles into people's feet affect what was happening in their kidneys, or their lungs? And where were these so-called meridans, or canals? Scientific tests had not been able to find them.

There might conceivably have been some sense to the method – doctors argued – if the acupuncture points had borne any relationship to the nervous system, as mapped by orthodox physiology. But they did not. In a book published here in 1962, the eminent pharmacologist Louis Lasagna reflected the prevailing medical opinion when he included acupuncture as a "lunacy" in his chapter on "Superstition and Ignorance", acupuncture charts were needed by practitioners, he jeered, because "hitting imaginary canals is not a job to be left to the imagination".

For the next 10 years acupuncture remained the medical profession's chief source of mirth whenever the absurdities of "fringe medicine" was discussed. Then, unexpectedly, the scoffers had their come-uppance. While on a visit to China in 1971, the *New York Times* political commentator, James Reston, developed appendicitis. Operated on in a Peking hospital, Reston was initially surprised when he was given only a local anesthetic, so that he was conscious throughout, but still more surprised when, subsequently, his post-operative pain was relieved with the use of acupuncture.

Pain relief using acupuncture

Acupuncture anesthesia, as it is commonly described (though purists insist it should be "analgesia" – insensibility to pain without loss of consciousness) had been a recent development. "Chinese medicine and pharmacology", Chairman Mao Tse-tung had pronounced in 1958, "are a great treasure-house, and efforts should be made to explore them and raise them to a higher

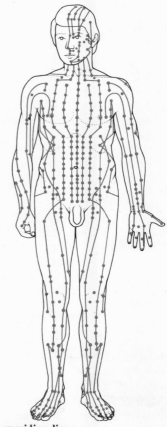

The meridian lines
If the acupuncture points of each of the 12 main groups are joined up, 12 meridians are produced. These carry the vital energy (chi) through the body. The number of points along each meridian varies – the heart, for example, has nine points on each side, while there are 67 on the bladder meridian.

level". And when it was discovered that acupuncture could be used to make surgical operations painless, Mao had not unnaturally been delighted. The Cultural Revolution too, when it swept the country, swept many doctors trained in western methods out of hospitals and teaching posts (they were seen as "experts" and "elitists" needed reeducation) and they were often replaced by acupuncturists.

Mao – or perhaps his foreign minister, Chou En-lai, who knew Reston and knew also how influential he was in the United States – realized that the despatch from Peking giving an account of Reston's hospital experience provided an unexpected and welcome opportunity to show the West that the Cultural Revolution, and the proletarian forces which had inspired it, were just as capable of stunning new advances in medicine as western technology. Distinguished American doctors were accordingly invited over to see for themselves that acupuncture worked. They were followed by television teams, and soon western viewers here were being treated to programmes showing Chinese patients undergoing serious operations while fully conscious; acupuncture needles providing the only anesthetic. And in spite of a few carping critics who suggested that it was too obviously part of a propaganda campaign (that the patients had either been given a discreet shot of a local anesthetic, or were only pretending not to feel pain), the general view was that unaccountably, acupuncture really worked.

Western medicine, however, though surprised and more than a little embarrassed, was not stunned. The fact that it happened to be acupuncture analgesia which had obtained the publicity gave the medical profession the excuse to concentrate on that aspect, rather than on acupuncture's general therapeutic potential. As always, the argument was put forward that more research was needed, so that the principles upon which acupuncture works could be better understood, before it could safely be used in the West. No serious attempt was made to introduce it into medical practice or medical education.

Inevitably, as a result, acupuncture in Britain was largely taken over by natural therapists. But Felix Mann, still hoping to persuade the medical profession to take it seriously, refused to train anybody who was not medically qualified. Only doctors could hope to practise it satisfactorily, he argued, as only doctors would have a good grounding in physiology and pathology. Acupuncturists "who do not know the basic principles of medicine", he feared, "all too often achieve results commensurate with their lack of knowledge".

Changing attitudes to physiology

This was a curious argument, given that the principles upon which acupuncture is based had so little connection with the

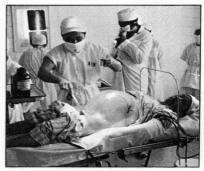

Pain relief during operations
Acupuncture was used as the "anesthetic" during this caesarian birth enabling the mother to remain conscious throughout the operation. This can also be of great benefit to the baby because he or she will not have been affected by any drugs which would otherwise have been given to the mother.

physiology which medical students were then taught. To become an acupuncturist, in fact, a doctor needed to put much of what he had been taught in physiology out of his mind. This view is now changing, as new attitudes to physiology emerge in the medical profession. But at the time, the result of Mann's policy was to perpetuate the split between the profession and natural therapists, which in turn led to the setting up of training schools for acupuncturists which lacked any support from the profession – except in the form of small but growing numbers of GPs taking the courses.

The decision to try acupuncture

People who decide they want to go to an acupuncturist often become involved in even more worry than if they had elected to try any other of the better known types of natural therapy – for a number of reasons. Acupuncture involves the acceptance of a set of assumptions alien to western science: the meridians remain an abstraction in the sense that they are not detectable in the way that, say, nerve channels are. The prospect of having needles inserted into the body until (as in some alarming illustrations) it looks like a pin-cushion, is also disturbing, particularly for anybody who shares the common phobia about medical injections and inoculations. And although newspaper and magazine articles, along with TV and radio programmes, have been familiarizing the public with what the acupuncturist does, a sizable proportion of first-time patients are likely to be nervous when they call up to ask for an appointment and even more so, when they arrive at the surgery.

Unsuitable cases

At this point it is worth mentioning that an acupuncturist will not necessarily regard yours as a suitable case for acupuncture treatment. The Chinese, after all, use other traditional methods, such as herbal remedies, where they seem more appropriate. There are also some disorders the therapist is not permitted to treat – sexually transmitted diseases for one. Others the therapists realize, can be more effectively treated by conventional means. Although acupuncture is an alternative (and in many ways rival) system based on very different principles, its practitioners here are as well aware as they are in China that conventional medicine can be more effective in dealing with some life-threatening diseases, such as severe infections, with accidents, and with certain deficiency diseases.

Most acupuncturists also have a personal list of the kind of patient they prefer to avoid. Hysterics, for example (though sometimes they can be helped) are often detected because they launch into venomous tirades against their doctor for his or her failure to appreciate their needs.

Acupuncturists and addiction

The "I am told you can stop me smoking (or eating, or drinking)" type of patient also needs to be judiciously handled. Acupuncturists who practise holistically like to make it clear from the start that theirs is not a form of treatment which depends simply on correct diagnosis and accurate positioning of needles during treatment, with the patient as passive onlooker while everything is done to and for him or her. On the contrary, all that acupuncture can do for many disorders is, in effect, to tune up the system; they emphasize the patient must do the rest.

Acupuncture can help in the early stages of giving up smoking, for instance, helping the former addict find the craving less powerful. But the actual resolution to resist the temptation to have "just one puff" (or to accept a proffered cigarette out of force of habit) must be summoned up by the patient.

Some experienced practitioners work largely on hunch, relying on what subsequently happens to the patient to guide them, if necessary, in a different direction; others require an elaborate accumulation of data relating to Chinese cosmology. Inevitably much will depend upon your general condition, and on whether the acupuncturist feels confident that your disorder can be simply treated, or decides that it is going to present problems.

Procedure

On your first visit to an acupuncturist, while obtaining routine information, such as a history of your past illnesses, the therapist will also be observing you very closely. The colour and texture of your skin; the glint, or fishiness, of your eyes; your breathing, whether deep and regular, or shallow and variable; the way you walk, stand and sit; your gestures and your tone of voice – all will be noted down for the build-up of a complete picture of *you*, which will form the basis of diagnosis. How your way of life and psychosocial problems are probed into depends on the degree of rapport established between patient and practitioner. Experienced practitioners are only too well aware that most patients are accustomed to regard medical treatment as being concerned only with their symptoms and that most people find it odd if they are asked what they feel like when they wake up in the morning – whether they feel great or unable to face anything until brought a cup of tea. And they may think it downright impertinent to be asked how they are getting on with the partner who brings it.

Following the taking of the case history, there usually follows a general physical examination. This will be more or less extensive according to what the acupuncturist has already found out about you. Often breathing and heartbeat are checked, and sometimes the temperature is taken. The tongue is given a particularly close inspection, and next comes the taking of pulses.

The 12 pulses

An acupuncturist's technique for checking pulses in quite different from that carried out by an orthodox doctor. For a start, it lasts much longer. This is because in acupuncture there are 12 pulses, one for each main meridian, six to each wrist. Each is identified with a vital organ, but the organ does not have exclusive dominion over it. An analogy some acupuncturists use is of a government with twelve separate and to some extent self-governing ministries each looking after its own, but subject to the doctrine of cabinet responsibility. While one ministry deals with drainage and clearance, another copes with nourishment – and so on. Mind and body, emotions and physical reactions, are held to be inextricably interlinked. The mind may need better nourishment as well as the body, or both may need a change of diet.

The pulses provide the acupuncturist with information about the meridians which need to have their energy balance restored, and about whether yin or yang is in the ascendant. Health is dependent on the equilibrium of yin and yang: yin tends to sedate and expand and is regarded as the negative principle; yang tends to stimulate and contract and is regarded as the positive principle. The rate of the beat is of less importance than the energy flow, strong or weak, regular or irregular. It is as if a qualitative, as well as a quantitative, element supervenes. The pulses can tell more about the individual patient than is to be found in acupuncture instruction manuals.

If you agree to take the course of treatment suggested, the acupuncturist may well defer beginning actual treatment until the next appointment. But in order to calm any fears, he or she may give you a demonstration to show that the needles really do not hurt. (Surprisingly, this is often true. Some acupuncture points appear to be the lineal descendants of the anesthetized areas which were looked for in olden times in the detection of witches: if needles were stuck into old women, and they did not yelp, it was considered to be one of the proofs of their guilt.)

Acupuncture needles

These are very fine and bear no resemblance to the hypodermic variety. In some points (or in some people) if the eyes are shut, the needles may not be felt at all. Other points are more sensitive. (Some authorities believe there should always be some sensation, as if to indicate the needle has "hit the spot".) Still, generally speaking, where pain is felt it is rather less than an accidental encounter with a pin, and the needle is felt only as it pierces the skin. Pushing it in deeper does not hurt, unless it comes up against an obstruction.

The other surprise for anybody who has not had acupuncture before is that the needles (sometimes a couple of them, sometimes half a dozen) may be inserted at points on the body which appear

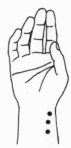

The meridian pulses
In acupuncture, the taking of the pulses plays a vital role. Each meridian has its own pulse and the therapist checks them all in turn. Each wrist has six pulses, as it is divided into three zones, all having a deep and a superficial position.

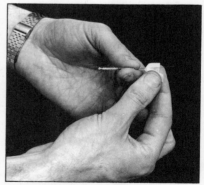

Sterilizing the needles
Qualified acupuncturists maintain high standards of hygiene and always sterilize their needles before use. Here, a needle is swabbed before being inserted into a point.

to bear no relationship to the symptoms – a headache sufferer may find that needles are inserted in the feet. The acupuncturist will explain that it is the appropriate meridian that is being treated, and will illustrate this by reference to a chart.

Inserting the needles

According to the position of the selected point, the needles may be inserted vertically, obliquely or almost horizontally. Sometimes

Consulting an acupuncturist

New patients are often surprised at the number of questions put to them at the first appointment. Besides being asked your own and some

of your immediate family's medical history, you may be asked about your emotional life, future plans, and so on. Your answers along

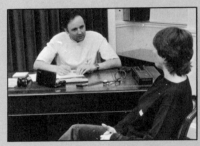

1 *At this first consultation, the acupuncturist talks to the patient about her illness and takes a detailed case history, including such data as her reaction to climatic changes and her food and drink preferences.*

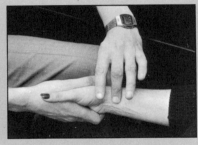

2 *The physical examination starts with pulse-taking. First the acupuncturist feels the quality and strength of the general pulse, then he takes each of the 12 pulses. Classical texts list 27 different pulse qualities.*

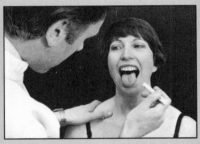

3 *Examining the tongue provides further clues to the patient's yin/yang balance. Its general condition, coating, moistness and markings are all indications of excess or deficient energy.*

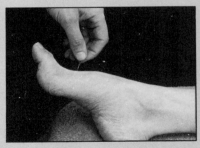

7 *Some needles are left in place undisturbed, but if the acupuncturist wishes to stimulate a point, he will gently rotate the needle, as shown here, or pump it in and out.*

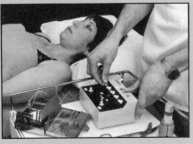

8 *Another method of stimulating a point is to apply a low-frequency electric current to the needle from a special instrument. This enables the practitioner to regulate the stimulus to the point.*

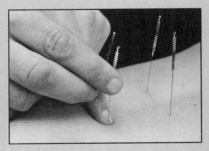

9 *Where more reinforcement of energy is required, "moxibustion", may be used. If the "heated needle" technique is used, the needles are inserted first in the appropriate acupuncture points.*

they just penetrate the skin; sometimes they are sunk to a depth of an inch or more. The acupuncturist will then "summon the energy" by twirling the needle (rotating it clockwise and anti-clockwise between finger and thumb), or using pumping movements (lifting and thrusting the needle) and sometimes by a combination of twirling and pumping. Some acupuncturists put a mild electric current through the needles, thereby enabling them to dispense with twirling and at the same time, they claim, to

with the taking of pulses and clues the practitioner picks up from your complexion, eyes, posture, and voice, will contribute to the over-all diagnosis and enable the acupuncturist to plan a suitable course of treatment.

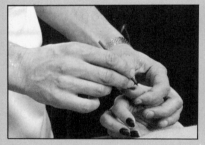

4 *In the* Akabane Test, *a glowing incense stick is repeatedly brought near the end point of each of the 12 main meridians, then withdrawn. Those with higher energy levels tolerate fewer applications.*

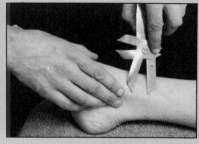

5 *Having determined the nature of the imbalances, the practitioner locates the points he wishes to treat – either by touch or with an instrument that measures the Chinese "inch", a measurement unique to each patient.*

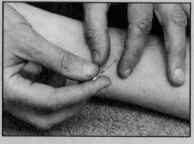

6 *He then inserts a sterilized needle a little way into the selected point. Normally the patient feels no more than a slight pinprick as the needle goes in; some people feel nothing at all.*

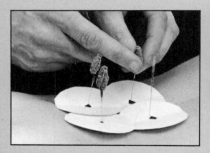

10 *Then a small cone of moxa (dried mugwort) is placed around the head of each needle. Discs of card around the base prevent any falling ash from coming into contact with the patient's skin.*

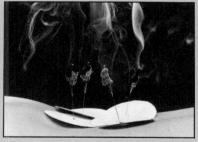

11 *Once ignited, the moxa burns with the right intensity to generate a pleasant heat down the needle and in to the point, clearing the channels and reinforcing the flow of energy.*

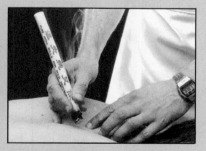

12 *Another way of applying moxibustion is by holding the glowing tip of a moxa roll close to an acupuncture point until it becomes too hot, then withdrawing it. This procedure is repeated a variable number of times.*

regulate the required energy flow with more precision.

The length of time for which the needles are left in depends upon their effect. In theory this is ascertained from the patient's pulses; in practice it may be based on what the acupuncturist has been taught, and on his or her experience of what works best for patients. Treatments usually take from 20 minutes to an hour.

A course of treatments

The number of treatments given inevitably depends on the nature and seriousness of the disorder and the patient's reaction to acupuncture. Occasionally a single treatment will give spectacular results; usually about six are required. By that time it should be possible for you to gauge whether they are producing results. If they are, they can be continued until you feel you have no further need for them or they can be resumed from time to time if the symptoms return.

How often treatments are given varies with the needs of the patients, and also with the number of entries in the acupuncturist's appointment book. Once a week is common, but some feel patients should initially come more frequently.

Moxibustion techniques

You may well be offered moxibustion as an adjunct to treatment with needles. One method was described by Sally Reston, as it was used with acupuncture when her husband was treated in China for his post-operative pain (see page 121): a foot-long roll of paper was filled moxa (*artemesia vulgaris*, the common mugwort), split in half, lit at both ends, and twirled just above Reston's stomach. But most acupuncturists prefer to put a cone of moxa on the needle over the selected acupuncture point and light it. In both cases, the aim is to clear the channel and promote the energy flow throughout the body.

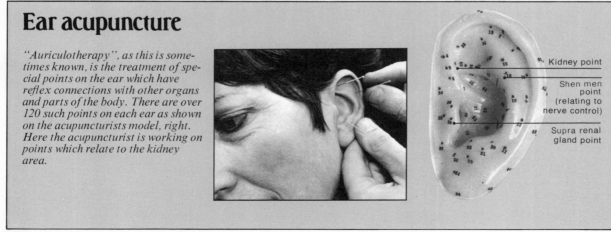

Ear acupuncture

"Auriculotherapy", as this is sometimes known, is the treatment of special points on the ear which have reflex connections with other organs and parts of the body. There are over 120 such points on each ear as shown on the acupuncturists model, right. Here the acupuncturist is working on points which relate to the kidney area.

Kidney point

Shen men point
(relating to nerve control)

Supra renal gland point

The immediate effects of acupuncture

Independently of the effects which acupuncture has on symptoms, it can also have some unexpected, not necessarily unwelcome, repercussions: many patients report a strange feeling of exhilaration "like walking on air" after their initial treatment. Others feel "woozy", or have a powerful inclination to sleep, but such effects soon disappear.

As with most types of natural medicine, a common consequence of an acupuncture session is temporary exacerbation of symptoms. Acupuncturists explain this in the same way as naturopaths and homeopaths. As the symptoms reflect the body's defence mechanism's struggle against the forces making for illness, when an ally arrives, in the form of needles put into the appropriate point on the appropriate meridian, the flare-up is an indication that the defences, reinforced, are at last gaining the upper hand. When they have gained it, the symptoms disappear.

There is also the possibility that when the flow of *chi* energy is restarted, its vigour may temporarily confuse the body's self-regulating mechanism, producing rashes or aches for a day or two. But there are never the kind of side-effects which result from the use of powerful drugs, acupuncturists assert, because with drugs, it is their toxicity which is responsible.

Ordinarily, any mishaps which may occur are the result not of acupuncture but of incompetence on the part of the acupuncturist. It must always be remembered that as the law stands, anybody can call himself an acupuncturist. If you choose to go to one who has had no training and has no qualifications, needles may be inadequately sterilized, or inserted incorrectly, perhaps even broken in the process.

Research

The bulk of the research into acupuncture has naturally been carried out in China and the countries of the Far East. Research in the West has chiefly centred on exploring acupuncture's potential value as a painkiller, apart from one or two projects designed (or so it would appear) to try to prove it would make no difference if the needles were stuck in at random.

Trigger points

The most assiduous investigator in the West has been the psychologist Ronald Melzack of McGill University, Montreal. It has long been recognized in conventional medicine that there are "trigger points" on the body which respond to pressure or stimulation by providing relief of pain elsewhere in the body. However, little use has been made of this therapeutically, doubtless because no satisfactory explanation has been provided for it and because of its inconsistency as a painkiller. In the mid-

1970s, however, Melzack and some colleagues undertook research to find whether there is any correspondence between these trigger points and acupuncture points as traditionally located on charts. "A remarkably high degree (71 percent) of correspondence was found", they observed in their report in the journal *Pain*, suggesting that trigger points and acupuncture points, "though discovered independently and labelled differently, represent the same phenomenon and can be explained in terms of the same underlying neural mechanisms".

Even temporary pain relief is welcome

Going on to compare acupuncture with electrical stimulation of trigger points, Melzack found that both can provide effective relief of some forms of pain. Though the differences were small enough to confirm Melzack in his impression that the two methods probably have the same underlying mechanism of action, acupuncture was the more effective. The time required for treatment, once the method has been established, is very short – only three minutes, in the trials he undertook. In half the cases, the pain was diminished not only at the time of treatment but for months afterwards; in others, the treatment had to be regularly repeated. But even then, "when it is recalled that many of the patients in this study had suffered pain for years, and several had

Acupuncture for children

Children too can be treated with acupuncture. The procedure will follow a similar pattern as for adults. However, it is important to explain to the child what is going to happen.

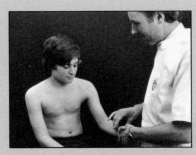

1 *After the case-history taking, the acupuncturist will begin by taking the pulses whilst continually reassuring the child.*

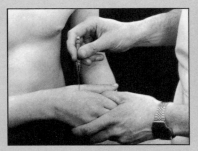

2 *If children are apprehensive about needles, the acupuncturist can massage the points by applying pressure with a blunt-ended "spring needle", which does not penetrate the skin.*

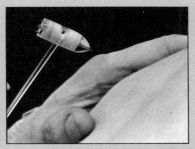

3 *Alternatively, the points may be stimulated by tapping them rapidly with a "Plum Blossom needle" – a small cluster of needles on the end of a flexible handle.*

undergone major surgery without relief, the value of a technique which brings partial relief for a few hours or days at a time is especially evident. It makes the difference between unbearable and bearable pain, between a sedentary, sometimes bedridden life and one that, for at least several hours or days a week, allows a normal social, family, or business life. Even a few hours or days of pain at tolerable levels permits some of these patients to live with more dignity and self-assurance, so that life in general becomes more bearable".

Acupuncture and infectious disease

Some of the research results which have been obtained will come as a surprise to anybody who thinks that acupuncture, however effective it may be against pain, cannot be expected to work satisfactorily in cases of infectious diseases. According to *World Health*, the magazine of the World Health Organization, "in 645 cases of acute bacillary dysentery, 90 percent of the patients were cured within 10 days, as judged by clinical symptoms and signs and the results of stool culture". A trial with similar numbers has shown acupuncture to be effective in relieving certain symptoms of heart disease in 80 percent of cases. And, in addition to its pain-relieving capacity, research has shown, acupuncture can control inflammation and fever.

Acupuncture and animals

One of the more remarkable results of research into acupuncture has been to show that it can be used successfully to resuscitate pets which are in danger of collapse while under anesthetic, or sometimes from other causes. In 69 cases where breathing became dangerously low in dogs or cats under an anesthetic, it was restored, in nearly all cases, to normal or near normal rates within 10 to 30 seconds, by insertion of a needle into the point marked on acupuncture charts *VG26: Jen Chung*. The recovery occurred in some cases even after the animals' hearts stopped beating, and they no longer showed signs of life.

Authenticating the existence of meridians

Recently, some sophisticated research has been undertaken to see if the meridians can be traced in ways which will finally convince orthodox physiologists that they exist and are not, as Louis Lasagna claimed, "imaginary" and "non-existent". In a recent issue, the Los Angeles *Brain/Mind Bulletin* reported that a machine had been invented in Japan which reads the meridians through electrodes attached to fingers and toes, providing information about the condition of the organs related to them – the criteria being established during research on 5,000 subjects. The inventor of the machine, Hiroshi Motoyama, emphasizes that the *chi* energy does *not* travel through the nervous system; his gadget demonstrates that "we possess non-physical properties and energies still largely unknown and uncharted by science".

Research is now in progress to discover whether lasers or ultrasound can be used in place of needles. But it will take time before clear findings are obtained.

Suitable cases

When acupuncturists are asked which diseases or symptoms they find particularly amenable to their treatment, they invariably reply that they do not treat diseases or symptoms – they treat people. They admit, however, that there are certain disorders for which acupuncture has acquired a particularly good reputation as a therapy, though inevitably these are apt to be the disorders which conventional medicine is *least* successful in handling.

A guide to acupuncture's best performance ratings has recently been provided by the members of an international seminar, organized by the World Health Organization in Peking. This was derived from clinical experience all over the world, rather than from research findings – and it did not attempt to assess just how efficient acupuncture is at dealing with specific disorders. Still the guide provides a useful list of the kind of illnesses which acupuncturists in general feel confident they can deal with. It includes:

● **Respiratory disorders**: Colds, acute sinusitis, acute tonsillitis, acute bronchitis, bronchial asthma.
● **Eye disorders**: Acute conjunctivitis, myopia (in children), cataract (without complications).
● **Mouth disorders**: toothache, post-extraction pain, inflamed gums, acute and chronic pharyngitis.
● **Digestive disorders**: Oesophagus spasm, hiccups hyperacidity, chronic duodenal ulcer (pain relief), acute duodenal ulcer (without complication), colitis (acute and chronic), bacillary dysentery (acute), constipation, diarrhea, paralytic ileus.
● **Disorders of the nervous system**: Headache, migraine, trigeminal neuralgia, facial palsy (early stage), peripheral neuropathies, Menière's disease, neurogenic bladder disfunction.
● **Bone and muscle disorders**: Low back pain, sciatica, osteoarthritis, "frozen shoulder", "tennis elbow".

It is only fair to add that many acupuncturists are uneasy, when they see lists of this kind, because they do not care for the emphasis to be put on the symptoms and the disorders from which their treatment is reputedly effective. Most patients, they argue, bring a "cocktail" of different symptoms which are treated separately in western pathology – in the sense that one specialist may be called upon to treat bone and muscle disorders and another, digestive disorders. To the acupuncturist, a link between the symptoms may be obvious, and they can be treated together.

This means, in effect, that acupuncturists are treating patients holistically, by restoring energy balance, in the expectation that the symptoms will then disappear.

Self-help

To a limited extent, it is possible for an amateur to practise acupuncture in the family, but as there is a well-established form of first aid, *Acupressure* (acupuncture without the use of needles), it seems more sensible to stick to this. (see *Shiatsu and acupressure*, pages 133 to 137).

Shiatsu and acupressure

Shiatsu is a Japanese word meaning "finger pressure". It was originally the Japanese form of Chinese acupressure, but like so many eastern therapies, it has developed characteristics of its own. Today in the hands of many of its practitioners, the technique has absorbed elements from both *Massage* and *Touch for health* (see pages 95 to 100 and 116 to 118). The traffic has not been all one-way, however, and several therapies, including these, have themselves adopted aspects of shiatsu.

Like *Acupuncture* (see pages 120 to 133), shiatsu is based on promoting health by stimulating *chi* (*ki* in Japanese) energy, using pressure on the skin at various points along meridians associated with the function of vital organs.

Acupressure is like acupuncture without needles. It is essentially a self-help technique in which the fingers are used to apply pressure to points known to be helpful for relief of various types of pain. In its western form, where it is sometimes known as G-Jo, acupressure has largely been overtaken by shiatsu. Although practitioners may insist that acupressure rates as a separate therapy from shiatsu, the differences in practice are hardly sufficient to justify making any distinction between the two.

Origins

Although shiatsu has been in use for hundreds of years, it only developed into a therapy in its own right half a century ago, when it was codified and taught by Tokujiro Namikoshi. In Japan today, where they view the therapy as a technique for early diagnosis as well as a disease preventative, many have shiatsu regularly every week. There, of course, it continues to be a simple home treatment and is often practised by members of a family on each other.

Acupressure originally developed in ancient China as a form of first aid for use in families. Today, the techniques can be learned so that it can be used for self-help purposes, or treatment can be sought from professional therapists.

Procedure

Unlike acupuncturists and masseurs, practitioners of shiatsu and acupressure use no equipment, machinery, or oils. Theoretically, therefore, these therapies can be practised anywhere, at any time. In reality, though, a firm surface, such as a carpeted floor, in a clean, quiet, warm room, are essential to treatment. Practitioners of shiatsu and acupressure often work in their clients' homes, though treatment is also often available at health clinics and therapy centres. You should always avoid wearing any tight-fitting, body-hugging clothes, as they will obstruct the practitioner's "touch", and they will undoubtedly be uncomfortable for you, too.

Ordinarily a shiatsu session can be expected to last an hour, or an hour and a quarter. During this period you will be part of the time on your back on the floor, part on your front, part sitting up for work on your shoulders, although not necessarily in that order. There is no fixed course of sessions as there is, for example, in *Rolfing* (see pages 133 to 137). Some people have shiatsu once a week, though most arrange for a treatment, or a course of treatment simply when they feel the need.

The first session of shiatsu treatment usually begins with case-history taking. This process follows the same lines as in acupuncture, including the all-important checking of the pulses. Professional practitioners are likely to want to take a substantial case history, at least on the first visit, particularly if they are being asked to treat some specific disorder, or for general ill-health, as distinct from a general toning-up of the system.

As with most manipulative methods, shiatsu does not lend itself easily to description in print. There is no set order, but most practitioners have a regular routine, say, starting with the body, moving to the head, then to the arms and legs, so that they can concentrate on the "feel" of what they are doing without having to think about the order in which they are going to do it.

Shiatsu treatment

The treatment itself is, in some respects, like massage, but with the therapist working on the acupuncture meridians; in certain respects it also resembles a much gentler form of rolfing.

Pressure is applied in a great variety of ways. Sometimes the bulb of the thumb is used, sometimes the fingers, the palm or heel of the hand, or a knee, an elbow or the soles of the feet – you may even be walked upon. This might sound alarming, but it is in fact a

Shiatsu treatment

There is no set order to a shiatsu treatment – each therapist devises his or her own routine according to your needs. If you feel pain when pressure is applied at a particular point, it may show that the flow of ki is impaired. After shiatsu treatment, the pain should be reduced as the ki flows freely again.

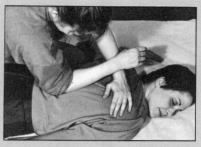

1 At the start and end of a session of shiatsu, the 12 pulses may be taken, as in acupuncutre, to reveal the state of the patient's energy before and after treatment.

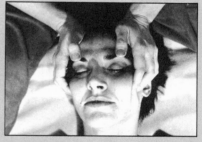

2 Elbow pressure down each side of the spine stimulates the points which influence such functions as respiration, circulation, and digestion. The pressure can be very deep but still enjoyable.

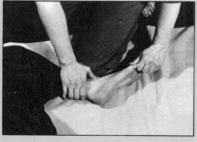

3 The patient's leg is bent out to the side to treat the gall bladder meridian which runs down the outside of the leg. The therapist is pressing an important point on this meridian, in front of the ankle-bone.

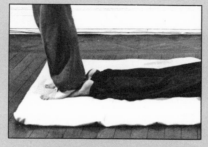

4 The patient lies on her stomach while the therapist walks on the soles of the patient's feet. This stimulates the kidneys and is very pleasurable besides giving the therapist a chance to relax.

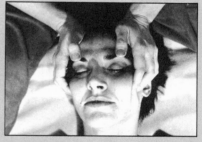

5 Pressing a small intestine point relaxes the jaw. Treating points on the head and face can be so relaxing that many patients almost fall asleep at this stage.

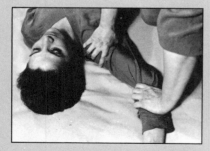

6 Here the therapist is working on the heart meridian on the arm. Limbs are often moved around in shiatsu to stretch the meridians and to loosen the joints so that energy can flow more freely.

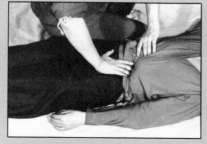

7 The "Hara" or abdomen is the centre of the body's life processes; the most important area for the diagnosis and treatment of imbalances. In Japan, therapists train for 12 years to work on the Hara.

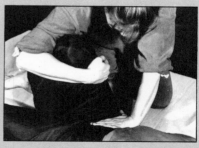

8 Gentle rotation and manipulation of the legs, combined with pressure on the appropriate part of the Hara, often relieves back pain and tension in the hip area.

very ancient technique which is pictured in classical texts and encountered in tribal communities; some patients find it oddly reassuring (see page 135).

The degree and type of pressure applied depends on many variables, but chiefly on the practitioner's estimate of how much is required (and whether a tonifying or sedating effect is required), and this in turn depends on where it is to be applied, and how you react. The pressure is applied at what the practitioner takes to be the appropriate points along the energy channels, roughly the same points as in acupuncture. But whereas the acupuncturist can stick the needles in, and leave them there, here it is a continuing process, with the pressure being applied lightly or forcibly, according to the "feel" of the therapist.

Pleasurable pain

Pressure is applied for a few seconds at a time, and may be repeated three or four times at each spot. As with massage, there are differences of opinion whether, and how much, pain should be caused. Some practitioners do not care to inflict pain, others feel that it can sometimes be desirable. The pressure, Namikoshi maintained, should produce a sensation lying between pleasure and pain, and patients quite often grope for words to express their feeling that though painful, the experience has also been pleasurable.

With acupressure, the points are stimulated in a similar way. The points are carefully located and pressure is applied with the fingers. Because people vary in their responses, the length of time for which relief lasts varies.

Suitable cases

Like acupuncture, shiatsu and acupressure can be used to relieve many kinds of chronic problems and disabling aches and pains. Working in London, shiatsu therapist Carola Beresford-Cooke has found that she obtains the best results with stress disorders, in particular migraine headaches. She finds that people who are high in tension are calmed down, people who are low in tension are revved up (so much so that for a few hours after a session they report the feeling that they are "walking on air"). Consequently, shiatsu is particularly welcome for anybody who is convalescing after an illness.

Acupressure is aimed at pain relief, and is suitable for a wide range of ailments including toothache, headaches of all kinds and backache. Depression, constipation, insomnia and diarrhea are also among the disorders listed as treatable in one book on the subject, *Relief from Pain with Finger Massage* by Dr Roger Galet.

There are, however, some contraindications. Shiatsu and acupressure are appropriately used for everyday disorders, not in cases of chronic illness. Handbooks also advise against combining these therapies with the consumption of medicinal or social drugs, such as alcohol, or their use during pregnancy. Always take advice from a trained therapist.

Self-help

To a limited extent it is possible for the lay person to learn how to apply finger pressure for first aid, in the sense that if, during sessions with a professional, you find that pressure on a certain spot relieves pain somewhere else, you can experiment with do-it-yourself treatment.

There are also a number of books providing instructions on do-it-yourself acupressure therapy. These provide a guide to the appropriate pressure points for different types of disorders, though to a considerable extent this is a matter of trial and error, as different people have different reactions. Estimating the amount of pressure required at any point is obviously a problem, but practitioners are agreed that it is not easy to apply too much.

Special exercises

Most shiatsu practitioners advise simple exercises, which can be used for common ailments. These exercises, which concentrate on stretching, rotating and moving muscles and limbs, can also be practised between treatments and are used to prevent *ki* energy stagnating in the joints. They are quite unlike most western exercises, which tend to help make the body hard and muscular; shiatsu exercises help to make it soft and flexible, in the same way that *Aikido* (see pages 147 to 149) does.

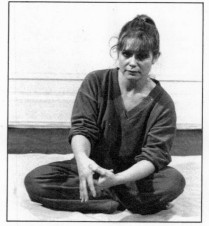

Pain relief
Squeezing hard on the web of flesh between the thumb and forefinger relieves many kinds of pain – from toothache or headache to constipation and period pains.

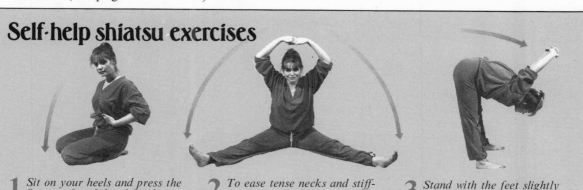

Self-help shiatsu exercises

1 *Sit on your heels and press the fingers of each hand firmly under the rib cage. Take a deep breath, then breathing out, bend forwards as far as you can go, digging your fingers into your solar plexus – this is for constipation and can be very painful.*

2 *To ease tense necks and stiffness, sit with the legs wide apart, keeping the knees on the floor. Clasp the hands, palms upwards, and pull up, straightening the back. Without twisting the torso, bend sideways as far as possible; repeat five times each side.*

3 *Stand with the feet slightly apart, the hands clasped behind the back. Bend forwards, raising the arms behind the head as far as they will go. Then straighten up and, bending the head back, raise the hands. This releases tense shoulders and opens up the chest.*

EXERCISE/MOVEMENT THERAPIES

Yoga, Aikido and *T'ai chi* may not, strictly speaking, be therapies, but they have better health as one of their aims. Also dealt with in this section is *Dance therapy*, which falls into two main categories: firstly, it is used by adults and children alike as an outlet for self-expression, for learning greater awareness of one's body and how it moves and works. Secondly, dance therapy is used with considerable success in special education, to treat a wide range of mental and emotional disorders.

Yoga

There are many varieties of yoga, and doubtless more will be appearing in the West as new gurus manifest themselves. They present a spectrum of disciplines with an emphasis on exercise at one end and on meditation at the other (though the two are often intertwined). Here we are mainly concerned with hatha yoga, which is the type most commonly encountered in the West. We deal with meditation separately, in the *Psychological therapies* (see *Meditation* pages 182 to 188).

Origins

To judge from archeological remains, notably sculptures and carvings, yoga must have been practised in India at least as long as 6,000 years ago. As it has come down to us, it was based on the theory of union of the self with higher consciousness. The word "yoga" comes from Sanskrit, from the same source as our word "yoke". According to yoga philosophy, body, mind, and spirit cannot be separated, and we must realize, too, that we are linked to all living creatures – even, indeed, to inanimate matter.

When westerners began to study Sanskrit, Hinduism, and Buddhism, it was for a time mainly for their historical and etymological interest. And those few who were tempted to explore the yogi path encountered problems. One was that the sources, in their recommendations for abstinence, included certain other moral imperatives. And although many, such as warnings against covetousness and theft, were in the Judaic and Christian traditions, others were not – not, at least, in the nineteenth century, when translators began to make these warnings known in the English language.

According to Patanjali, whose *Yoga Sutras*, written in the fourth century BC, remain a cornerstone of yoga teaching, among the essential precepts were "abstention from causing pain at any time, in any way however small, to any living thing", even to insects. As for the observances, many of them – ritual bathing in

Yoga is relevant to our age because, far from being mystical or other-wordly, it is a teaching firmly grounded in physiological reality and can be understood in contemporary terms. We know that our experience of the world depends entirely on the state of our nervous system. This in turn is influenced by a host of factors – heredity, diet, environment and so on. If the nervous system is fresh and rested, the body will be healthy and the mind alert and comprehensive.

Alistair Shearer
Effortless Being

ashes, for example, or in the dust raised by sacred cows – were remote from western culture.

As a consequence, new schools of yoga have developed, that are better adapted to western attitudes and habits.

The mind-body relationship

All gurus, or instructors, insist that the basic aim of exercises, both physical and mental, is to create a healthy mind in a healthy body. Whether people elect to pursue more esoteric goals, such as those associated with yogi in the final contemplative stage of development, is up to them. For the rest, it is enough if they learn to bring mind and body into sufficient harmony to discover how to enjoy life to the full, in whatever circumstances they happen to live and work – whether as dukes or dustmen. Good health, the belief is, arises out of this harmony.

For over a century after yoga had been introduced to the British public, its therapeutic potential was not taken seriously, partly because of resistance to the idea that meditation could have any real influence physiologically, partly because the stories about fakirs being able to exercise "miraculous" powers – lying on beds of nails without injury or submitting to being "buried alive" for days – sounded bogus. The first man of any eminence within the medical profession to insist they deserved attention was Henry Sigerist, Professor of the History of Medicine at John Hopkins University.

Meditation and physical disorders

In 1961, in the second volume of what, had he lived to complete it, would unquestionably have become the world's standard medical history, Sigerist challenged the established notion that the mind played little part in healing. "Every cell of our organism is controlled by the nervous system which conveys impulses of the mind", he asserted. Determination to get well is, in many cases, a decisive healing factor – so "how much more potent must be the effect of a mind concentrated in meditation. We may think of autosuggestion, autohypnosis; but whatever the mechanism may be, there can be no doubt that a philosophy such as that of Yoga has great medical potentialities". And he cited the evidence of the German anthropologist Edward Erkes, who had learned a Taoist technique of meditation in China and found that even as a beginner, he could apply it to cure everyday disorders such as colds and headaches.

Sigerist was writing his history at the height of the "wonder-drug" era, when the idea that meditation of any kind could be effective in treating disorders of the body was not taken seriously. In the next decade, however, interest in its healing potential began to mount, thanks partly to the publicity obtained by the Beatles for the Maharishi Mahesh Yogi and his *Transcendental medi-*

A Tibetan Buddah
Yoga has been a way of life in the East for thousands of years – a means of promoting health and spiritual development. This Tibetan Buddha is in a typical Yogic pose.

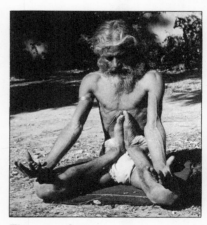

The yoga adept
In Kanda Pindasana, pressure exerted by the feet on the navel and chest regions results in improved functioning of the abdominal organs, thus aiding digestion.

tation (see pages 186 to 187). And during the 1970s, yoga groups, some owing allegiance to gurus, some offering down-to-earth physical courses with hardly a hint of any mystical element, began to be a commonplace in the western world.

To try to distinguish here between all the forms of yoga now available to the public would present difficulties, as the differences can be of a kind which, important though they may seem to devotees, are not readily apparent to the rest of us. Still, it is certainly true that some forms of yoga are more flexible than others in their approach. At one extreme are those cults in which the guru's word is law; at the other is "clinically standard meditation" (CSM), recently imported from America, where the only instruction the beginner is thought to need is provided for him on a single tape which, it is claimed, sets him on the road to effective meditation – and the next tape – within a week.

Here we are concerned primarily with hatha yoga, as it is the most familiar form of yoga in the west, largely for historical reasons. According to the French writer Félix Guyot, who investigated the subject between the wars, hatha yoga was the most accessible to westerners because it is "open to all, without distinction of sex, nationality, caste or religion". Less pretentious than other forms, too, it is chiefly concerned with exercises designed to improve posture and breathing, on the principle that these not only lead to better physical health but to greater self-confidence and serenity, because stress and tension are removed.

Procedure

Yoga courses concentrate on three main aspects: posture, breathing and meditation. What you can expect from your first class will vary according to the type of yoga chosen and the preconceptions of the yogi, or the instructor. But ordinarily the emphasis in the initial stages is on achieving mind-body control with the help of exercises which, after they have been demonstrated, can be practised at home.

Yoga and beginners

Asked how the complete beginner should approach yoga, Dr M.I. Gharote, one of the directors of the Kaivalyadhama Institute near Bombay, has emphasized the following: posture exercises should be done very slowly and smoothly; they should be maintained for a comfortable time; they should be released in a slow and sustained manner; if you ever feel fatigue, you should overcome it with one of the relaxation postures; while you are doing your postures, try to be aware of your breathing; and always devote your entire concentration to what you are doing. Gharote, unlike some other yoga teachers, does not consider the sequence of postures to be of great importance.

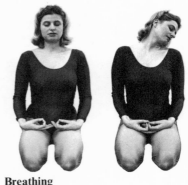

Breathing
Kneel down with your thumbs and index fingers touching, as shown above left. Completely empty the lungs. Now, gently breathe in to the count of seven and out to the count of seven. Repeat for about three minutes morning and evening.

Neck roll
Kneeling in the same position, let your head fall towards your chest, then rotate it slowly and smoothly clockwise three times and anti-clockwise three times, as above right. Move only your neck, not your shoulders. This relieves tension in the neck area.

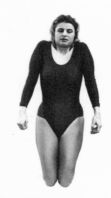

Shoulder roll
Kneel down, but keep your hips up and your arms down by your sides. Slowly rotate each arm clockwise three times and anti-clockwise three times. Then repeat the exercise, rotating both arms simultaneously.

The salute to the sun

Prayer *Stand with your feet together and your hands palm to palm.* Salutation *Breathing in, lift your arms above your head.* Prayer *Bring your hands back to the prayer position.* Ostrich *Breathing out, bend forward and drop your arms down. If you can, rest your hands by your feet.* Praying Mantis *Breathing in, bend the right leg and bring the left leg back. Rest the fingertips on the floor, level with the right foot and arch*

back *as far as possible.* Cheetah *Breathing out, lean forward and place your hands down flat on the floor.* Lizard *Breathing in, bring the right leg back and curl the toes of both feet under.* Giraffe *Breathing out, lift your hips up as high as you can.* Caterpillar *Bend your knees to the floor, push your head forward and flatten your chest, with your hips still raised up.* Cobra *Breathing in, bring the hips down and lift the chest area up.*

Giraffe *Breathing out, curl both feet under and raise the hips up again.* Praying Mantis *Breathing in, step forward with the right foot and lean back.* Ostrich *Breathing out, bring your feet together and come up very slowly to the* Prayer *position. Now start the sequence again, bringing the right foot back instead of the left in the* Praying Mantis *and* Cheetah *positions and finish in the* Pose of the Child.

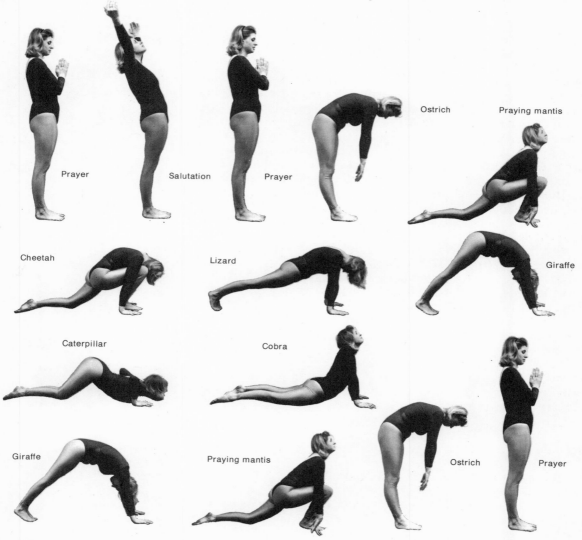

Prayer

Salutation

Prayer

Ostrich

Praying mantis

Cheetah

Lizard

Giraffe

Caterpillar

Cobra

Giraffe

Praying mantis

Ostrich

Prayer

Learning to breathe

Although everybody knows that breathing is related to emotional states, breath coming faster in alarming situations, the converse, that regular, slow and deep breathing may banish tension, has not been so generally recognized. An example of this kind of exercise designed to promote tranquility is one which goes under the name of "rhythmic cleansing breath". As a simple relaxation technique this has several advantages, not least of which is the fact that it can be done almost anywhere, even in public, without drawing the attention of other people.

The postures

These are primarily designed to keep the body supple and to promote mind-body harmony. The significance of *asana* (the attitudes and positions of the body) has been emphasized by the eminent anthropologist Professor Mircea Eliade in his book *Pantanjali and Yoga*. "It is only with the practice of *asana* that yogic technique, properly so-called, begins", he claims. It is better demonstrated, he admits, than described. But "what is important is the fact that *asana* gives a rigid stability to the body while at the same time it reduces physical effort to the minimum. Thus one avoids the irritating sensation of fatigue or of the numbness of certain parts of the body; one controls the physiological process; and thus one makes it possible for one's attention to be occupied exclusively with the fluid part of consciousness".

At first, the *asanas* are bound to be uncomfortable, but in time, and with practice, some postures begin to become natural. "The posture becomes perfect", as a manual of instruction from the seventh century put it, "when the effort of achieving it vanishes". This is the first step towards what Eliade calls "the isolation of the consciousness" which may ultimately be achieved by people who are prepared to go all the way to the removal of all sense of the physical presence and limitations of the body, which also provides control over its functions.

The importance of relaxation

After completion of a set of postural exercises, it is considered of great importance that you should spend at least five minutes relaxing. Again, there are various methods, one of the most popular of which is the "corpse" position.

Research

From time to time, the Yoga and Meditation School in Copenhagen publishes a pamphlet, *Medical and Psychological Scientific Research on Yoga and Meditation*, and an English translation of it published recently gives an idea of the amount and range of the research work that has been done so far. It contains references to

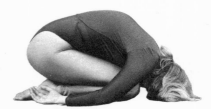

Pose of the child
Kneel down with your head in front of your knees for this relaxation pose. To come out of the posture, very slowly uncurl the head as you straighten the spine.

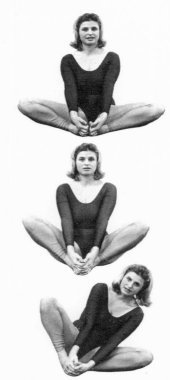

Butterfly
Sit with your knees bent and the soles of the feet together. Clasp the feet and draw them in to the body. Breathing in, open the legs as wide as possible, then breathe out and lift the legs up towards your arms. Repeat 3–4 times. Now rock from side to side on your buttocks.

nearly 500 reports, many of them from established medical and pyschological journals throughout the world.

Many of the reports deal with research into the physiological and neurological effects of meditation, and they show an interestingly consistent pattern. No matter the type, meditation appears to be effective in reducing tension, as measured by skin resistance, blood pressure and other indicators.

In general, recent research confirmed these findings. Thus Dr Michael A. West, of the University of Kent, divided volunteers into two groups: the members of one practised meditation regularly for six months, and periodically presented themselves for skin-resistance tests, the members of the other simply attend for tests. The experimental group showed a significant decrease in spontaneous skin conductance responses over the six-month period, West reported in the *British Journal of Social and Clinical Psychology*. "The comparison group, and a small group of subjects who gave up meditation early in the experiment, exhibited no significant change".

The chief value of yoga, however, is in prevention of illness, and little research has been done in this area. Nor will it be easy to do. As Dr Gharote once remarked "we want to see how people are progressing, but once they have gone away they tend to forget about it – they are not interested in reporting to me for two years, five years".

Yoga exercises during pregnancy

During pregnancy, yoga exercises are extremely beneficial and will keep you supple and relaxed. Obviously, certain positions will be physically impossible but, conversely, there are some which are particularly effective.

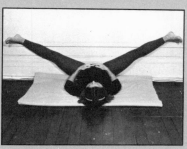

Legs apart on a wall
Lie with your buttocks against a wall and your legs straight up, then slowly open them as far as they will go. This strengthens the inner thighs and helps varicose veins.

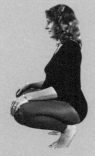

Squatting on toes
This position can't be maintained long without support. It helps to prevent and relieve backache, muscle cramp, constipation and varicose veins.

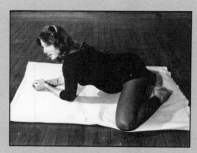

The "frog" position
Sit on the heels with the knees apart and gradually bend forward on to the elbows, with a straight back. This relieves backache and the heavy feeling of pregnancy.

Suitable cases

According to Dr Gharote, experience at the Kaivalyadhama Institute suggests that "all the chronic diseases are specially amenable to yoga treatment" – diseases, that is, of the digestive system, such as dyspepsia, ulceration, constipation, and diseases of the nervous system, such as multiple sclerosis. In particular, yoga is effective in dealing with stress disorders through body-mind interaction.

In the introductory pamphlet *Yoga* issued by the Friends of the Healing Research Trust, Jenni Adams lists the conditions which most commonly respond to yoga: arthritis; asthma; backache; breathing difficulties; bronchitis; constipation; dysmenorrhea; dyspepsia; hypertension; nervous disorders; obesity; and sinusitis.

Some exercises are more valuable than others for people suffering from a particular disorder, but most yoga teachers feel that it is wise for beginners to take the prescribed course and then find by trial and error which of the postures is most effective in warding off a headache – or whatever the symptoms may be.

T'ai Chi

T'ai chi has been described as "meditation in motion". It can be regarded as a civilian version of the some of the ancient eastern martial arts such as kung fu, and it has some affinities with dance therapy. Unlike dance therapy, however, it is ritualized into a succession of flowing movements, with relatively little scope for individual variations. Each movement or exercise has a symbolic interpretation, and emphasis is laid upon the psychological or psychic element involved. All the movements are circular and aim to develop muscular control, rather than muscular bulk.

Origins

The early history of t'ai chi is obscure. One story is that it originated in Taoist institutions as a game for children, to keep them occupied; another, that it developed out of exercises derived from the martial arts, but adapted for the benefit of patients convalescing after illness. There are many elements in it of Taoism, and some of Buddhism. Until the mid-nineteenth century t'ai chi was hardly known outside China, and it was regarded there as an esoteric pursuit. And although it then began to spread, it remained suspect in the eyes of those who were to take over in China after the Long March (1934–5).

This hostility abated, however, and when America's President

⟨ In aiming for subtlety, not physical strength, the movement exercises and explores all aspects concurrently without strain, coordinating mind, body, breath and spirit into harmony . . . the body rides easily through the constant shifting of weight, linked fluidly via the waist with the circular movements of the arms. The slow, peaceful but dynamic flow of forms reflects the continuity of the life force . . . developing awarement throughout the body, and teaching the containment and distribution of energy. ⟩

Beverley Milne

Nixon visited China in 1972, some of the newsreel films taken showed demonstrations of t'ai chi. By this time it had also begun to spread out from "Chinatowns" in the United States. And in Britain, Gerda Geddes, who had lived for some years in the East and had learned t'ai chi from a teacher in Shanghai, began herself to teach the techniques. Many of her pupils have become teachers.

Procedure

All teachers of t'ai chi, and indeed all pupils, emphasize the impossibility of adequately describing it in print. "The only way to get an authentic impression", as Stephen Annett puts it in his *The Many Ways of Being*, "is to watch it being performed".

T'ai chi, he explains, "is very simple, with no frills, decoration, or superflous movement. It is about finding the centre of balance, with the physical centre gradually leading to the spiritual centre. It teaches the individual containment, the way to build up energy in the body, and then to direct and control its release through movement".

T'ai chi movements

The secret of t'ai chi is tranquillity. All movements should be performed with a relaxed mind and body. Maximum effect comes from minimum effort. Keep your weight mainly on one foot and rely on balance and alignment, rather than using any structural support. The correct posture will naturally result in your breathing well, ensuring perfect coordination.

| 70% weight | 30% weight |

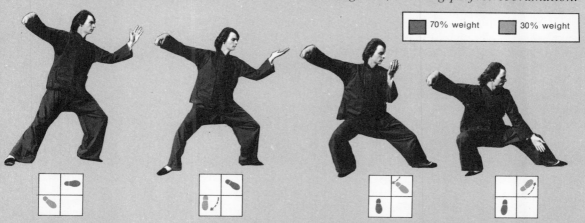

Squatting single whip
Also known as "Snake Creeps Down to the Water", this whole sequence is performed on an inbreath. Turn your right foot 25° to the right, then draw back and lower your body, transferring your weight to the right foot, and turning your left foot 25° inward to the right. Now draw your left hand back to the chest and, as you lower the body further, sweep the hand down to touch the left knee. Simultaneously, turn your left heel 50° to the left. keep your right hand hooked to maintain balance.

At first glance, the martial arts element still features, with "pushing hands", one of the movements, visually suggesting a kind of shadow boxing. But, as Mrs Geddes has explained, "slowly the body is transformed, the movements become smoother and more flowing, the breathing becomes freer and deeper, and your thoughts clearer", until "there eventually develops a sensation of calmness, stillness and non-attachment".

There are two forms of the movements, one protracted, with over 100 movements, which take 20 minutes to complete; the other shorter, with 37 movements, taking less than 10 minutes. When performed by an expert, what strikes observers most is the absence of any sign of effort. "Most Westerners attack daily exercise as though they were wrestling with a bear", Walter B. Dudley observes in Bricklin's *Natural Healing*. "They don't really enjoy doing it. Up and down, puff, puff, back and forth". By contrast, t'ai chi requires total relaxation: "eventually you will experience a sensation almost as though you were floating".

"Eventually", however, can mean a long apprenticeship, 10 years, or so. As with so many natural therapies, one school of traditionalist thought strongly resents the spread of what it regards as a very superficial version of t'ai chi, as taught in most classes. Teachers in this mould refuse to take pupils except on a long-term basis, and require them not just to learn the dance, but also to study Taoism, the *I Ching*, and their general philosophies.

Tuning in to *chi* energy

It does not, however, require such a long apprenticeship to appreciate the difference between t'ai chi and most western forms of exercise, and to reach at least the beginning of an understanding of the signficance, in this context, of *chi*, the life force, which in Chinese metaphysics is held to permeate the atmosphere. The aim is to tune in to *chi*. In Chinese metaphysics, the assumption is that mind and body in combination can be opened up to it, so that the energy itself takes over, as it were. Instead of having to go through the motions, the dancers find the motions going through them.

Suitable cases

T'ai chi has come to be prescribed by some cardiologists for patients who have had, or are threatened with, heart disease – patients with palpitations, angina or hypertension – because it is a form of exercise which imposes no strain. Some general practitioners, too, have been recommending it to "type A" patients – those who drive themselves too hard, as an alternative to tranquillizers. But most teachers emphasize its value as a general conditioner, toning both mind and body so that, unless you are unlucky, you will remain immune to everyday disorders.

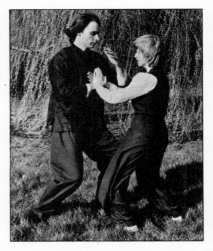

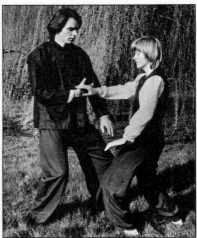

Single and double push hands
According to the classical texts, to understand the Tao of self, you should practise the solo form of t'ai chi; to understand the Tao of others, you should study "push hands". As your partner pushes forwards, you yield backwards, twisting the hips and transferring your weight to your back foot. When the push is over, you return it with your own push, straightening the hips and shifting your weight to the front foot.

Aikido

Aikido is a form of martial art from Japan. It can most easily be visualized as a form of weaponless fencing, or wrestling, where the objective is not so much to overcome one's partner but to use his or her force in self-defence in the way that, traditionally, wrestlers in the ju-jitsu tradition do. As a therapy, it has developed into something more than this – a kind of ritual dance in which, though there appears to be a contest, the two people involved are in fact together seeking to exploit *ki* (the Japanese word for the life force) much as the individual does in *T'ai chi* (see pages 144 to 146). The central aim, according to the British Aikido Federation is "self-realization through discipline".

Origins

In its modern form, aikido was invented by Professor Morihei Uyeshiba, a leading exponent of the martial arts in Japan between the wars, although its origins can be traced back as far as the twelfth century. By Uyeshiba's own account he had a vision which was to change his entire attitude: while in the grip of exaltation he realised that he should not want to *win*: "a martial art should be a form of life". His aim was, through aikido, to promote harmony and love, first on an individual, and ultimately, on a universal scale. For a while he taught only disciples, but a few years after the Japanese defeat at the end of the Second World War he decided the time had come to spread his gospel; in the 1950s and 1960s, he sent some of his disciples off to Europe and the United States to make aikido known.

The art of non-resistance

Aikido is partly devoted to training in the art of self-defence, although perhaps it would be nearer the mark to say that it teaches the art of non-resistance. The primary aim being not to overcome an attacker so much as to disarm him or her in the emotional as well as the physical sense, if possible. But it goes on to convert the "contest" into something more positive, with students learning that winning means nothing. To quote Uyeshiba, "if I win today, the time will inevitably come when I must lose". As a result, the movements become a form of cooperation with each other.

"The teacher of aikido speaks about harmony, and then throws the student to the ground!" – according to a teacher cited by Chris Popenoe, manager of the celebrated Yes! bookshop in Washington, DC, and author-editor of *Inner Development*. Popenoe explains why: "Our training teaches us that by alternately throwing and being thrown we are expanding our spirit, increasing our ability to both give and receive". Thrower and thrown may appear to be fighting, but what they are really doing is learning the art of give and take.

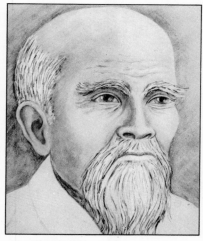

Morihei Uyeshiba
O-Sensei Morihei Uyeshiba (1883–1969), the founder of modern Aikido, a form of combat which he saw as a dance of exceptional beauty.

The concept of a vital force

As in t'ai chi, the element of the vital force is strongly emphasized. The assumption is that when the "wrestlers" are in full harmony, their powers are increased, and not just their physical strength. The *ki* is thought to extend awareness, so that the practised performer can sense where any adversaries are and what they are doing, even if they are behind his or her back or at a distance, and can take the appropriate moves to anticipate them.

Interestingly, this ties in with what the mesmerists reported from their research during the nineteenth century. Certain susceptible subjects, when mesmerised, could "see" objects held behind their backs, and react to signals from the mesmerist even when he was out of their sight. The mesmerists also had the same explanation; animal magnetism was simply another version of *ki*, or *chi*. Later James Braid, who introduced the concept of *Hypnotism* (see pages 166 to 173), claimed that there was no need to think in terms of any such vital force: it was simply that individuals in the trance had an increased physical awareness, and some aikido teachers today prefer to think in these terms.

Procedure

Aikido is taught to classes of about 20 to 30 people in a special *dojo* or practice room. The sessions, at beginners, intermediate, and advanced levels, usually take place weekly, though often people attend several different ones if they are really keen, and are led by a trained instructor.

Etiquette is strict, and visitors who come simply to watch are expected to fit in with the rules of the *dojo*. There are proper procedures to follow from entering the *dojo*, to leaving. Classes usually last about an hour, and are graded according to proficiency. A short period of meditation is usually followed by

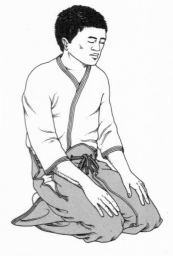

Aikido meditation
The shout, "Kiai" is the yell of combat and is seen in Aikido as a whole art in itself. It is necessary first to adopt this meditative posture for anything between five minutes to an hour, gathering all your reserves of energy so that they can be unified in "Kiai".

Irimi-Nage
Irimi-Nage, *the exercise shown on the right is one given to beginners but it does, in fact, demonstrate the principles of Aikido perfectly. The technique is based on the idea of the bamboo, swaying in the wind. In the same way the Aikido defender employs* Irimi, *the capacity to absorb and take over the aggressive energy (*Nage*) of his opponent. In an apparently effortless, gentle movement, the defender overpowers his attacker.*

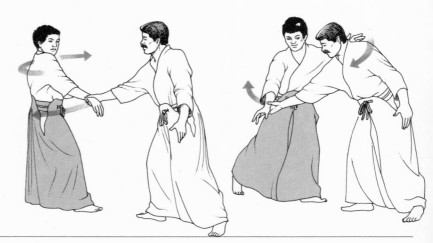

limbering-up exercises before beginning the serious business of learning new throwing or holding techniques usually working in pairs. The overall effect is of graceful, circular movements.

The movements used follow the principle of non-resistance: the participant turns away when pushed, enters when pulled. All the techniques consist of both these elements of motion. The Aikido postures maintain great stability both in stillness and in action.

In practising these techniques, you must unbalance your partner by circular movements centred in and around your hips and this diverts the direction and impetus of his attack while producing a centrifugal or centripetal effect. To quote the Aikido Federation's pamphlet: "There is no dualistic opposition, but the partner's body, while under control of one's own, is in complete unity with it. When the continuity of such circular or spherical motion is maintained, the grace and rhythm unique to Aikido appears".

Suitable cases

People do not as a rule go to aikido class with therapy in mind, but the teachers claim that the exercises help liberate joints, tendons and muscles that have seized up. This in turn, they believe, improves the circulation of the blood and benefits the nervous system in general. Obviously, people with serious mechanical disorders – back troubles and the like – should consult their therapists before embarking on aikido training.

The main emphasis tends to be on the value of aikido as a mental, moral and spiritual training, as well as a physical one, the combination helping to ward off most everyday disorders. General overall fitness is often claimed to be a by-product of going to classes regularly, and women are said to be especially good at aikido; children, too, seem to love it.

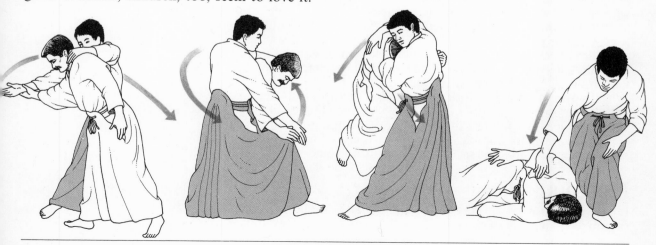

Dance therapy

Movement and dance are used as therapy in a number of different ways. Young children, of course, have always learned dance at school, where it is taught for a variety of reasons – one being that it is good for them in terms of posture and movement control, another that it can be used to help them learn to give outward form and expression to inner feelings. Dance or "movement therapy", however, in the form that it has taken in the United States and is now taking in other countries, aims at more specific and positive health promotion for all ages, and can be adapted to treat mental and emotional conditions.

Origins

The use of dancing as a therapy in tribal communities is almost universal and is commonly linked with progression into the trance state. A witch doctor may dance himself into convulsions, in which he looses control of his body and becomes possessed, or he may put members of the tribe into a similar possessed condition with the help of music, drumming and dancing. In the trance state, the assumption is, the spirits which possess the body can heal it or renew its vitality.

Medieval dancing mania

In the civilized world this tradition lingered on, for a time. Fits, even outbreaks of mass hysteria, such as the "dancing mania" of the early Middle Ages, were taken to be divine visitations, and had their own patron, St Vitus. But when fits came to be regarded as a form of mental illness, dancing survived, like so much else, only as a ritual or pastime purged of its therapeutic content.

There have always been individuals, however, who have felt that dance has a place in therapy, not just as an exercise for the body, but as an outlet for the emotions. Rudolf Laban, a German who emigrated to Britain, regarded dancing as a way of restoring mental health, and taught it between the wars as an adjunct to psychotherapy.

After the Second World War, another form of dance therapy was introduced in the United States by Marian Chace, when she was invited by a psychiatrist to work with patients at a Washington mental hospital. Other dance therapists started up, going their own ways, until in 1966, the American Dance Therapy Association was founded in the hope of bringing about some standardization in qualifications. Nevertheless, dance therapy must be considered to be still in its exploratory stage.

Procedure

Dance and movement classes for the general public are often organized in a series of six to eight weekly sessions. No two dance therapists offer the same formula, but anybody attending a session for the first time will probably find a group small enough to enable the teacher to give each member personal attention.

Classes often begin with simple movement exercises which are designed to loosen up the body. A typical dance therapy session has been described by Esther C. Frankel in Bricklin's *Natural Healing*. "The formation most commonly used is a circle, because it creates a feeling of security and oneness. For withdrawn people, merely holding hands and facing other members of the group are healthy steps in the right direction". Music, if any, may be selected by the therapist or the patients themselves, though often music is abandoned, and the dancers use their own rhythm. "One by one, each body part moves to the rhythm – head, shoulders, arms, hips, knees, ankles".

Another account by Claire Schmais, in Kaslof's *Wholistic Dimensions in Healing*, describes the group as "not necessarily looking at or talking to one another, but connected by a kinetic bond through the sound of the music and the movements of the therapist", a cohesion which, "stemming from common rhythmic action, nurtures new roles and supports spontaneous dance dramas. Latent fears, angers and sorrows become visible within the confines of this magical circle".

Dance therapy techniques

Dance therapy aims to encourage you to discover your own rhythm and flow of movement and to find ways of expressing yourself through "dance". Sessions normally last about 2½ hours and are held once a week. They are open to both men and women. Classes begin with exercises designed to warm up and stretch the body.

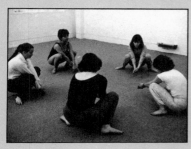

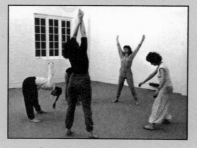

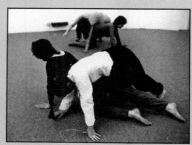

1 *Squatting is often used as a warm-up because it requires minimal muscular and skeletal exertion, promotes mobility in the pelvic region, and encourages relaxation and openness.*

2 *After a short set of guided warm-up instructions, you will be asked to find ways to stretch and complete your preparation for the session; classes often develop out of material emerging at this point.*

3 *In this particular exercise, called "rolling over bridges", the person below acts as a bridge, supporting the other person's weight. The person on top is encouraged to explore moving over the bridge.*

As already noted, most therapists develop a method unique to themselves, whether working with groups or individuals. Therapy may take the form of acting out or recreating inner states through the experience of movement and dance which help release inhibitions and clarify experience. "Barely recognizable feelings are brought to fruition by the therapist's reaction and the group's reinforcing responses", Claire Schmais explains. Emotions are expressed in movement: "fragments of expression evolve into actions and then into interactions. Closing fingers may change to a fist and then to a punch, leading the patient towards the source of his or her anger".

Some teachers concentrate on motor activities and bodily techniques while others encourage free improvisation. Words and song are often evoked spontaneously in this way. As in most other therapies, it is not always possible to have a clear picture of what your experience will be until you have tried it yourself.

Dance therapy in special education

Many handicapped (particularly autistic) children have very little sense of their own bodies and it is believed by many in special education that dance and movement can be used to help them improve body awareness. A greater understanding of self will also help them in their dealings with other people and the world around them. Simple physical skills such as walking, running, sitting, and lying will also be improved incidentally – and this will *also lead directly to greater self-confidence. Self-expression and the release of emotions which are encouraged in these sessions can also help the handicapped learn more about themselves and the way they react to the outside world. The aim always is to help children to gain a greater understanding of themselves and their relationship to the environment around them and this it is hoped leads to a greater independence and ability to affect the life around them.*

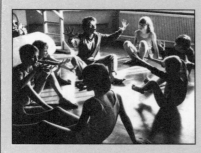

1 A group of children with autistic tendencies responding to "Every one stretch your hands out". This relatively simple movement meets with varying degrees of success from total involvement to total indifference.

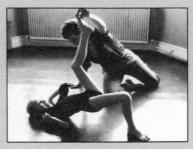

2 One of the children – a girl of eleven who has been undergoing treatment for some time – is asked by the therapist to stretch a little further. Her delight in her achievement is obvious.

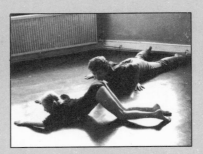

3 The same child is pretending to be a balloon, while her teacher "blows her up". Not only is her body awareness growing, but so is her ability to concentrate and sustain an idea in play.

Suitable cases

Many people attend dance classes simply to unwind and use them as a less strenuous, non-competitive alternative to sport, as a means of keeping fit and lessening the physical effects of tension. In terms of disorders, dance therapy is slowly being recognized by those working in mental hospitals, training centres, residential institutions and clubs. All types of human conditions which result in people having difficulty in coping with day-to-day living could benefit from individual or group-based therapy.

Marion Chace had her initial success with mental patients suffering from the then common symptoms of what has since come to be known as "institutional neurosis". Mental hospitals used to be full of patients sitting or standing around in a catatonic state, and it was found that music and dancing roused some of them who had gone beyond the reach of verbal psychotherapy. And although the locked doors, padded cells, and other characteristics of the old snakepit lunatic asylums have, for the most part, been banished, making institutional neurosis less common, experience has shown that patients with mental disorders which tend to cut them off from the community, but not seriously enough to require hospital treatment, can respond well to a programme of dance therapy.

In particular, success has been reported with handicapped or retarded children, autistic children, and adolescents with neuroses which tend to make them withdrawn. In addition, stroke patients, the blind and the physically disabled have also been found to respond well to the dance therapy approach. Adults recovering after an accident or serious operation can also benefit, though in their case the therapy is undertaken more for the restoration of a full range of movements.

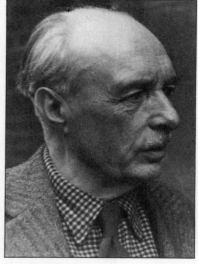

Rudolf Laban
Laban (1879–1959) believed passionately in the therapeutic value of dance on the mental and emotional state of the individual.

SENSORY THERAPIES

Over the past few years there has been a growing feeling that even when the psychological and psychosomatic aspects of health and illness are recognized and given their due, too much attention is focussed on the "mind" in the restricted sense of the source of our thoughts and emotions. Not enough attention is paid to "mind" as an aborber of impressions of other kinds (visual, for example) much as those of colour and shape. That noise can create health problems has been recognized; yet little attention has been paid to the possibility that agreeable noises, such as music, may be exploited therapeutically, though there is plenty of historical evidence of its use in that role.

To a limited extent, admittedly, some sensory therapies such as art therapy, have been employed for health purposes, but this has been the case chiefly in mental hospitals, though the tendency has been to use them as a way of keeping inmates from boredom. Only very recently have some of these therapies begun to achieve wider recognition in their own right. Owing to the financial straitjacket imposed on public medicine by successive governments, however, their development has been slow.

Colour therapy

The potential value of colour therapy is perhaps best illustrated by imagining what it would be like to have to live in a room painted scarlet, or mud colour, or black, or any colour for which you happen to have a particular aversion. The converse then suggests itself: if the thought of a hideous colour, or any combination of colours can be depressing, may not a colour or combination of colours which we like be used therapeutically to give us a lift – or, for that matter, to tranquillize or sedate us?

In a sense, colour therapy is an everyday, though hardly recognized, practice in conventional medicine, for pharmaceutical companies have long tried to make their products look alluring by choosing popular colours. Colour is coming into use increasingly as an adjunct to natural therapies: sometimes as a therapy in its own right. Interestingly, blind people can also be treated as colour changes manifest themselves on the skin's surface as well as on the eyes.

Procedure

Colour therapy takes many forms. Some psychotherapists explore their patients' colour preferences by, say, noting what colours they are wearing, and getting them to note down their likes and dislikes. From these it is possible to make certain deductions which can influence the course therapy will take. Others may use the test of Dr Max Lüscher, who in the 1940s researched the correspondences between people's colour preferences and their psychological make-up. As a result of this research, he devised a colour-based personality test that became widely used, even in some cases as a basis for job selection.

Research

Experiments in many countries have shown that most of us find certain colours stimulating and others tranquillizing. Different colours are also known to affect our perception of temperature. For example, a Norwegian study recorded that people in a blue room set a thermostat three degrees higher than people in a red room. And there are other studies supporting the notion that hue affects our perception of time and even our ability to concentrate and memorize. The knowledge thus gained of common ways in which people experience colour has been used by architects and designers in, for example, decorating hospital wards and libraries.

The effects of red light

Elaborate colour charts are now available in which the colours of the rainbow, and some of the intermediate blends, are allotted their particular characteristics. Nick Humphrey, Assistant Director of the Department of Animal Behaviour at the University of Cambridge, includes the following physiological reactions amongst the accepted findings: "Large fields of red light induce physiological symptoms of emotional arousal – changes in heart rate, skin resistance and the electrical activity of the brain. In patients suffering from certain pathological disorders, for instance, cerebellar palsy, these physiological effects become exaggerated. In cerebellar patients red light may cause intolerable distress, exacerbating the disorders of posture and movement, lowering pain thresholds and causing a general disruption of thought and skilled behaviour. When colour vision is impaired by central brain lesions, red vision is most resistant to loss and quickest to recover".

The effects of colour in the nervous system

Specialists in colour therapy are now beginning to speak out and claim that there is a great deal more to colour than simple psychological reactions to visual stimuli. For it appears that the non-visual system must also be sensitive to shifts and changes in colour. It seems, for example, that red and blue light produce changes that parallel those that are known to take place in the sympathetic and parasympathetic divisions of the autonomic nervous system, it is aroused by the effect of red light, or calmed through the effect produced by blue light. Some researchers are going even further and saying that we may be sensitive to minute changes of colour such as those that occur between daylight and artificial light, and that these differences can affect our health. But although we do know that our moods and mental health are affected by diurnal and seasonal changes in the light cycles (for example, lack of sunlight in winter is linked with suffering from a particular type of depression, and the research is well documented on the affect of light on women's hormonal cycles and thus moods), there is still controversy about the evidence on the different effects of natural versus artificial light. Whilst some people argue that artificial light is harmful, others enthuse over its benefits in the treatment of a variety of disorders, from psoriasis to jaundice in newborn babies.

Suitable cases

It seems that we are all suitable cases for colour treatment in that far more attention needs to be paid to the colour design of the places in which we live and work. Further than this, though, it can only really be left up to individuals to decide on what is appropriate. Whether, for example they feel that a particular colour environment may be of help for their ills. Or it may be that colour healing from a psychic who purports to be able to "read" auras and "see" what colours are appropriate is more suitable, or perhaps phototherapy (the use of artificial light in therapy) will provide the answers.

Art therapy

The basis of art therapy is that patients draw or paint pictures, or make models. The aim here is not to create an accurate representation of objects, as it would be at a drawing class for instance, or of producing something "artistic". Rather, it is designed to enable people to express themselves in a way which may be easier for them than verbal expression. The belief is that this process is not merely therapeutic in itself, but that if the inner meaning of the pictures or the models can be interpreted, it also aids diagnosis.

In Britain, art therapy is still a young profession. Courses for therapists (usually art graduates) were only introduced in the early 1970s and it was not until December 1981 that their organization, the British Association of Art Therapists, was at last admitted to the status of one of the Professions Supplementary to Medicine. Henceforth members will be in the paramedical category.

Origins

Among the forms of occupational therapy introduced into mental hospitals when they began to break out of the custodial "lunatic asylum" era, were simple drawing, colouring and modelling, such as a child might do at a nursery school. Freudian psychoanalysts then realized that their pictures and shapes could give useful clues to what was going on in the patients' unconscious minds, and began to encourage them to express themselves in this way. But the absence of any agreement among the psychiatrists on the basis for the interpretation of pictures has meant that it has been regarded mainly as a relatively easy and inexpensive way of keeping patients from boredom.

By-passing words

In the United States, however, Freudian teaching won greater acceptance than in other western countries, and art therapy has been extensively employed outside mental hospitals. According to its protagonist, Margaret Naumberg, it facilitates the treatment of mental and emotional disorders by allowing patients to express their dreams and fantasies as they see them, rather than have to put them into words. This, she believes, means that they are more likely to be able to evade what Freud described as "the censorship of the ego". The pictures also provide a record which can be monitored for progress, or to reveal where patients have contrived to forget or hide some unwelcome idea. Rapport between patients and the therapist, too, is facilitated because they can be encouraged to contribute to the interpretation of what they have drawn.

Procedure

At present, there can be little universally accepted procedure in art therapy: the discipline is too young and has not, as yet, established a theoretical framework from the variety of other disciplines that it draws upon: education, psychiatry, psychology, anthropology and the arts. Much more research is therefore needed to understand the ways in which art is of therapeutic benefit. Until that happens, the way into therapy can only rest with the inclinations and intuitions of the individual practitioner. For example, Benjamin Walker feels that to be effective "the patient must allow himself to drift into a kind of automatism, or free association with pen and brush, so that material from the unconscious has the chance to rise to the surface". The material which emerges may be straightforward, or it may be symbolic, requiring an experienced interpreter. As the interpretation is apt to vary according to the preconceptions of the therapist, it is likely to be different according to whether, say, a Freudian or a Jungian

Art therapy is a tremendous way for me to release and learn to understand my inner life. At the very beginning I used it simply to get out my rage at the world – scrubbing at the paper with brush or crayon in violent colours and movements . . . What a relief it is to get it on paper after all this time of damping it down with too much medication, and to discuss the meaning of each one of these pictures with my therapist . . .

Now I am calmer, more in control of myself, especially of my anger, not frightened to explore further – in fact, looking forward to seeing what comes up.

analysis is used. Still, whatever the type of analysis, it can help to uncover what your problems are.

Another therapist, however, might feel that helping a patient begin to observe and record, say, some object with the use of drawing will have effect by helping relate that patient to the outside world. Or that the use of a particular technique, such as the Creativity Mobilisation Technique developed by J.H. Schultz will be the best way in to therapy.

One of the leading practitioners of art therapy in Britain was Rita Page Barton, a psychoanalyst who trained under Jung in Zurich. "Art", she wrote in an article published shortly after her death in 1980, "can be of great value when applied diagnostically on the individual level". Paintings by patients, too, she believed, could often be put to therapeutic use: "the therapeutic value of the arts in eliciting the patients' own healing powers is constantly shown and never fails to be awe-inspiring".

Art therapy, Rita Barton found, often works through enabling a patient to take the first steps towards detachment, when more rational methods fail, by "exteriorization of the unconscious contents of the mind". How treatment proceeds from there depends upon the training and beliefs of the therapist and the needs of the individual patient.

Art therapy
Vera Diamond, art therapist, is seen here in action – demonstrating the tremendous release of emotional energy in this technique.

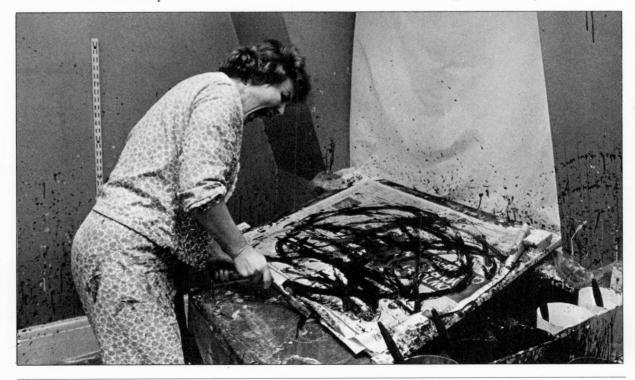

Facing our "inner monsters"

As an example, she cited a theme which often recurs, the painting of a monster. A patient may then paint over it, as if to blot it out from the mind, unless the therapist is quick to rescue it. "These 'rescued' monsters from whom we hide behind flowers, or pieties, or what you will, are most interesting and improve upon acquaintance", Rita Barton found. "They have value and significance, and tolerance of the monster on paper may well be the first step towards an inner reckoning with the dark side."

Suitable cases

"In the treatment of illnesses such as anorexia nervosa, alcoholism and drug addiction", an article in the then London *Times Health Supplement* has claimed, art therapy "has effected obvious lasting cures". But the writer admits that it is not possible to assess its value in objective terms, such as a statistical success rate, "apart from the difficulty of defining mental health and quantifying mental illness, there is the problem that the benefits of therapy are subjectively felt, but not always observable in clinical symptoms".

Anybody who suspects that some unidentified repressed conflict is the source of neurotic symptoms can experiment with art therapy as a means of tracking it down to its source. Some psychiatrists feel, however, that it is unwise to use it in cases of schizophrenia; it might reinforce the split in the personality.

Music therapy

Music therapy is based on a two-fold premise: that the ability to respond to music is innate in each one of us, and that this ability is not lost as a result of, and may indeed exist in spite of, physical or mental handicap, injury or psychological disorder.

In Britain, the music therapy profession is still in its infancy, and only about 60 trained therapists (with qualifications recognized by government departments) are practising within the public health service at present.

Origins

In tribal communities, music and dancing were employed to induce fits, the aim being to help sick members of the tribe to literally shake off their ills, both physical and psychic. Our literary heritage is full of references to the power of music. In the "Book of Samuel" in the *Bible*, for example, there is a description of how

❛ Music is therapy and has always been so . . . But only in our own very methodical and ailing world have we rediscovered the techniques, the specific means of applying music to the rehabilitation of (people) suffering from any of the crippling affections which prevent them from leading a normal, active life. ❜

Yehudi Menuhin

when an evil spirit possessed Saul, the young David played to him on a harp. Saul was refreshed, "and the evil spirit departed from him". And again, in Homer's *Odyssey*, when Ulysses was wounded during the seige of Troy, Autolycus sang a magic melody to staunch the flow of blood.

Like so many other early forms of therapy, however, music lost its hold during the era of the great plagues, when it was resorted to in desperation as a preventative, with predictable lack of success. An attempt was made to revive it during the eighteenth century by Richard Brocklesby, one of Samuel Johnson's doctors, who argued that in view of the failure of other methods of treating insanity, the ancient practice of employing music, "which was attended with such surprising and salutary effects", would be worth reviving. But when J.G. Millingen published his *Curiosities of Medical Experience* in 1839, music was among them – a joke. Discarded as a therapy, for the next 100 years music was seen as little more than a standard way of quietening babies.

In *Wer Heilt hat recht* published in 1958, Heinz Graupner (one of the earliest European writers to attempt to rescue alternative

Working with mentally-handicapped children
The little boy, below left, has Lowe's syndrome and is unable to talk. He is, however, very musical and can be seen here listening intently to the music played by the therapist. After several months work with music therapy his vocal sounds and pre-speech babbling are increasing. The teenage girl, below, is severely retarded and only partially sighted but she can become completely absorbed when working with the therapist. Here she is singing while she plays the Greek bells; notice her pleasure and involvement.

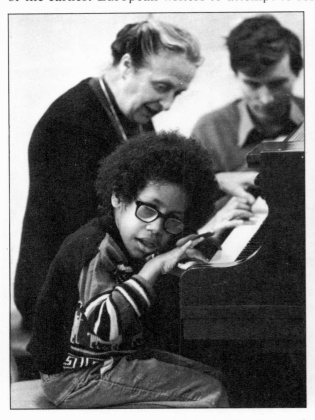

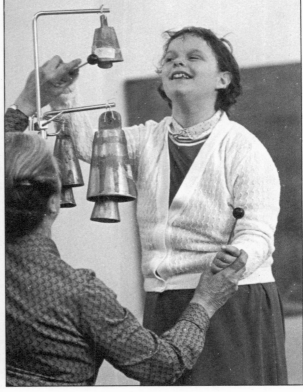

therapies from the discredit into which they had fallen) stated that some of the credit for the revival of music therapy should go to the Schüssler Sanatorium in the Hartz mountains. The doctors there had been using Schultz's *Autogenic training* (see pages 178 to 181), but found that for some patients it was not enough. When music sessions were suggested, they were at first "rather chary of the notion, but when they began to see what they could achieve with the help of music, they included it in their daily schedule of treatment. Today, they speak of the amazing results which have been obtained".

Procedure

Although the aim of music therapy is clear: to achieve an interaction between patient and therapist that can lead to a therapeutic outcome, the actual procedures followed will vary according to the training and individual experience of the therapist. A broad division may be drawn between therapy based upon responding to music, whether through singing, dancing, imaging or just quietly listening, and that which emphasizes teaching the patient how to make and improvise his or her own music. The purpose here is to develop nonverbal skills of communication and creative expression, an approach which has been found to be particularly helpful for the mentally and emotionally disabled.

Suitable cases

Music therapy can be used in a variety of settings for a variety of people – from geriatric wards, institutions for the mentally ill and community centres, to groups or individuals in private psychotherapy sessions. Its application to the problems of severely handicapped children can cover those that are mentally retarded, physically disabled, emotionally disturbed, autistic or suffering with speech difficulties.

PSYCHOLOGICAL THERAPIES

For convenience, psychological therapies are commonly divided into four categories: *Psychotherapies; Behavioral therapies*; *Humanistic psychologies* and *Transpersonal psychologies*.

Abraham Maslow, President of the American Psychological Association from 1967–8, describes them in a paper he wrote at the time: "First is the behavioristic, objectivistic, mechanistic, positivistic group. Second is the whole cluster of psychologies that originated in Freud and in psychoanalysis. And third there are the humanistic psychologies or 'third force', as this group has been called, a coalescence into a single philosophy of various splinter groups in psychology". The third group, Maslow insisted, included the first and second. And, he added "as a matter of fact I am developing what might be called a fourth psychology of transcendence as well".

Although it is convenient to have these four categories, in practice the therapies cannot easily be kept in separate compartments. A man who describes himself as a psychotherapist may adopt some behavioral techniques, as well as some from humanistic psychology, and some from transpersonal psychology. Individual therapies often straddle the boundaries, or while originating in one camp, later begin to spread out into another.

There is a further source of confusion, particularly for a work of this kind which is primarily intended to provide a survey of therapies not ordinarily available from the medical profession and its associated organizations. Many of the psychologists who provide the services listed in these four groups of psychological therapies do not think of themselves as practitioners of alternative medicine. The fact remains, however, that the therapies have tended to develop beyond the territory of orthodox medicine.

Letter from a clinical psychologist

"Psychologists are, and always have been, a profession independent of medicine. . . . Clinical psychologists have practised psychotherapy since psychotherapy first came into being. Rogerian psychotherapy was the brainchild of a psychologist – not a psychiatrist. Behavioral psychotherapy is . . . based entirely on psychological principles – not medical. Freud, the ultimate authority, argues cogently in *Essays on Psychoanalysis*, that a medical training is not only unnecessary for the practice of psychotherapy but also that, in some ways, it could be a positive disadvantage in successful practice. . ."

From E.L.R. MacPherson, Principal clinical psychologist, Inverness, to the journal *World Medicine*.

PSYCHOTHERAPIES

The term "psychotherapy" can be used in many senses: narrowly, to describe a type of therapy initially derived from the work of Sigmund Freud; broadly, to take in almost any type of therapy which relies for its effects on the ability of the mind to sort our physical, as well as mental and emotional problems, and by so doing to promote health and remove symptoms. Here, we have grouped in this category those therapies which have a common source in eighteenth-century mesmerism and nineteenth-century hypnotism. The first is "psychotherapy" in the narrower sense of the term.

Psychotherapy

Psychotherapy can be defined as being the treatment of the mind, or rather the psyche, by psychological means. According to Boris Semeonoff of the Department of Psychology at the University of Edinburgh in his introduction to a series of books on the subject, psychotherapy is commonly understood to be a process "whereby a patient is helped to understand and, ideally, to solve his problems through talking them over with a 'doctor'". Such treatment normally involves a personality change and puts a great deal of pressure on the emotions of both patient and therapist.

Nowadays, it is often equated, at least by the lay person, with psychoanalysis. But what really distinguishes psychoanalysis from less structured forms of psychological therapy is its contention that patients are unlikely to be aware of the basic nature of their problem, so that any "talking over" takes on a special character.

Origins

It was Sigmund Freud who gave psychotherapy its special character. Following visits to France towards the turn of the century in order to gain experience in hypnosis, among other things, he began to use it for the indirect treatment of symptoms by exploring the recesses of his patients' unconscious minds. Under hypnosis, he found, they could recall traumatic episodes which they had "repressed" – blotted out entirely from their conscious memories. These "repressions", Freud realized, were often the source of neurotic symptoms. It was as if the buried toxic material was leaking to the surface, manifesting itself in symptoms ranging from facial tics to formidable obsessions. By bringing the repressed material to the surface of consciousness, Freud found, the pent-up feelings connected with it could be released and the symptoms would disappear.

' I've been in therapy since 1964. I've had lots of shrinks. I've felt great greyness in my life, long bouts of depressions, and the feeling I wasn't driving my own train. I know it's viewed with a lot of scepticism, but therapy is very important. I've met some very helpful, insightful people through it. It's always a joke in England, or considered a rich man's pastime. But group therapy is cheap and most useful. I love the American attitude to psychology, its everydayness. In the past few years I've come out into realistic sanity. For me, therapy is the most important thing in life. It has made my professional life blossom, I can use what I have learnt. '

Dudley Moore
(from an interview in the *Sunday Times Magazine* 13 December 1981)

Freud's analytic method

Freud also found, however, that hypnosis was not a satisfactory way to bring the repressions to the surface. It was as if the patients needed to come to terms with the repressed material themselves, rather than have it extracted by the hypnotist, like a lanced abscess. As a result, he developed his analytic method in which the patients bring themselves back to the traumatic repressed episodes. This method is still used by analysts in the Freudian tradition and, modified, in the tradition of C.G. Jung, who developed his own brand of analytical psychology after his break with Freud.

Freudian and Jungian analyses, however, are sufficiently well established (though not always highly regarded) within the medical profession not to be considered as alternative psychological therapies. Psychotherapy, as it is most commonly given, is a rather different matter, however. It has developed as an abbreviated version chiefly because analysis is so time-consuming and so expensive. Since, theoretically, it is also available on public health schemes both in mental hospitals and, to a limited degree, from psychiatric social workers, psychotherapy is not, strictly speaking, in the alternative camp.

Nevertheless, practitioners who style themselves as psychotherapists and who have no medical qualifications have some justification when they say that they owe their existence to the fact that members of the public often cannot obtain psychotherapy without paying for it, whether from psychologists or from psychiatrists. The average GP has no time to offer it (even if trained to provide it, which is unlikely, except in very rudimentary ways). As a rule, when a doctor has patients whom he or she feels need psychotherapy, they will be sent to a psychiatrist.

Psychiatrists rarely recommend psychotherapy; they are more likely to prescribe drugs for the less serious cases, and admission to a mental hospital for the more serious. People who have wanted to try psychotherapy consequently have to shop around, and psychotherapists who are not medically qualified are usually less expensive to consult than those with qualifications.

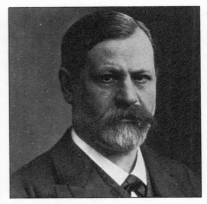

Sigmund Freud
Freud (1856–1939), the father of psychoanalysis, the forerunner of psychotherapy. Psychotherapy has made radical changes not least that of promoting a close relationship between therapist and patient.

Procedure

The mind's eye picture of psychotherapy is still drawn from the procedure which Freud used, and his followers adopted. The patient lies on a couch, with the psychoanalyst just out of sight behind the head, and in this position talks for an hour, five days a week, for two or three years. These days, the tendency has been for the number of sessions a week to be reduced, and the number of years to be increased. Five-year analysis is now common, 10 years is not unusual, and a few people, if they can afford it, settle for it for life.

Outside formal psychoanalysis, though, psychotherapy is a more pragmatic affair. You are less likely to be directed to a couch – the psychotherapist will probably sit facing you – and, departing from the strict Freudian tradition, he or she is likely to intervene more to direct your thoughts, help with interpretation of dreams, perhaps to encourage you to express your feelings, and even to offer you a shoulder to weep on.

To Freud, the idea of such contact was anathema. But increasingly over the past few years even some of his formerly dedicated disciples have been coming to the conclusion that this was his own hang-up, and that better results are achieved if the therapist can achieve rapport with subjects by direct touch, as well as through verbal interaction.

Regular weekly sessions

How the sessions are conducted depends so much on the training, development and whims of the psychotherapist that it has become impossible to present a simple picture of what you can expect. But most practitioners hold to the "50-minute hour" (the final 10 minutes are for writing up their notes, having a cup of coffee, and so on), once, twice or three times a week, according to your need and your ability to pay. The sessions continue until you feel either that they are no longer productive, or that you do not need to attend them any more.

Research ·

As its results depend so greatly on the degree of rapport established between therapist and patient – a highly subjective matter – research designed to find out how effective psychotherapy is has not proved easy. Some trials have been set up in mental hospitals to compare, say, psychotherapy with *Behaviour therapy* (see pages 196 to 197), by dividing the patients into two groups and allotting them at random to one or the other. But as they take no account of the quality of the therapy or the ability of the therapists, such trials give only some indication of the effectiveness of the psychotherapy in particular clinics.

Suitable cases

"Who should receive psychotherapy?" Professor Ian Stevenson of the University of Virginia asked in an article in 1954, when it was just beginning to dawn on the medical profession that the psychosomatic theory of disease could no longer be dismissed as a passing fad. "Since everyone's illness contains an emotional component, every sick person needs some psychotherapy. And it should be dispensed according to the size of the emotional contribution to the disability".

The person best placed to dispense it, Stevenson realized, should be the general practitioner, who is in a position to provide minor psychotherapy much as he or she can provide minor surgery by lancing a boil, for example. But Stevenson's hope that doctors would become better equipped to perform this function has not been fulfilled.

Self-help

This should be indicated by the psychotherapist. But a useful beginning is to get hold of a copy of Dr Anthony Storr's book *The Art of Psychotherapy* which, though conservative in approach and dealing only with "straight" psychotherapy is a very sound and balanced survey of the subject.

Hypnotherapy

Antonia Carr, a practising hypnotherapist, has described her technique as "psychotherapy using hypnosis as a tool". But nobody has yet succeeded in providing a generally acceptable definition of the state which is described as "hypnosis". It is commonly described as an altered state of consciousness, similar in many ways to the condition known as somnambulism.

Somnambulists are in a condition somewhere between being asleep and being awake. They are not consciously aware of their surroundings, yet unconsciously they must be, as they avoid obstacles and often perform certain tasks as if in full possession of their faculties. Hypnosis differs from somnambulism chiefly in that it is usually induced by a hypnotist (self-hypnosis is a technique which may be taught by a hypnotist) and in the fact that the control to a large extent passes to the hypnotist. It is as if hypnotized subjects hand over responsibility for their actions, and to some extent their thoughts, to the hypnotist, who uses this power for therapeutic purposes.

Inducing a trance state

At the outset, however, it needs to be said that a trance state can sometimes be induced without hypnosis, i.e., without deliberately inducing it. In this it is similar to mediumship, where the trance may be either induced or come spontaneously. An interesting attempt to account for hypnosis has been put forward by the distinguished Australian psychiatrist Ainslie Meares. He regards it as atavistic regression, that is, a return to the state of nature when instinct was allowed more scope than it is in our consciousness-dominated society. Meares relates the hypnotic trance to the condition which the yogis seek, and which can be the outcome of other practices such as *Visualization therapy* and *Transcendental meditation* (see pages 184 to 186), in which the psyche's own recuperative powers are liberated (see also *Yoga*, pages 138 to 144 and *Meditation*, pages 182 to 188).

Origins

There are many travellers' tales about tribal shamans which suggest that they must have exploited hypnotic powers, and there is also some evidence that hypnosis was employed by the priest/therapists in the temples of Aesculapius in ancient Greece.

Mesmer's "animal magnetism"

The first clear case of the use of hypnotherapy of the kind commonly practised today was described less than two centuries ago. It was a spin-off from "animal magnetism", a healing method invented by Franz Mesmer in the late eighteenth century. Although mesmerism and hypnotism have often been used as if they were loosely interchangeable terms, Mesmer's therapy bore a closer resemblance, to healing as practised by shamans and by the "strokers" (see *Hand healing*, pages 241 to 254). He would often demonstrate that he could control patients' movements simply by his gestures, but he appears to have done this chiefly to show the way in which "animal magnetism" was transmitted to them through him. The aim of Mesmer's treatment was to induce in his patients a loss of control of mind and body, with convulsions, dissociation and catatonic states.

Hypnosis and pain relief

Mesmer's followers soon found another feature of the induced trance state. If it were suggested to the subject that he or she would feel no pain, no pain would be felt. By the 1820s, they were giving demonstrations of these techniques, and working with medical practitioners for purposes of treatment of patients. A "magnetizer" would put patients into a trance (following assurances that they would feel no pain), enabling the surgeon to perform operations while the patients lay quietly, feeling nothing. The medical establishment, however, refused to believe it was genuine. Even when such operations were performed in front of doctors, to try to prove they were genuine, the explanation was that the patient must have been trained (and paid) to pretend he or she felt no pain. Animal magnetism, the surgeons argued, was spurious – a superstition. So how could its painkilling properties be genuine?

In the 1840s the Scots surgeon, James Braid, investigating mesmerism from the standpoint of a sceptic, came to the conclusion that it was not, after all, spurious – but that it was not

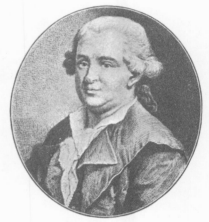

Franz Anton Mesmer
Mesmer (1734–1815), was an Austrian physician who developed animal magnetism or mesmerism, an early form of hypnotherapy.

animal magnetism which was responsible. Braid coined the term "hypnosis" to give the trance state a fresh start, with no occult links. It was a condition, he argued, of the nervous system, and the function of the hypnotist was simply to trigger it off.

Braid produced his explanation, however, just as ether, chloroform and other anesthetics were introduced in the United States, enabling surgeons to put animal magnetism out of their minds. "This Yankee dodge", Robert Liston crowed after the first British operation with the patient under an anesthetic had been conducted in 1846, "beats mesmerism hollow". For a time it looked as if the dispute had been settled, not by demonstration but by default. Whether or not there was such a thing as a state of hypnosis had ceased to matter.

The relief of pain, however, was not the only use to which hypnosis could be put. A French country doctor, A.A. Liébeault, more impressed by Braid's work than his compatriots had been, began to try it out in his practice near Nancy. He was able to gain experience by offering to treat his patients, most of them impoverished peasants, for nothing, if they allowed him to try "Braidism". So successful was he at removing their symptoms by simple suggestion under hypnosis that his results converted the initially suspicious Professor Hippolyte Bernheim, who introduced hypnosis as standard practice in his Nancy hospital.

At the same time Jean-Martin Charcot, who had established himself as a leading neurologist in Paris, was investigating hypnosis by trying it out on his hysteric patients from the Salpêtrière hospital. Early in the 1780s he managed to convince the deeply sceptical members of the Academy of Medicine that his patients really did go into trances, losing control of mind and body to the hypnotist.

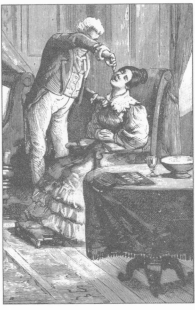

Hypnosis in dentistry
This drawing dating from 1836, shows a Doctor Oudet extracting a tooth from a woman while she remains in a hypnotic state, unconscious of the pain.

Organicism and after

Acceptance of hypnosis, however, came too late to ensure that hypnotherapy, as it now began occasionally to be called, would become part of a medical student's training. This was the era when the medical profession was beginning to accept the dogma that only organic disorders are "real". Hypnosis was assumed to be a form of induced hysteria, and although a committee despatched by the British Medical Association to observe Bernheim and Liébeault at work in Nancy reported back very favourably, its recommendations were ignored.

Freud began to hypnotize patients, following a spell working under Charcot, and a visit to Nancy. "I witnessed the moving spectacle of old Liébeault working among the poor women and children of the labouring classes", Freud was to recall. "I was a spectator of Bernheim's astonishing experiments upon his hospital patients". Both men profoundly impressed him. Later, however, Freud came to the conclusion that hypnosis only impeded satisfactory psychoanalysis, because patients did not themselves get through to the material repressed in their unconscious minds. Many of his followers still accept that judgment.

The decline of hypnotherapy

So it came about that hypnotherapy, accepted in the 1880s, went into a decline in the 1890s and by the turn of the century had all but disappeared from orthodox medicine. No one repudiated hypnosis any longer, no one denied the influence of suggestion on hypnotized patients. "People simply ceased to talk about them", the great French psychiatrist, Pierre Janet, who had done some of the most impressive research into the subject later recalled. Hypnotherapy came to be identified with quackery, practised by charlatans with no medical qualifications, who preyed on the gullible with the help of mumbo-jumbo.

The occult image persists

Hypnotherapy need no longer be an outcast today, but it has never quite shed its "occult" image, and although growing numbers of doctors use it, these numbers are still very small.

Regretting this, the *Lancet* has recently commented that as a consequence, the revival of medical interest in hypnotism "is likely to be parallelled by an increase in treatment by lay therapists". It urges that legislation is needed "if the public is to be protected from potentially dangerous non-medical hypnosis". If such protection is needed, it surely is the profession's own fault for its failure to incorporate hypnosis into conventional medicine. Having for a century dismissed hypnosis as bogus, and then for a further century almost ignored it, the profession's claim that only medically-qualified practitioners should be permitted to practise hypnosis – as some Members of Parliament have been arguing on the BMA's behalf – is yet another illustration of professional myopia at its silliest.

Procedure

Broadly speaking, there are two main types of hypnotherapy. In one, the kind practised by Liébeault, the hypnotist puts patients into a trance and suggests that their symptoms, physical or emotional, will disappear. In the other, they are put into a trance to facilitate whatever form of psychological treatment is being used – for example, to enable the therapist to explore what is going on in their subconscious minds.

Whichever type is to be used, the initial procedure is likely to be similar. It has been described recently in the *Journal of the Royal Society of Medicine* by J.B. Wilkinson. He is medically qualified, but hypnotherapists generally follow a similar course.

The initial session "involves the taking of a full history,

including questions designed to produce information about the patient's psychological state, especially with regard to anxiety and depression, and of the degree of motivation towards recovery" – and also as a check to ensure that some organic condition is not responsible for the symptoms, whatever they may be. If hypnotherapy is indicated, the therapist will give you a full description of what it will entail: "more treatment failures are due to lack of this than to any other cause, as misconceptions about hypnosis are common". Only if you have had previous experience of hypnotherapy, and require less of a briefing, is it likely that you will be put under hypnosis in this first session.

In the second session, hypnosis will be induced by whatever

Consulting a hypnotherapist

Hypnotherapists work in different ways but whatever their method the effectiveness of a course of hypnotherapy depends largely on your level of trust, receptivity, cooperation, and motivation. It is therefore vital to establish a good rapport between the two of you and to create a calm, relaxing atmosphere during sessions.

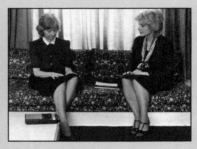

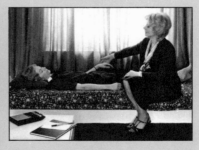

1 *At the first session, this therapist takes a case history and tries to discover any deeper causes for the patient's problem; if the patient has underlying fears of hypnosis, these are discussed and allayed.*

2 *She tests the patient to find out how she will respond to hypnosis. In a calm, quiet voice, she tells her that her eyes are becoming tired and closing, then asks her to concentrate on whichever hand she uses least.*

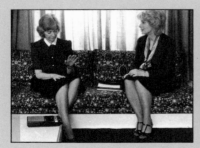

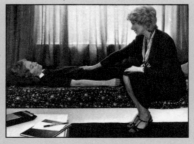

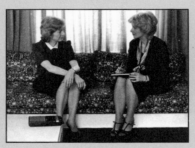

3 *Then the therapist suggests to the patient that the hand is getting lighter and rising up. If it does, the therapist knows that the patient will allow herself to be guided into a deeper state of relaxation.*

4 *On the second visit, the patient is asked to lie down, breathe deeply, and think of a time and place when she was relaxed happy. The therapist rests a hand on her stomach to relax and reassure her.*

5 *Before starting to work directly on the patient's problem, the therapist checks the depth of relaxation by lifting her arm. At the end of a session, she will either count or talk the patient out of the trance.*

method the hypnotherapist favours. In the one most commonly used, the patient sits opposite or close to the hypnotherapist, who slowly talks him or her into the trance state, sometimes using an object upon which the patient focuses his or her eyes. When it is felt that the time is ripe, the therapist can either begin to use direct suggestion to the effect that the symptoms are going to clear up, or he or she can begin to explore, with the help of probing questions, why the patient's health problems have arisen.

Wilkinson regards the main purpose of hypnotherapy as assisting relaxation and lessening tension, giving increased confidence and ability to handle problems. To suggest while patients are under hypnosis that their symptoms will simply go away "tends to strain the patient's credulity", he finds, whereas if the level of tension can be lowered, the symptoms may disappear at the same time.

Direct and indirect suggestion

How long the sessions last, and how many are needed, depends on some obvious variables, notably the degree of rapport established between therapist and patient, which can affect how long it takes for patients to become entranced (ordinarily the first occasion is the difficult one; later the hypnotherapist may only have to snap his or her fingers to induce the trance). A minority of patients cannot be put into any trance at all. They remain in possession of their faculties, though they appear to come under the hypnotist's control to the extent of doing automatically what they are told to do; a few go into so deep a trance that, if they are told to, they will remember nothing of what transpires while they are in it.

Common fears about hypnosis

A question often asked by people contemplating trying hypnotherapy is whether it is "safe". Doubtless unscrupulous hypnotists could extract damaging secrets from their patients and use them for blackmail. There have been rumours of hypnotists using their control for sexual satisfaction. But patients are normally protected by the fact that the hypnotic trance is not an entirely stable condition. They may come out of it suddenly, into full awareness – particularly if the hypnotist asks them to do something they would not think of doing if they were awake.

The other common fear is of the mind being in some way tampered with by "post-hypnotic suggestion", which is quite commonly used in hypnotherapy. Patients are told while still in a trance that symptoms will disappear after they awake, and will not return. In theory a hypnotist could implant dangerous suggestions. Again, though, such malpractice would only need to be detected once to ruin the practitioner's entire career.

One other hazard is often brought up by those doctors who still disapprove of hypnotism: that when suggestion works, it works by suppressing the symptoms, and not by removing the causes. This argument would have more force if it were not so often presented by doctors who themselves prescribe drugs which suppress the symptoms without removing the causes – sedatives, tranquillizers, anti-inflammatory drugs, beta-blockers and the rest. All sensible hypnotherapists tell the patient that the removal of symptoms is likely to be temporary, and that other ways need to be looked for if they are not to return. The chief benefit of straight suggestion under hypnosis is simply the revelation of the power of the mind over the body. Once this is grasped, patients can take up whatever other kind of therapy appeals to them.

Research

A great deal of the research reported in the 1880s – the decade when interest in hypnosis was at its height – has been repeated in recent years, and certain facts about the power of suggestion under hypnosis are now well established. This does not, unfortunately, mean that treatment is ever 100 percent effective, as its effectiveness depends upon subjective factors, such as the degree of rapport and the depth of trance achieved. But it does mean that certain effects have been observed again and again in trials by researchers. Among the commonest are: the removal of warts; the healing of burns; pain and allergic symptoms relief.

Perhaps the most striking achievement of all in research into hypnotherapy has been an experiment conducted by Sydney Fogel and Charles R. Knight in Saskatoon, Canada, and reported in the *Canadian Medical Association Journal*. It is notoriously impossible to graft skin from one patient to another – the graft simply sloughs off. Fogel and Knight took some skin from a man and grafted it on to the body of a woman – not related to him, who had been hynotised and given the suggestion that the graft would "take". At the same time, as a control, her skin was grafted on to the man. In the man's case, the graft was rejected in a couple of weeks, as is normal. But the graft was still there on the woman, and apparently stable, after eight months.

Unluckily the experimenters were unable to repeat this success. As they admitted, it might have been the result of exceptional circumstances: the woman, for example, had suffered from schizophrenia, which has long been known to exercise anomalous influences on physical health. The fact that the graft "took" can nevertheless be regarded as an indication of hypnotherapy's as yet largely untapped potential.

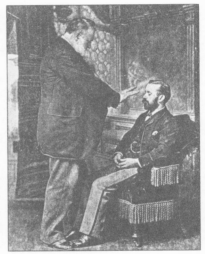

The magnetic pass
The hypnotist makes what was known in the last century as the magnetic pass over his patient's eyes, to produce or deepen the mesmeric state.

Suitable cases

Hynotherapy is most effective in dealing with disorders which in medical parlance have an "emotional overlay", and with psychosomatic and stress disorders – high blood pressure, asthma, migraine, insomnia and ulcers of the digestive tract. It is particularly valuable in helping to bring addiction – to cigarettes, alcohol, drugs, and to sugar – under control. Post-hypnotic suggestion cannot break addiction on its own. But it can help tide addicts over the difficult stage when craving is at its height. To be effective in such cases, though, requires cooperation of the patient and a strong underlying wish to "kick" the habit.

In his South London practice, Dr Ryde has found hypnotherapy most useful in cases where conventional treatment is notoriously least effective: "afflictions such as blushing, enuresis, phobias, insomnia, sexual upsets and problems with relationships, school, auditions, exams, work and nerves have received varying degrees of benefit, often from just one session".

Self-help

If your therapist considers that you could usefully learn auto-hypnosis during hypnotherapy sessions, "this simple technique can be used in nearly all cases of psychosomatic illness", Wilkinson claims in his *RSM Journal* article – particularly of asthma. The advantages are obvious, as self-hypnosis is less time-consuming, lessens dependence upon the therapist, "and lastly (and perhaps most importantly) it is a form of self-help which raises the morale and increases the confidence of the patient, which must surely be the aim of all treatment in this field". Self hypnosis should only be practised on the advice of a therapist.

Autosuggestion/couéism

Couéism, William A.R. Thomson observes in his *Faiths that Heal*, "deserves a chapter to itself – if only a short one": partly because "of the simplicity of his (Coué's) advice – 'technique' or 'system' is too strong a word; partly because of his innate goodness and charity that were never affected by the world-wide fame which he achieved".

Emile Coué is remembered now, where he is remembered at all, for the tag that won him world-wide fame: "Every day, in every way, I am getting better and better". But the philosophy behind it was, and is, extremely important – that all of us have largely untapped reserves of health-giving energy which can be liberated by the use of simple autosuggestion. Although practitioners of straightforward Couéism are not now often encountered, what he taught is incorporated in many psychological therapies, and is indeed one of their vital ingredients.

Origins

Working as an apothecary – midway between GP and chemist – in Provence, in the late nineteenth century, Coué became interested in the role of the mind in treatment when he analyzed a newly marketed patent medicine which had cured one of his patients of a long-standing disorder and found it was little more than coloured water. To study the subject further he went north to Nancy in the 1880s to observe Liébeault and Bernheim treating patients by hypnosis. From his observations he came to the conclusion that the decisive factor in hypnotism is not *hetero*-suggestion – what the hypnotist induces in the patients' minds – but *auto*-suggestion.

This did not run entirely counter to the theories about hypnotism. Cures, Charcot wrote, where they occur are engendered "by special disposition on the part of the patient; a confidence, a credulity, a receptivity to suggestion". But so far as the public was concerned, hypnotism owed its power to hetero-suggestion – because this was what it looked like in demonstrations, with the hypnotist bringing his subjects under his control, so that they obeyed his every whim.

The will to live

Coué did his best to turn this tide. What is vital for hypnotherapy, he argued, is what goes on in the mind of the patient. And here he added a new dimension: the importance of the imagination.

In the battle against illness, Coué claimed, far too much attention had been paid to the will, "the will to live", say, being considered all-important by those who still upheld the mind's power over the body. All too often, he protested, people who had the will to get better, feared in their imaginations that they were *not* going to get better, and, "when the will and the imagination are at war, the imagination *invariably* gains the day".

To illustrate this thesis, Coué would call attention to the fact that we cannot will our bodies to perform various desirable functions, but we can use the imagination to stimulate performance. For example, we cannot will ourselves to salivate, but we can make our mouths water by imagining a favourite dish.

Again and again, Coué reiterated this argument. "Above all, the will must not intervene in the practice of auto-suggestion", he wrote. "What we have to work for is the *education of the imagination*. It is thanks to this difference of method that I have often been able to attain success where others, persons of conspicuous ability, have failed".

How can we educate the imagination? Coué advocated adherence to the principles of *Yoga* (see pages 138 to 144): a search for concentration (though not of the kind usually associated with that term, as when we tell ourselves, I *will* concentrate on this, or that). The aim should be to clear the mind of all thoughts, and of

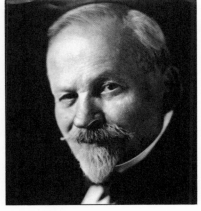

Émile Coué
As a way of helping people to heal themselves, Coué (1857–1926) advocated repeating the mantra: *"Every day, in every way, I am getting better and better."*

all concern about job prospects or family worries. To facilitate this process he suggested the use of sacred words – the "mantras" from Hindu teaching – to try to ensure that the mind remains "spontaneously immobilized".

Coué's mantra

It was for this purpose that Coué introduced *his* mantra, "every day, in every way, I am getting better and better". It would serve, he thought, as a combined operation for health, both as an incantation, to assist in the "spontaneous immobilization" process, and as a spur to the imagination, when it seeped through to the unconscious mind.

In one sense, it was an unfortunate choice of mantra. The great majority of people who picked it up on its spectacular journey through the world, in the 1920s, were not aware of the philosophy behind it, and many thought it was a way of helping them to consciously *will* themselves better – the very opposite of what Coué intended.

In all probability this mistaken belief contributed to Couéism's decline to little more than a music hall joke in the 1930s. But that decline was also hastened by the implacable hostility of the medical establishment. Doctors, ironically, were prepared to concede that the *will* could do something, even if very little, to assist recovery, or delay the end. But the idea that the *imagination* could exercise control over the nervous system, and in doing so prevent disease, was dismissed as fantasy.

Now that the power of the imagination and autosuggestion has been so conclusively demonstrated, the validity of Couéism has been reestablished, and there is no reason why his recommendations should not be adopted – provided that his mantra is recognized rightfully – an incantation rather than an exhortation.

Procedure

Couéists do not use any form of therapy, they simply help subjects to learn how to follow the master's advice. In these times you are more likely to find a teacher of *Autogenic training* (see pages 178 to 181), which incorporates Couéism (though not all of its teachers recognize this). But if you do come across a pure Couéist he or she is likely to recommend you to follow the advice of Coué's disciple Charles Baudouin, Professor at the Rousseau Institute, and author of *Suggestion and Auto-Suggestion*.

"Regularly, daily, without a single exception we must practise concentration in the morning and the evening. It must bear on the general and extremely simple formula (day by day, *in all respects*, I get better and better"). Each sitting will require a few minutes only. Through regular performance, it will become a confirmed habit, and its technique will be steadily perfected".

Suitable cases

Coué emphasized that the mantra was not designed for use to treat specific disorders; and Baudouin italicized "in all respects", as the translators of his book put it ("in every way" became the common English usage) to underline the importance of regarding symptoms as mere nuisances which will go away provided that the imagination recovers control.

Self-help

Charles Baudouin did, however, allow that autosuggestion can be used to help get rid of pain or worry: "Sit in a comfortable armchair, motionless, with the muscles relaxed and eyes closed. Localizing the suggestion, so to speak, the matter in question, we say (inaudibly if needs must, but at least making the appropriate movements of articulation with tongue and lips) these simple words, 'It is passing off', reiterating them rapidly until the trouble, if not cured, is at least sensibly relieved".

Again, as Coué used to insist, these words are an incantation, *not* a command. They must be repeated rapidly ("there is no harm in gabbling") because they are aimed at the imagination, not at the conscious mind, which may be dubious about the success of so apparently infantile a technique – much as "buying" a wart or treating it with dandelion juice may impress a child, but make a grown-up feel silly.

Physical movements of the hands can be used as an adjunct to this form of self-treatment. "Each time we utter the words, we shall do well to pass the hand rapidly over the affected part", Baudouin recommended. Whether or not the "magnetizers" were correct in their assumption that these "passes" transmitted a healing fluid, he pointed out, "they unquestionably aid the fixation, the materialization, of our thoughts". By their very monotony, too, these so-called passes also tend to promote autohypnosis.

Silva mind control

This meditation technique is designed to exploit what is known about brain-waves as an aid to the development of greater mental discipline, so that the power of the mind can be used more effectively. It combines some of the elements of Coué-type *Autosuggestion* (see pages 173 to 176) with *Meditation* (see pages 182 to 188), but the emphasis here is on the need to expand intuition and extrasensory perception.

Origins

This type of meditation is the brainchild of José Silva, a Mexican-American who in spite of having no formal education, let alone qualifications, became an electronics engineer. Picking up some knowledge of psychology and hypnotism, Silva found the formula he needed to launch his "mind control" ideas when he surmised, from his work in electronics, that as the best electrical circuits are those which have the least resistance, the human brain as a receptor might be at its most effective at certain wavelengths. For a while, Silva experimented with hypnosis, but he found that although it improved receptivity, it blocked reasoning power. Silva has since concentrated on getting patients to think at the "alpha" level, a wavelength of ten cycles a second – the level associated with day-dreaming (see also *Biofeedback*, page 189).

"Mind control is dynamic meditation" Silva recently told Marie Herbert, author of *The Snow People*, in an interview published in the magazine, *Here's Health.* "By teaching you to think and analyze your problems at 10 cycles, using visualization and imagination, it enables you to draw on senses and faculties other than the five physical senses". Yoga, transcendental and other types of meditation go deeper, to five cycles, the "theta" level; and this can give control over the systems by which the body automatically regulates breathing, heartbeat and so on. At 10 cycles, "we can learn not only to control and regulate these same involuntary systems, but we gain control over our psychological systems also. Mind control, unlike any other meditative discipline, teaches you to have control over your mind. . . ."

Procedure

In an appendix to his book the *Silva Mind Control Method*, José Silva gives an outline of his standard four-day course. Day One gives students an opportunity, after an introductory lecture, to practise entering the "alpha" level of meditation (and past it, to "theta", to notice the difference). On Day Two, the students learn how to apply his dynamic meditation, with exercises similar to those of *Autogenic training* (see pages 178 to 181). Day Three carries the students on to exercises designed to develop their intuition and perception. The faculty for extrasensory perception, by which Silva sets great store, is worked on in particular to see if the students can project themselves to other places, or backward and forward in time. And on Day Four, they are given detailed instructions on how to progress on their own, or preferably in groups, now that they have realized "at first doubtfully, then with growing assurance, and finally with an exhilarating realization, that they have been successfully trained to call on Higher Intelligence and function psychically whenever they wish".

Suitable cases

So far as Silva and his disciples are concerned, anybody and everybody can be expected to benefit from a course on his method. But two psychiatrists in Philadelphia have explored the possibility that it might be dangerous for people who are emotionally unstable. Their findings are given in an appendix in Silva's book. Of 75 patients who took the course at different times, they reported, only one became more disturbed; the others all benefited to some degree, a few of them markedly. "There was a greater relaxation and lessening of anxiety. Patients learned to rely on their own inner resources to understand, cope with and solve problems, and being able to do so gave them more self-confidence".

Autogenic training

Autogenic training is first cousin to Couéism. Both had the same original source, hypnotism, and both developed into *Autosuggestion* (see pages 173 to 176). To quote Dr Malcolm Carruthers, who brought autogenics to Britain from Canada in the 1970s, it consists of "a series of easy mental exercises designed to switch off the stress 'fight or flight' system of the body, and switch on the rest, relaxation and recreation system".

Recognizing the fight or flight response

The importance of acknowledging, and learning how to handle, the instinctive "fight or flight" response was lucidly explained by Dr A.T.W. Simeons in his book *Man's Presumptuous Brain.* Prehistoric people met emergencies with the help of a number of automatic reactions. Their hearts beat faster, their appetites disappeared, their bowels prepared to evacuate themselves, and so on, in readiness either for a struggle, or for running away. Today, civilized people still have these reactions, but they often cannot work them out of their systems by either fighting them or escaping from them.

Where the source of the tension is in the unconscious mind, a person may be unaware of the reasons for his or her physical reactions, attributing them to illness. "The once appropriate clenching of his back muscles which have to hold him erect while running he calls lumbago. The increased heartbeat becomes palpitation, the rise in blood pressure he notices as headache, the sudden elimination of waste matter he calls diarrhea or a urinary disorder, and so forth".

Dealing with stress reactions

It is not always possible to avoid this type of reaction, and it is sometimes difficult even to recognize it for what it is. The purpose of autogenics is to provide a simple way to deal with it through – as Carruthers describes them – "gentle exercises in body awareness and physical relaxation", designed to induce a state of "passive concentration" – the same state that Coué's incantation promoted. The ability to do this at will "breaks through the vicious circle of excessive stress, whatever the origins".

The term "autogenic" (generated from within) refers to two aspects of the process. First, the basic shift from the stressed state in which most people now live, to a specific, restorative, healing "autogenic state", similar in some ways to that of being under hypnosis, which is designed to move the body "from a state of war to one of peace". And second, the active participation of each individual involved, provided he or she is regarded as suitable for the training. "Given the basic techniques and a degree of advice and encouragement, the trainee can proceed safely to apply the method for himself and make it part of a health-promoting lifestyle".

Origins

At around the same time as Coué was developing his theory and practice of autosuggestion early this century, Johannes Schultz, a Berlin neurologist, was proceeding along an almost parallel track. Schultz had read about yoga, and had studied hypnosis; putting the two together, he came to much the same conclusion as Coué, giving autohypnosis the credit for the results of *Hypnotherapy* (see pages 166 to 173).

At this point, however, Schultz took a different course from Coué, and began to develop a method of training the mind to influence the body by exercises. He knew that under hypnosis, it was easy to persuade patients that their limbs felt heavy, or that their fingers were warm. And he surmised that if patients could learn to put themselves into the auto-hypnotic state, they could bring about the same impressions in themselves. At the simplest level, this would be a way of warming up the tips of the fingers on a cold day. But it could also represent the start of a voyage of discovery through the range of mind-control of the kind that yogis practise, but adapted to western needs – and limitations.

The incantations Schultz taught had some similarity to Coué's, but they were more specific: "My right arm is heavy"; "my left arm is warm", and so on. Schultz's method, however, did not begin to establish itself in the public eye until one of his disciples, Wolfgang Luthe, working in Montreal, described "autogenic training" in books, and provided courses for those who wanted to learn the method.

Procedure

For simplicity, Carruthers likens autogenic training to learning to drive a car. There is a starting procedure – getting into a comfortable position, banishing distractions. There are gear changes – moving from bottom (the state of mind we tend to be in during a working day) to top ("passive concentration"). And there is a stopping procedure – preparatory to returning to worrying about job or family or whatever it may be.

Again as with Couéism, autogenics can be done anywhere, at any time: in bed or in the bath; sitting up or lying down. It can be self-taught, though most people take an eight-week course, one

Learning autogenics

Before embarking on a course you will be screened for physical and psychological suitablity Then you will be taught the three best postures for autogenics – sitting on a comfortable or an upright chair, or lying on your back. The training itself consists of six

basic exercises; you will for example, be asked to imagine that your arms are heavy or that your forehead is cool and to repeat the instruction to yourself three times. Learning how to come out of a practice session properly is also very important.

Sitting in an upright chair
In order to carry out the exercises in an upright chair, sit bolt upright and imagine you are being pulled up. Then flop forward on to your knees and carry out the exercises. Finally stretch up in the usual way to come out of the sequence.

Coming out of a session
After each sequence of exercises (left), first open your eyes, clench your fists and bend your arms (below left), then, stretch your arms up and give a big yawn.

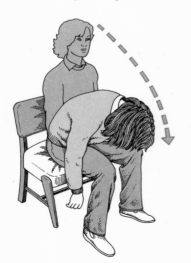

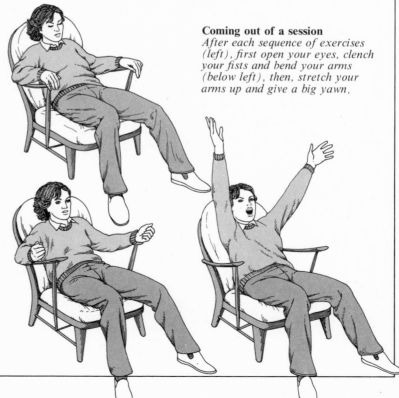

hour a week of instruction and exercises three times a day, eventually learning, in effect, to put themselves into a state of deep relaxation. To aid the process, visualization is used of the kind described in the section on *Meditation*, in connection with the work of the Simontons and Ainslie Meares (see pages 184 to 186) It sounds ridiculously simple, but acquiring the art of passive concentration is not so easy – and when it has been acquired, it can give quite a shock to a system unused to being instructed in this manner.

A few people experience startling reactions during autogenic training – abreactions, as they are usually described. It is as if barriers which have been put up to suppress or repress emotions are suddenly removed, releasing them in the form, say, of tears, or laughter, or a mixture of the two; sometimes of pain.

Suitable cases

Hundreds of research papers have been published on and around autogenics and there is no longer any doubt about its effectiveness as a technique for promoting relaxation, and thereby getting rid of, or relieving, stress disorders. How useful it is, though, must depend on the individual. Inevitably it works better for some people; only by trying it can its effectiveness be judged.

In a note *Applications of Autogenics*, The London Centre for Autogenic Training lists some of the commoner stress-related disorders for which it has been found effective: "It can relieve tiredness and insomnia, lessen anxiety and examination nerves, and reduce circulatory disturbances, including migraine, high blood pressure and the effects of stress on the heart. Many 'diseases' of psychosomatic origin can be corrected by sustained practice of autogenic training, including being overweight or asthmatic, having skin problems, nervous sweating, disturbances of gastro-intestinal functions, speech disorders, writer's cramp and some allergies".

"Autogenic training can help people who have problems with alcohol or tobacco, feelings of depression, inferiority, hostility or tension. Gynecological problems respond including pre-menstrual tension, and menopausal difficulties. Autogenic training has been shown to reduce dependency on anti-depressants, tranquillizers, sleeping tablets, blood-pressure-lowering drugs and medication of all kinds".

Self-help

The chief need is to learn and master the basic exercises, practising, if possible, two or three times each day, as indicated below. Then, if wished, it may be possible to learn techniques for dealing with specific disorders.

Meditation

Meditation cannot be fitted neatly into the psychotherapy category, as it owes some of its initial acceptance in the West to research conducted by behaviourists, and is incorporated in both humanistic and transpersonal psychologies: it straddles our four categories of psychological therapy. Meditation techniques have also begun to take a prominent place in those physical therapies where relaxation is considered desirable. But when employed as a means to reach an altered level of consciousness, meditation has obvious links with nineteenth-century *Mesmerism* and *Hypnotism* (see pages 166 to 173), and it is very much a part of *Auto-suggestion/couéism* and *Autogenic training* (see pages 173 to 181).

In a sense meditation is a misleading term, as in its common colloquial sense it implies thinking about a problem, whereas in its therapeutic role the aim is to bring the mind under control and focus it in such a way that, as the Friends of the Healing Research Trust pamphlet puts it, "one frees it from its enslavement to discursive thoughts with their attendant feelings, which together dissipate energy and cause stress and suffering".

Origins

In the Indian subcontinent and in many parts of Asia, meditation has been practised as far back as recorded history, and some tribal communities have similar practices which suggest that its origins may lie in the attempts of shamans and witch doctors to find ways to facilitate entry into the trance state for purposes of divination. Initially, the commonest method was to stare at some object until the imagination took flight, as it were, and began producing pictures, as in crystal-gazing. But at some stage "mantras" (sacred words which the meditator would try to concentrate on in order to get rid of intrusive thoughts) came into use.

The development of meditation techniques

In the East, the practice of meditation developed into *Yoga* (see pages 138 to 144) and became the central feature of the yogi's way of life. In the West, however, it took a different turn: prayer. Although in Christian communities prayer was, and in some religious orders still is, a form of meditation, it gradually ceased to be a way of abstracting the self from conscious thought, and became instead a way of communicating with God, or Jesus, or Mary, to confess sins and plead for forgiveness (an exception is the "Jesus prayer" in the Russian Orthodox tradition). And although a few individuals in the West practised meditation techniques derived from the Buddhist model, they did not begin to attract more general interest until the advent of the Maharishi Mahesh Yogi and transcendental meditation (T.M.). His mantra technique has been the most successful form of meditation to come to the West in recent years. He became famous almost overnight when, in the 1960s, his crusade took root in Europe and America, for a time scooping up the Beatles, among other well-known personalities. T.M. played an important role in establishing meditation as a form of therapy, because it was trials with its devotees that convinced Professor Herbert Benson and his colleagues at Harvard of its value, as he was to describe in his best-selling book *The Relaxation Response*. Since then, meditation has been incorporated into treatments of many kinds, so that patients may find it recommended as an adjunct to physical therapies like say, osteopathy or acupuncture, as well as to any of the psychological and psychic ones.

The goal of meditation

In his book *How to Meditate*, the New York psychologist Lawrence LeShan points out that there are now many schools of thought holding different and even apparently contradictory views about the goal of meditation, and still more, about the right paths to it. He lists four main paths: *through the intellect* – the assumption being that knowledge and wisdom can be developed through meditation to the point of transcendence; *through the emotions* – as in the Christian "God is love" concept (and in some cult teachings); *through the body*, in exercises such as those offered by the teachers of *Hatha yoga* and *T'ai chi* (see pages 138 to 147); and *through action*, as in the developments from the martial arts such as *Aikido* (see pages 147 to 149).

There are also techniques of meditation designed for specific diseases, and two of them, visualization therapy and intensive

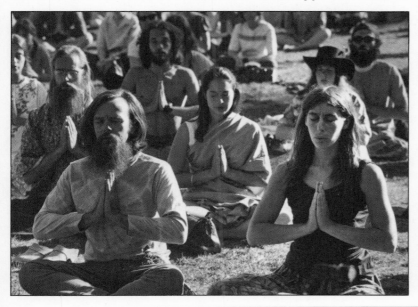

The meditation boom
In the Sixties and Seventies, meditation became immensely popular. "Earth Rebirth", a spiritual festival at the University of California was one of many such events. Here, festival participants are practising meditation under the tutelage of Swami Satchidanarnda.

meditation, directed to cancer patients, have attracted interest even in orthodox medical circles, though they have not as yet been accepted by cancer specialists.

Visualization therapy

Carl Simonton, a doctor practising radiotherapy at Fort Worth, Texas, became impressed by the accumulation of evidence that cancer is related to personality – the more so because he himself had had cancer as a young man, and looking back, realized that he had fitted into the category of people who "bottle-up" emotions, and whose cancers are often precipitated by some stressful event. It was not the event itself, Simonton now felt sure, that was the precipitant of the disease, so much as the individual's reaction to it. Although he continued to use radiation to try to destroy established cancers, he began to train patients to use the power of their own imaginations to restore health.

Treatment for cancer

He has described the method he evolved as relaxation and mental imagery – a variant of autosuggestion. In his own words, "In the regular sessions with a patient I ask the patient to practise simple muscle relaxation, focusing on breathing. Then I have him mentally picture his cancer – picturing it the way it seems to him – and the way he views the treatment, how he sees the body and body-cells operating against the malignancy, and so on. I try to get him to produce mental descriptions of all aspects of the disease. Through these techniques, the patient begins to activate his motivation to be well and to arouse emotions and problems into consciousness".

Simonton's first patient simply visualized healthy cells attacking and overcoming the cancer cells, with immediately striking results. Subsequently he encouraged patients to visualize whatever kind of conquest would most appeal to them – a football fan, for example, might be encouraged to think of the cancer cells as an opposing team.

Simonton kept records to compare how those patients fared who elected to try visualization therapy with those who did not. These showed that the survival time of the visualizers was, on balance, about twice as long; in a few cases, their cancers ceased to spread, and they could return to active life.

Visualization therapy has since been carried on by his wife Stephanie, and taken up by other doctors, notably Bernard Siegel, an assistant professor of surgery at Yale University Medical School. In his practice, Siegel tries to draw out the intuitive or clairvoyant element in dreams from his patients with the help of a variety of techniques. One way is to have them draw pictures which, he finds, are often unconsciously revealing of what is the matter with them.

The will to live

One cancer patient in five, Dr Siegel has found, does not really *want* to live. About half the patients would like to be cured – but they think in negative terms of simply looking for something, or somebody, to cure them. The remainder say, in effect, "I'll do anything I have to do to get well: just show me". It is with these "exceptional cancer patients", as he describes them, that he gets results. As he put it in a recent interview in the journal *New Age*: "We all have the ability to heal ourselves. Our brains know, but we've forgotten on an intellectual level. On the primitive level we still know . . . but on the intellectual level we don't know how to take charge and control the healing process".

Intensive meditation

A type of meditation introduced by the psychiatrist Ainslie Meares in Melbourne, Australia, is derived from his theory of "atavistic regression", which in turn derives from his early work in hypnosis. The hypnotic state, Meares came to believe from his research, represents a throwback to the state of mind which existed long before the development of reason. It can be valuable in therapy, he decided, because before the development of reason, people, like animals, relied on instinct for health guidance. Instinct worked very well – then, much better than reason does now, in fact. Similarly, under deep hypnosis some people can actually diagnose what is the matter with them and prescribe for it, though they may have no knowledge of medicine.

Atavistic regression

Yoga-type exercises and meditation, Meares decided, could also be used to induce "atavistic regression", particularly for the treatment of cancer. Removing patients' immediate worries and fears, he has argued in an article in *The Practitioner*, has the effect of liberating instinct to do its work. "If the reduction of anxiety is sufficiently profound and sufficiently sustained, there will come about a state of affairs in which the host's capacity to cope with cancer cells is significantly enhanced".

The techniques of meditation which Meares uses differ from the standard yoga procedures in that he does not ask his patients to contemplate some particular idea, because he feels this interferes with his aim. He wants to eliminate conscious activity. Patients adopt a posture which initially involves some slight discomfort, but as they relax the discomfort is transcended, so that they have nothing to distract them from achieving the aim of a totally empty mind – emptied, that is, of everyday distractions.

Removing the fear of dying

This form of therapy, Meares emphasizes, is not designed to *cure* cancer. Most of the patients who come to him have been warned that they have only a short time to live and that nothing more can be done for them. Often in his experience cancer is simply the way by which their lives are being terminated – "there is a time for living and a time for dying". For such people the treatment is mainly designed to remove the fear of dying. If they can come for treatment often enough to acquire the technique of losing themselves in meditation, he has found, nearly all of them can achieve a significant reduction of depression "together with much less anxiety and pain". But a few patients actually recover.

Procedure

Each of these paths to meditation may be incorporated, to some extent, in others. The most straightforward way to learn about meditation is to join a local group, preferably on the recommendation of friends. If you are going to a meditation group for the first time, particularly if it is for therapeutic purposes, you are most likely to start off with the mantra method, or a technique of concentrating on breathing – counting the breaths taken, visualizing and "feeling" them.

These are no more than expedients to enable you to learn to abstract yourself from your ordinary level of consciousness. And as LeShan emphasizes, the particular method you happen to encounter first may not be right for you. "Most schools tend to believe that there is one right way to meditate for everyone and, by a curious coincidence, it happens to be the one they use", he complains. But it is obviously stupid "to give the same meditational programme to two individuals differing widely in the development of the intellectual, emotional and sensory systems and in the relationship of these systems to each other".

Transcendental Meditation

The initial training provided by the disciples of the Maharishi Mahesh Yogi is straightforward and surprisingly simple. It is commonly taught in four hour-long lessons, on four successive days, the aim being to show students how to use their mantras or chants to achieve progressively quieter levels of thinking until a stage is reached when thought itself, in its everyday sense, is transcended. Simple though it sounds, exponents of transcendental meditation insist that this preliminary stage cannot be picked up from a manual of instruction because "the teacher must not only show the aspirant how to experience the subtle stages of thinking, but should also be responsible for checking his experience as he proceeds on that path".

Though it is possible to take the preliminary four-day courses at any of the centres which have been set up by the International Meditation Society without further commitment, T.M. has really developed into a cult. Even the initial course has cult overtones;

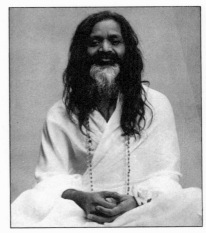

Maharishi Mahesh Yogi
Founder of the International Meditation Society, the Maharishi claims that T.M. can develop your creative intelligence, raise your level of consciousness, and enable you to make fuller use of your mental potential.

each student is given a mantra which he or she is told must be kept secret, and those students who do stay on to take further courses immediately immerse themselves in what is clearly not a straightforward therapy.

In *Freedom in Meditation*, Patricia Carrington, a clinical psychologist and lecturer in the Department of Physiology at Princeton University, surveyed some of the alternatives available to anybody who is contemplating taking up meditation; she includes her own. This is in some ways similar to T.M., but a simplified version, shedding some of the esoteric side: you can choose your own mantra and learn enough in a couple of lessons to be able to continue on your own.

Research

Regarded simply as a therapeutic aid, the value of meditation appears to be that it is a solvent of stress. Because the mind is allowed to relax, the body calms down too, and the homeostatic mechanism is given a chance to recover its authority. And although the ways in which this is done have yet to be elucidated, a great deal of information from research projects has become available to show that meditation does have significant physiological, as well as mental, effects.

When the first results of research into the physiological effects of meditation began to appear in the early 1970s, showing striking changes in heart rate, respiration and skin conductivity, they were greeted with some incredulity. Surveying meditation in the *British Journal of Psychiatry* in 1979, however, Dr Michael West of the University of Kent showed that subsequent research has broadly confirmed the initial findings, and has also demonstrated positive effects in connection with the reduction of hypertension. There are considerable difficulties in assessing results, West observed, because – among other things – so much may depend upon the interest aroused. It is difficult to distinguish the effects attributed to meditation "from the effects of merely treating (no matter what the treatment)". Nevertheless the work which has been done, he felt, "has provided grounds for cautious optimism".

Patricia Carrington has written in *Freedom in Meditation*, that one of the reasons why she came up with her "clinically standardized meditation" was that when she inquired about research into transcendental meditation, she was informed by the organization that the Maharishi would not sanction it on the grounds that he believed that forms of meditation other than his own were damaging to those who practised them. As local T.M. bodies must obtain the permission of the organization's central research department for any experimental work, this has meant that trials, "the lifeblood of scientific inquiry", to compare T.M. with other forms of meditation, have been banned.

Suitable cases/Self-help

It is possible to argue that all of us are suitable cases for meditation, to promote relaxation of mind and body in order to reduce tension and ward off stress disorders. Patricia Carrington has pointed out that although the techniques of meditation may differ, there are some ground rules common to those derived from the mantra tradition, which are generally followed:

- **Plan the sessions** so that you will not be meditating immediately after a meal or after taking stimulants.
- **Avoid distractions;** use a quiet room, and make sure you silence the telephone.
- **Meditate seated** before some pleasant object, such as a vase of flowers, in subdued light.
- **Sit in a comfortable position** and do whatever you need to do to stay comfortable.
- **If interrupted**, try not to jump out of your meditation: surface slowly. And, after it ends, allow a couple of minutes to return to your everyday preoccupations.

Some teachers of meditation who do not regard themselves as proponents of the "more rigorous forms of meditation" nevertheless suggest that a certain amount of discomfort may be desirable in the early stages, while you are learning to meditate – either because you should be learning to sit in a more correct posture (rather than slouch) or to demonstrate to yourself that moving into an altered state of consciousness removes awareness of your discomfort – or both.

Biofeedback

Anybody who takes his or her temperature and, on finding it is above 100°F, decides to go to a doctor (or to bed) is using biofeedback; as is anybody who looks at his or her tongue in a mirror, and decides he or she needs some medicine. The term has come to be used recently in a more specialized sense, employing gadgetry to measure bodily changes of a kind of which we would not normally be aware. These include changes in the resistance of the skin, as measured by variations in an electric current; changes in the brain-wave pattern, shown on an electroencephalograph (EEG); changes in blood pressure; changes in visceral responses, such as acid secretion in the digestive system, and so on.

Biofeedback, then, is not in itself a therapy, but as it has played a significant part in developing techniques of relaxation and meditation, it has come to be thought of as such. In their book *Beyond Biofeedback*, Elmer and Alyce Green make a distinction

❛ It isn't biofeedback that is the power within the human being to self-regulate, self-heal, rebalance. Biofeedback does nothing to the person; it is a tool for releasing the potential. ❜

Elmer and Alyce Green
Beyond Biofeedback

between the biofeedback process and biofeedback training. The process involves "getting immediate ongoing information about one's own biological processes or conditions, such as heart behaviour, temperature, brain-wave activity, blood pressure, or muscle tension". Information is usually fed back "by a meter, by a light, or by sound; or subjects simply watch the physiological record as it emerges from the monitoring equipment". Biofeedback training "means using the information to change voluntarily the specific process or response being monitored".

Origins

Researching into hypnosis a century ago, several investigators reported finding physiological reactions accompanying emotional changes. But when hypnotism fell out of favour again, these discoveries were not followed up – with one exception.

Variations of mood, the French neurologist, Charles Féré had shown, are accompanied by fluctuations of skin resistance to a mild electric current. Because tension increases perspiration, electrodes placed on sensitive areas of skin and attached to a monitoring device can reflect changes of mood. And Swiss psychiatrist Carl Jung exploited this discovery, for a while, in word-association tests on patients. He would recite a string of words, and watch to see which of them caused the current to jump.

Brain waves and medical diagnosis

The technique, however, did not establish itself in psychiatry. It was chiefly used, when it was employed at all, by detectives in "lie-detector" tests. Not until the 1960s was the potential of biofeedback for the treatment and prevention of illness realized by a number of researchers in the United States, working independently of one another – among them Joe Kamiya, Neal Miller and Elmer Green.

Kamiya, a neuropsychiatrist working in Chicago, followed up the discovery of brainwaves by the German scientist Hans Berger. By attaching electrodes to the scalp, Berger had found it was possible to "tune in" to the brain and obtain electrical signals at different wavelengths. This had attracted little but ridicule when he announced it in the 1930s and when, after the Second World War, it came to be used, it was chiefly for diagnosis of mental disorders such as epilepsy. Kamiya surmised that if physical states were related to brainwave activity, it might be possible to alter the physical state by learning how to tune in to a different wavelength. To assist in this effort, Kamiya arranged that whenever a bell rang, students should guess whether they were mentally on the brain's equivalent of long, short or medium wave. In time, he found, not merely could the students guess correctly, but they could learn to shift their brains from one channel to another.

Controlling the autonomic nervous system

Working with laboratory rats, Neal Miller, Professor of Psychology at the Rockefeller University, New York, obtained even more startling results. Like all medical students up to that time, he had been indoctrinated with the belief that the autonomic nervous system, regulating heartbeat, blood pressure, temperature and so on, is regulated by the body's own homeostatic mechanism; and that although heartbeat or blood pressure can be raised temporarily by some emotional activity – as when we get tense or angry – we cannot learn how to alter the setting of the homeostat, say, by lowering blood pressure and keeping it low.

Miller was able to show with the help of "operant conditioning" – pellets of food and electric shocks – that rats could learn. As Lewis Thomas, President of the Sloan Kettering Cancer Institute in New York, put it in his fascinating book *The Lives of a Cell*: "Rats, rewarded by stimulation of their 'pleasure centres', have been instructed to speed up or slow down their hearts at a signal, or to alter their blood pressures, or switch off certain waves in their electroencephalograms and switch on others". One of Miller's rats even managed to "blush" in one ear at a time – the ear becoming warmer than the other.

If rats, why not humans? The problem with humans was that consciousness could get in the way of a message such as "reward available if blood pressure lowered" and prevent it from being passed to the autonomic nervous system. But Elmer and Alyce Green of the Menninger Foundation knew of Schultz and Luthe's *Autogenic training* (see pages 178 to 181) and of Kamiya's technique of biofeedback, and they combined the two. Through straightforward autogenic training, subjects could gradually learn, for example, how to raise the temperature at their fingertips. But the learning process was greatly speeded up if the initial small rise in temperature – too small to be felt – could be relayed back to them, indicating to them that they were beginning to move into the required autohypnotic state of relaxation.

Blood pressure and biofeedback

At Harvard, Professor Herbert Benson had been working on blood pressure with baboons, when a group of students who practised transcendental meditation (see pages 186 to 187) came to him to suggest he should use them for his trials instead. Benson originally rejected the proposal, but after reading about biofeedback and about Miller's experiments, he changed his mind. And very soon, in a series of tests, he found that using the relaxation technique which the Maharishi's followers employed, patients with high blood pressure could learn to reduce it, and to keep it low.

In Britain, the chief exponent of biofeedback is Maxwell Cade, who describes himself as a "biophysicist". "If through the use of

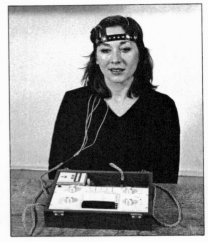

Uses of biofeedback
Biofeedback can be used on its own or in conjunction with other therapies to reach relaxation. It has been found to be useful for, amongst other things, headaches, high blood pressure, insomnia and anxiety.

some device one can become aware of an internal event of which one is not normally aware – such as the production of alpha rhythms in one's brain", he explains, "then one can learn to control some aspect of that event".

Procedure

There are two main types of biofeedback course, according to whether it is the process (to use the Greens' distinction) which is being taught – to show you how to use one or more of the gadgets – or whether biofeedback training is simply part of the therapy, as it can be in *Autogenic training* (see pages 178 to 181) or *Yoga* (see pages 138 to 144).

Biofeedback instruments

Feedback can be provided in many ways: usually either by sound – a tone which varies according to the changing mood – or visually, the rise and fall of a needle on a chart, or by colour

Biofeedback equipment
There are several kinds of biofeed-back machines which can be based, for instance, on reading ESR (electrical skin resistance), brain wave patterns or muscle tension. The appropriate feedback will be selected for each complaint.

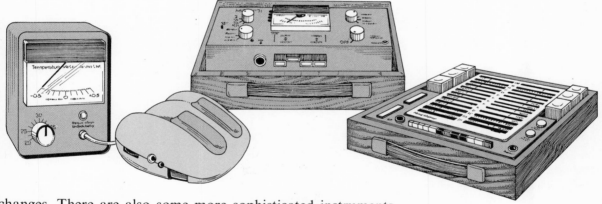

changes. There are also some more sophisticated instruments, such as the "mind mirror", which gives a picture of what is going on in both hemispheres of the brain (or in the same hemisphere of two people) at one time.

Skin resistance is normally measured by attaching electrodes to the palms of the hands, which happen to be particularly sensitive to mood (as has long been known, in the traditional link between "sweaty palms" and nervousness). This was the principle that Féré discovered, Jung used, and is still employed for lie detection by some police forces, recruitment agencies and so on.

The electroencephalogram (EEG) for biofeedback purposes shows brain-wave frequencies, measured in cycles per second, reflecting different levels of consciousness: beta, the normal waking rhythm; alpha, the "relaxed awareness" state; theta, drowsiness, day-dreaming; and delta, deep sleep. Hopes that the discovery of these different relationships would simplify the process of relaxation have not been wholly justified, as there are complex interactions, and different individuals give different readings. For some people, however, the feedback is invaluable.

Research

By one of the weird paradoxes that give orthodox scientists nightmares, Miller's research with rats, which did most to establish that control of the autonomic nervous system is possible with the help of biofeedback, has not been successfully repeated since, although it was repeated initially by a few other researchers. This is mystifying, because research with humans since that time has repeatedly demonstrated how effective biofeedback can be.

The researchers have been looking for the answers to three questions. Can people be trained to control their autonomic nervous systems? If so, how is it accomplished? And how can it best be used for preventing and treating illness?

The answer to the first of these questions is not now in dispute. Tens of thousands of people have found out for themselves that they can alter the temperature at their fingertips, or reduce their blood pressure, after a course of training. But how this is accomplished has yet to be satisfactorily answered. And what it can best be used for is not a question which can easily be answered in the abstract, because biofeedback is not a therapy, only an adjunct to therapy.

An aid to relaxation

Biofeedback, for example, does not in itself lower blood pressure. The process of attaining a state of relaxation, in which blood

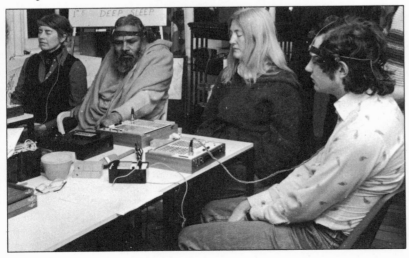

The effects of meditation
With each subject connected to a "mind mirror" (a type of encephalograph), Maxwell Cade conducts an experiment to monitor the effects on consciousness of a "Divine Love" meditation with Swami Prakashanand Saraswati. The board defines eight levels of consciousness, from deep sleep to "cosmic consciousness".

pressure is lowered, is facilitated by biofeedback – as Chandra Patel, a Croydon GP, has demonstrated in a series of trials. In the first of them, she divided patients into two groups – one taking a course in yoga, with biofeedback from a skin resistance meter, the other group being simply encouraged to relax.

The results showed that the yoga/biofeedback group did decidedly the better of the two. And this is only one of scores of trials all over the world where biofeedback has been shown to assist relaxation therapies.

Suitable cases

Any illness where tension is a component may be treated by using one of the therapies which reduce tension, and a biofeedback instrument should be used to facilitate that process. In a recent survey, Professor Erik Peper, President of the Biofeedback Society in the United States, claimed that biofeedback has been found "extremely useful" in the treatment of headaches, irregular heartbeats, high blood pressure, stroke, backache, and many other disorders.

Biofeedback's chief role, however, is – or should be – in prevention. The proof of the power of the mind over the workings of the body impresses upon people who use biofeedback both the need for self-help, and how easy it is to put into practise. "Using biofeedback for stress reduction and relaxation responses ultimately leads to change in a person's life-style", Peper points out. "The training is useless unless the patient is ready to incorporate the newly-learned skills into his everyday life."

Self-help

After the technique is learned, it can be exploited for whatever purpose the learner wants. In *Beyond Biofeedback*, the Greens describe an interesting example from the early days of their work in this field. A woman journalist who had picked up the fairly elementary technique of warming her hands with biofeedback from a thermometer decided to experiment, on her own, to see if she could lower her blood pressure.

"If she had been a relatively sophisticated medical student, she might not have attempted it, but she reasoned that since blood pressure involves control of blood flow, there might be a connection between blood pressure and warmth in the hands". So she stopped taking the valium her doctor had prescribed, and did her autogenic hand-warming exercises instead. When she next went for a checkup, her blood pressure was normal. The explanation, the Greens feel, is that the autogenic exercise had worked for her because, in achieving the autohypnotic state, she had released the tension responsible for her hypertension.

Dream therapy

Psychoanalysts use their patients' dreams to facilitate the analytic process; dream therapy is a group version of the same procedure.

Origins

Dr Montague Ullman, a psychoanalyst with a particular interest in dreams and founder of the Dream Laboratory at the Maimonides Medical Center in New York, initially followed the Freudian method of interpreting dreams. But he came to realize its limitation, and hearing a colleague use the term "dream appreciation", he latched on to it and began to apply it in therapy.

Appreciating dreams

"We appreciate art and we can learn to appreciate our dreams", he wrote in his book *Working with Dreams*. A psychoanalyst can *help* us appreciate a dream "but he cannot, regardless of the accuracy of the interpretation, appreciate it *for* us". The significance of this point of view became clearer as the scepticism grew about Freudian, and to a lesser extent about Jungian dream interpretations. As Ullman says "A snake may mean a phallus in a dream interpreted along Freudian lines, or an archetypal reference to the Fall in the Garden of Eden when interpreted along Jungian lines. But neither may be the place the dreamer is at in his selection of a particular image". Seeking for ways to help people understand their dreams through their own appreciation, rather than a therapist's interpretation, Ullman hit upon the group idea.

Procedure

The group, where possible under the guidance of somebody with previous experience, meets at specified intervals. Each member brings along a record of a recent dream, or dreams, and relates

' The Dream is a law to itself; and as well quarrel with a rainbow for showing, or for not showing, a secondary arch. The dream knows best, and the Dream, I say again, is the responsible party. '

Thomas de Quincey

Dream patterns
Even if we can't remember when we wake up, we do dream every night. Dreaming occurs during the lightest sleep and it is usual to pass through this level four times in a night's sleep.

them to the group. One by one, the other members of the group provide a commentary, an appreciation of the dream as if it were *their* dream. The dreamer consequently receives a range of views. Sometimes these may not fit his or her own appreciation (if any), but if they do, or any one of them does it can be fitted in.

Interpreting dreams

Suppose a woman member of the group has dreamed about a snake. She may be told (and probably will be) roughly what each member of the group would think if he or she had had this particular dream. The advantage is that all of them can present their own opinions without giving themselves away, after all, it is not *their* dream. The dreamer can listen, and decide which, if any, of the views fit so far as she is concerned, also without giving this away if she does not care to admit, at the time, that one of the group has confirmed her ideas on the subject.

Suitable cases

Dream therapy has the advantage that any group of people who are having, or contemplating having, psychotherapy, can come together, at regular or irregular intervals, with or without a therapist – though obviously it will be an advantage to find somebody with previous experience, to fill in the background and structure the proceedings.

BEHAVIOURISM

The behaviourist theory derives from the experiments which the Russian scientist Ivan Pavlov made with animals, especially dogs, at the turn of the century. Pavlov showed that they could be given a "conditioned" or required reflex, such as salivating at the sound of a bell which rang when they were about to be fed. They also became "neurotic", he found, if they were given contradictory forms of conditioning – if, for example, the food was then accompanied by electric shocks (this induced neurotic state could be put right by further conditioning).

If this happened with animals, he reasoned, why not with humans? The behaviourists, as they came to be known, insisted that neuroses, being conditioned reflexes, can be unlearned. J.B. Watson, and later B.F. Skinner, in the United States, Professor Hans Eysenck in Britain, and Joseph Wolpe in South Africa became the leaders of a campaign to promote "learning theory" as a replacement for Freudian and neo-Freudian principles.

Behaviour therapy

In its oldest and simplest form, and still to most people, its only form, behaviour therapy consists of punishing a naughty child and rewarding a good one. The assumption is that conditioning of this kind, if correctly and systematically applied, can get rid of neurotic symptoms (which they take to be learned habits), first by de-conditioning, and then, if necessary, by reconditioning to substitute other habits.

Procedure

Behavioural treatment can take many forms, of which *aversion therapy* is the most familiar. Alcoholics, for example, may be given a drug which will ensure that if they take alcohol in any form, they will be violently sick. Not all of the techniques involve such unpleasant experiences; sometimes the emphasis is on "reinforcement" – the equivalent, for humans, of the morsel of food which a rat in a cage receives when it learns to press the right lever. And with some neuroses the method can be effective – as when people who have a terror of spiders are weaned from it by being brought gradually into proximity with them.

Rejecting the concept of "mind"

The behaviourists, however, have brought ridicule on themselves by succumbing to the temptation of thinking that human beings act and react just like laboratory rats. This has meant rejecting the human "mind", in the sense that the term is commonly used.

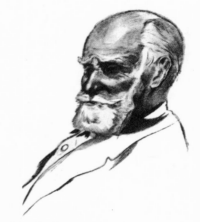

Ivan Pavlov
Ivan Petrovich Pavlov's (1849–1936) experiments on dogs and their conditioned reflexes led to the theory of behaviourism.

How are poems written? "We get them", Watson explained "by manipulating words, shifting them about until a new pattern is hit upon". As with Pavlov's animals, in other words, the poet's eye rolls in a fine frenzy until by chance the right pattern of words emerges. "Right" in this case meaning that it is going to win approval, which in turn provides the "reinforcement" which makes it the more likely that the right pattern of words will be hit upon again. Such concepts as "mind" and "idea", Skinner has claimed are spurious; they cannot be accepted because they cannot be scientifically demonstrated.

Partly because of the ludicrous lengths to which the behaviourists have taken their theory, and partly because of the element of physical discomfort or pain which has been associated with "negative reinforcement", behaviourist-oriented therapies are not in common use other than by some psychiatrists and clinical psychologists. The fact remains, however, that non-medical practitioners of other forms of psychological treatment use them, to some extent, without being aware of their behaviourist source.

The behaviourists themselves have recently been tending to move away from Skinnerian excesses, and whereas in the 1960s, polls of psychology students used to name Skinner as the most influential psychologist, his followers of that era are embarrassed at the recollection. The discoveries of Neal Miller and Herbert Benson in connection with mice and men, too, have thrown a bridge over what used to be an impassable divide between them and practitioners of *Humanistic psychology* (see pages 198 to 219).

One of Pavlov's Dog Experiments
Pavlov's most famous experiments were those concerning conditioned or acquired reflexes. He also found that contradictory signals such as electric shocks given at the sight of food produced neuroses but that, by further conditioning, these too could be cured.

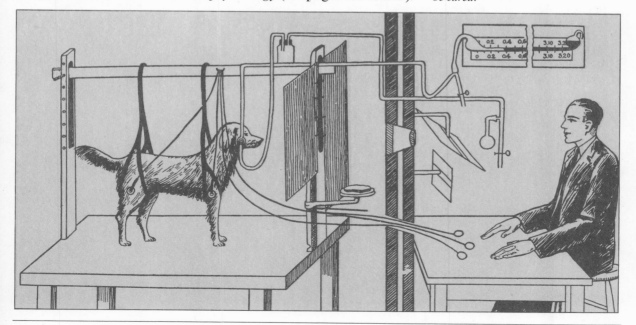

HUMANISTIC PSYCHOLOGY

Humanistic psychology is not one therapy, rather it is a chest-of-drawers holding a range of therapies, and it has often been described as the third force in modern psychology, after psychoanalysis and behaviourism. It can also be regarded, as Thomas C. Greening puts it in Kaslof's *Wholistic Dimensions of Healing*, as providing "a theoretical context, a loose but widespread confederation of explorers, and a forum for the sharing and integrating of findings".

As a concept humanistic psychology owes much to Abraham Maslow, who sees "high-level wellness" as the aim of psychology, rather than a simple escape from emotional blocks and neuroses. In practice, humanistic psychology derived a great deal of its impact from the "growth movement" of the 1960s, which it suited so much better than conventional psychology. It has encouraged the adoption of psychological ideas and practices from many different sources, appropriating some from Freud, Jung and Reich, some from the behaviourists and some from Assagioli's

Human potential: the growth movement

"Why do these methods work? What is the mechanism through which fantasy, dramatic and non-verbal techniques bring about release and joy? . . . . what potential is it that these methods help the individual to realize? Perhaps it's the potential for being more of a person than I thought I could be; for being more significant, competent, and lovable; for being a more meaningful individual, capable of coping more effectively with the world and better able to give and receive love. . .

William C. Schutz
Joy

We are developing ways to make our bodies more alive, healthier, lighter, more flexible, stronger, less tired, more graceful, more integrated. We have ways for using our bodies better, for sensing more, for functioning more effectively, for developing skills and sensitivity, for being more imaginative and creative, and for feeling more and holding the feelings longer. More and more we can enjoy other people, learn to work and play with them, to love and fight with them, to touch them, to give and take with them, to be with them contentedly, to be happily alone, to lead or to follow them, to create with them. . . Our institutions can be improved, can be used to enhance and support individual growth.

The underlying philosophy behind the human potential thrust is that of openness and honesty. A man must be willing to let himself be known to himself and to others. He must express and explore his feelings and open up areas long dormant and possibly painful, with the faith that in the long run, the pain will give way to a release of vast potential for creativity and joy".

Psychosynthesis (see pages 220 to 222). It has also brought in many physical forms of treatment, such as *Massage* and *Rolfing* (see pages 95 to 103), and paid much attention to nutrition and other aspects of *Nature cure* (see pages 16 to 44).

The British Institute for the Development of Human Potential states that "Although eclectic in nature, there are certain common themes".

- **First**: Personal growth, responsibility and self-direction.
- **Second**: Life-long education.
- **Third**: full emotional functioning.
- **Fourth**: The need to learn, or perhaps to relearn, what play and joy are about.
- **Fifth**: Recognition of a person's spiritual dimension; there is an acknowledgement of human capacity for altered states of consciousness.

From this list it will be clear why the structure which we have been using up to this point in the book to assess the different therapies needs to be modified. Many of the categories of humanistic psychology, though their history can usually be traced, and a rough idea of their aims extracted, can now rarely be separated into distinctly different therapies. There are still individuals who would identify themselves as "Rogerians" or "gestalt therapists", but you are much more likely to find a practitioner who interprets "humanistic" loosely, and uses a variety of methods. Terms like "gestalt therapy" in fact now have little meaning, except as an indication of their roots. Consequently, we have been more concerned to fill in the background, than to tell you precisely what to expect.

Rogerian therapy

For many people, the name Carl Rogers is synonymous with a new era in the psychological therapies, the Growth Movement of the sixties and seventies. It was during this period that psychoanalysis was brought out from the clinics and consulting rooms into everyday life, and developed into numerous techniques and activities affirming, as the Irish psychiatrist Anthony Clare wrote in *Let's Talk About Me*, "the essential goodness and equality of man, the curative effects of understanding and love", and man's natural tendency towards personal growth.

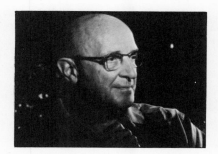

Carl Rogers
Carl Rogers was the founder of Rogerian Therapy, in which the therapist intuits the patient's needs.

Origins

Rogers was one of many American psychoanalysts who, in spite of a debt to Freud as a thinker and innovator, came to be disillusioned with analysis as therapy. One defect, he realized, was that Freud had tried to fit it into the prevailing clinical pattern, with the doctor in charge, conducting rigidly structured sessions along strictly scientific lines – or as close to scientific lines as psychotherapy could get. So, during the 1940s and for the next 25 years or so, Rogers began to develop a very different approach, abandoning the medical model, with its questions about how to "treat, or cure, or change this person" and replacing it with questions of how to provide "a relationship which this person may use for his own personal growth".

In Freudian psychoanalysis, analysts kept their distance from the patients or "analysands". They were out of sight behind the head of the couch, out of reach, "out of touch", in fact, Rogers began to think – in both senses of "touch". Freud had striven to maintain strict, scientific detachment, so that he could provide expert guidance. But for Rogers and his followers, the "experts" are the patients themselves. It is they who know, intuitively, what is the matter with them, and it is they who can find what to do about it if the therapist, or counsellor, cooperates, intuitively not intellectually. As he has said, "To try to get inside the world of that other person, to sense and feel it as if you were inside that world, is a very rare thing, but a very powerful thing".

‘ (Our) attitude is one of involvement, in contrast to a theoretical or detached attitude . . . A self which has become a matter of calculation and management has ceased to be a self. It has become a thing . . . You may have a precise, detached knowledge of another person, his psychological type and his calculable reactions, but in knowing this you do not know the person, his centred Self, his knowledge of himself. Only by participating in his Self, in performing an existential breakthrough into the centre of his being, will you truly know him. ’

Paul Tillich
The Courage to Be

Procedure

Although there are no set techniques and no set procedures to follow in Rogerian therapy, there are certain conditions that both client and counsellor have to meet for growth to take place. It is crucial for the client to accept him or herself – warts and all, and to trust to the genuineness and uniqueness of his or her own experience. But this will be impossible if the counsellor fails to demonstrate an openness, an "unconditional positive regard" for the client, and plenty of "under the skin" understanding or overt empathy.

Rogerian counselling does occur on a one-to-one basis, though a considerable amount of it takes place in a group setting, within the framework of what is known as the "encounter group". Clients meet together regularly with a counsellor who acts as a guide, and is often described as an "active listener". When the encounter process is under way, people gradually find themselves able to let go and begin to express how they really feel about themselves and each other.

Fairly early on in the development of his approach to counselling, Rogers outlined seven stages which he had observed clients to pass through in search of growth or what he called "self-actualization". Stage one consists of almost no awareness of anything other than present concerns and actions, while stage seven is one of trust in and responsibility for one's own inner development and growth. Rogers considers that this "journey" from stage one to seven takes years to complete, which in part explains why the Growth Movement becomes a total way of life for so many of those involved in it.

Suitable cases

Both aspects of Rogerian therapy – the encounter group and one-to-one counselling – have been and are still applied in a variety of therapeutic and growth settings and situations, from therapeutic communities to school and university counselling, and so on, even to courses in management training and group behaviour. More often than not, though, participants may be unaware when they are involved in Rogerian-type methods.

Encounter

One development from *Rogerian therapy* (pages 199 to 201) which has had a striking and not always beneficial influence is encounter therapy—a development from group therapy. Aware of the limitations of psychoanalysis imposed by the one-to-one relationship of analyst and "analysand", Carl Rogers and other analysts had begun to put patients into groups, consisting of half a dozen and a dozen people with the emphasis on getting the participants to express their feelings.

There was a curious similarity, here, between Rogerian methods and those which had been introduced by the American evangelist Frank Buchman, who founded the "Group" or Moral Rearmament Movements between the wars. But the Buchmanites were Christians, and as such, encouraged to confess their sins. Rogers insisted that there should be no question of compelling participants to think in terms of "sins" or to make disclosures. The aim should be rather to give them the chance to express whatever feelings and thoughts disturbed them, knowing that in the group they would find a sympathetic, or empathetic, audience which would be neither mocking nor censorious.

It was at Esalen, which lies on the Pacific coast between San Francisco and Los Angeles, that encounter therapy began to take a different course. Here, gurus preached to their disciples, and they, in turn, moved away to found new colonies, or new, rather different courses. Esalen was the Mecca of the Growth Movement, the spiritual home of the counter-culture, a cross between a rest camp and, as psychiatrist Anthony Clare has described it, "a particularly twentieth-century version of the religious retreat house, a place for the recharging of spiritual batteries, out of the

❛The expression of self by some members of the group has made it very clear that a deeper and more possible encounter is possible, and the group appears to strive intuitively and unconsciously, towards this goal. Gently at times, almost savagely at others, the group demands that the individual be himself, that his current feelings not be hidden, that he remove the mask of ordinary social intercourse.❜

Carl Rogers
Encounter groups
London 1971

hurly-burly of the mainstream of life". But whereas in the religious retreat, the self is disciplined, in Esalen it is to be "discovered, liberated, fulfilled". To this end, all manner of therapies have been adopted, adapted, modified and sometimes altered almost out of recognition, as they spread out through the United States in the 1960s, and out to other countries throughout the world in the ensuing decades.

Rules for groups

The leading exponent of encounter has been William Schutz, whose book *Joy* was published in New York in 1967. The rules he laid down for groups were:

- Pay attention to your body.
- Stay with the here and now.
- Express yourself physically, rather than verbally.
- Speak for yourself – and always directly to the person you are expressing feelings about; do not generalize.
- Take responsibility for yourself and for your decisions.

Citing these rules in the best recent introduction to self-help therapies, *In Our Own Hands*, its authors Sheila Ernst and Lucy Goodison describe encounter as, "based on the assumption that we live in a society which alienates us from our bodies and our feelings". Writing primarily for women, they claim as one of encounter's virtues that "it can help a woman to recognize the strength of her own feelings, and to open up dramatically the feelings towards others which we have found hardest to show", the release of energy being therapeutic in itself. "The difference between an *encounter* and lovers' brawl in the street", they explain, "is that in the encounter group the two people scream out their anger and hatred with the understanding that they are not trying to win a battle, but rather that they need to express the angry and hateful feelings and to understand and move on. . . ."

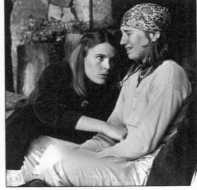

At an encounter group
Encounter groups often release emotions that have long been repressed, whether of anger, joy or grief. For participants to be able fully to explore and experience their own personal blocks, it is important that there is a caring, supportive atmosphere.

The negative side of encounter

It is here that encounter has all too often failed in its purpose and what has emerged has been an ugly form of emotional asset-stripping, with members of the group being encouraged by the leader to humiliate each other, physically as well as verbally, in ways which suggest that the gratification of sadism, rather than therapy, is the object of the exercise. In some cases, what has appeared to be very effective use of encounter has degenerated to the point where it has been scarcely recognizable as such.

Procedure

Groups now come in a bewildering variety of shapes and sizes. They may follow the relatively mild Rogerian lines, or they may be of the "ordeal" type. Some group leaders like to have their flock together for a succession of short periods, some prefer sessions during which members of the group spend a couple of days and nights literally locked in each other's company. The only way to find out what kind of encounter you can expect is from somebody who has been through it.

Some therapists believe in setting two of their clients at each other; others take on individuals themselves, and revile them. Some keep the session on a more intellectual, or at least verbal, plane. Some prefer short sessions, and so on. Johnny St John's account of his experience gives an idea of what might happen, (see box text) though in fact, it is impossible to give an adequate picture of what to expect simply by describing a session, because the description can hardly begin to convey the feelings aroused.

Painful and embarrassing though St John had found the encounter experience, "as we hugged and kissed goodbye I felt I had fifteen new friends whom I knew in a curiously special way", he concluded. "They'd helped me not only to begin to understand a little more about myself but also to be more aware of the immense hidden tracts and spaces inside me that were waiting to be discovered".

One man's experience

Johnny St John, a director of the publishing company Heinemann, who in his late fifties decided to explore this, to him, wholly strange world, described it, sympathetically but not uncritically, in his book *Travels in Inner Space*.

In his first "encounter", 16 people, strangers to each other (except for two married couples), came together in a slummy room in London furnished only with a carpet and cushions, a record player, an old tennis racket and the chamber-pot. They were to be there for 48 hours, and to do and say whatever they felt like, except that they must not use physical violence.

They introduced themselves, and after some "eyeball-to-eyeballing" to bring out instinctive likes and dislikes, were told to say what they thought about each other, as lovingly or bitchily as they cared to. When rage took over, they could pound cushions, shout and scream obscenities, or beat the cushions with the tennis racket. Hatreds spewed out freely, as did tears; people cursed each other, hugged each other.

Games were played. After a brief release for a walk, they were called upon to undress and move around amongst each other, embracing each other (without differentiation by sex), massaging each other. There were intervals for "feedback" – comments by the leader or participants, the session ending with "positive feedback", in which they were encouraged to give constructive, and even kindly, comments on each other.

Gestalt

Gestalt therapy is one of Esalen's progenies (see *Encounter*, page 20). Its guru was Friedrich (Fritz) Perls, who began his career as a psychoanalyst in Berlin, but later became discontented with orthodox Freudian methods, and worked for a while with the psychiatrist Wilhelm Reich. After the Second World War, Perls became interested in the ideas put forward by Max Wertheimer in the late nineteenth century concerning form and shape – (*gestalt*, in German). His idea was that we can have a number of apparently unrelated ideas or feelings which, taken separately, may be meaningless, and even confusing, but which given some overall shape, may begin to make sense.

The dangers of turning on

Perls set to work to try to fuse into gestalt the useful elements from psychoanalysis, along with existentialism. But he grew worried by the excesses at Esalen. "It took us a long time to debunk the whole Freudian crap", he explained in *Gestalt Therapy Verbatim*, "and now we are entering a new and more dangerous phase. We are entering the phase of turners-onners: turn on to instant cure, instant joy, instant sensory awareness". To Perls, psychoanalysis did little to the patient "except for making him deader and deader", but at least it was well-intentioned. Turning on was too often "a dangerous substitute activity, another phony therapy that *prevents* growth".

Gestalt therapists were therefore to concentrate on getting people to think in existential terms, in terms of the "here and now". This does not mean a search for instant cure, Perls insisted. It takes time. It means constant self-examination, not just of the "self" in psychological terms, but of everything we do, in particular of our gestures.

Humanistic hedonism

In what he describes as "an impressionistic notion" of Gestalt's injunctions, the therapist Claudio Naranjo has listed:
- **Live Now**: Be concerned with the present rather than with the past or the future.
- **Live here**: Deal with what is present rather than what is absent.
- **Stop imagining**: Experience the real.
- **Stop unnecessary thinking**: Rather, taste and see.
- **Express rather than manipulate**, explain, justify or judge.
- **Give in to unpleasantness and pain**: just as to pleasure. Do not restrict your awareness.
- **Accept no should, or ought**, other than your own. Adore no graven image.
- **Take full responsibility for your actions**, feelings and thoughts.
- **Surrender to being as you are**.

The essence of gestalt, in short, is self-discovery and, through it, self-liberation, or (Naranjo's term) "humanistic hedonism".

The gestalt prayer

❝*I do my thing, and you do your thing.
I am not in this world to live up to your expectations
And you are not in this world to live up to mine
You are you, and I am I,
And if by chance we find each other, its beautiful.
If not, it can't be helped.*❞

Fritz Perls
Gestalt Therapy Verbatim
(New York 1971)

Procedure

The combination of the flexibility required to allow each individual to achieve the here and now, and Perls' own objection to techniques ("a technique is a gimmick") makes it impossible to pin the therapy down for the purpose of a description of what you will be likely to find on joining a gestalt group. "Gestalt therapists develop different styles rather than using specific, potentially mechanistic techniques (fixed gestalten)", his wife Laura Perls has explained. Many other activities – "movement and art therapies, bioenergetics, primal and transaction methods" – are being incorporated into gestalt therapy: it is not fixed, "but an ongoing innovative process on the boundary of actual and potential experience".

Psychodrama

The idea behind psychodrama is that we can "act out" our problems because the fact that we are playing a part, not being ourselves, enables us to throw off inhibitions.

Drama therapy – an eclectic approach to the understanding and alleviation of social and psychological problems which uses theatre, dance, mime and psychodrama – is not included; it is still in the process of becoming a therapy.

❛Give a man a mask and he will tell the truth ❜

Oscar Wilde

Origins

Psychodrama was founded by Jacob Moreno, a remarkable character of uncertain origin who became a psychiatrist in Vienna after the First World War, and who dabbled in avant-garde production in what he called the "theatre of spontaneity" (one of the actors, apparently, was Peter Lorre). Moreno found that an actress who had been a harridan in her private life while playing "sweetness and light" roles in the theatre, became all "sweetness and light" in her private life when given "bitchy" roles in the theatre. This led him to develop the theory of psychodrama as a form of psychotherapy.

A number of techniques have been developed to structure psychodrama: "soliloquy", in which the actors describe their feelings in connection with some traumatic event – the death of a parent, for example; "mirroring", in which one person's behaviour is imitated by another, the "double", so that the actor expresses the emotions which the performer feels, but has been unable or unwilling to release; "role reversal", where one person tries to *become* another.

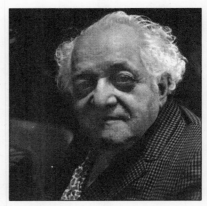

J.L. Moreno
A contemporary of Freud's, Moreno (1892–1974) developed psychodrama as an alternative to the primarily verbal, one-to-one approach of psychoanalysis.

The uses of psychodrama
The London psychodrama teacher Dr Joel Badaines has summed up possible uses of this therapy in the *Encyclopedia of Alternative Medicine*; choices of life situation are increased because of the exploration of alternatives. The spontaneity removes inhibitions and develops creative response. Through identification with other performers, empathy is improved. Individuals are brought into touch with feelings, thoughts and imagery. Flexibility is increased, giving "a greater sense of mastery over a variety of roles (parent, lover, student, friend, etc)". For people who find it hard to relate to friends or family, or who feel inhibited, psychodrama offers the prospect of a more fulfilled and healthier life.

Transactional analysis

Transactional analysis resembles *Gestalt* (see pages 204 to 205) in its dedication to unmasking what we really think and feel, but it is more structured, concentrating on the ruses we are endlessly employing to avoid coming to terms with uncomfortable realities. As its name implies, Roger Kreitman has explained, "T.A. concerns itself largely – though not exclusively – with the social realm of transactions between people; so inevitably attention is focused on the client's relations with his family, his workmates etc. T.A. therapists are very aware of the importance of involving the client's intimates in the therapy process".

Origins

In the 1950s, Eric Berne, like so many of his psychiatrist contemporaries, became dissatisfied with orthodox psychoanalytical concepts, and gathered around him a group in San Francisco to explore what he initially described as social psychiatry. Out of this grew transactional analysis (T.A.), and Berne's book *Games People Play*, describing his theory, became an international bestseller on its publication in 1964.

The "ego state"
Basic to transactional analysis is the concept of the "ego state". Every person carries a child, an adult and a parent self within him. The child in a person "feels, wants, demands, plays, adapts, fights"; the adult "thinks, computes, analyses"; the parent "believes, protects, controls, directs, nurtures". Any one, or more, of these ego states may be called into play by a social interaction, and of course, the states may match, or as more usually happens, a particular state in one person will attract a

❛ There are times when I look over the various parts of my character with perplexity. I recognize that I am made up of several persons and that the person that at the moment has the upper hand will inevitably give place to another. But which is the real one? All of them or none? ❜

William Somerset Maugham

different state in another. So, to choose a typical stereotype, the husband who comes home tired from work and flops down, exhausted and calls for his wife, may – if he is in luck – elicit the parent in her, who will come and pour out the drink, and cook the meal for the child in him.

Procedure

Again, like gestalt, the procedure varies according to the views of the therapist and the nature of the people he or she is dealing with. Some therapists stick closely to the original Berne formula, the sessions being primarily devoted to picking up, exposing and analysing the structure of the ego states, the transactions that go on, the events acted out, the "games" that are played; but many combine T.A. with other growth ideas and practices.

The first thing to be learned in T.A. is how to recognize and understand the ego states. From this initial work a person may go on to observe how he or she uses this information (known as a script) to obtain "strokes" – ways of receiving attention, that are not necessarily self-enhancing – and to analyze the results or pay-offs of different behaviour.

The aim of T.A., according to Berne, is to "attain social control", to learn how to bring the "adult" in each of us into situations that require it. As people learn how to achieve this aim, they are encouraged to set up and obtain some concrete goal, and, in fact, many people are expected to make a specific contract for a change in their behaviour before they take part in T.A. Although some T.A. can be undertaken in individual sessions, on the whole the work takes place in groups.

Suitable cases

Any case deemed suitable for psychotherapy, according to Berne could be treated with infinitely greater speed using T.A. Teachers and other people involved in communications are becoming increasingly interested in the possible applications of T.A.

One striking development to come out of T.A. has been pioneered by American psychologists Jacqui and Lee Schiff, and described by Jacqui Schiff in her books *All My Children* and *The Cathexis Reader: Transactional Analysis in the Treatment of Psychosis.* They took in a paranoid schizophrenic youth and proceeded to treat him as if he were reborn, putting him through all the experiences he would have had if he had been their baby. The experiment worked; they took on more psychotics; and although there were many frightening times and some failures, within four years they had brought 17 apparently hopeless cases back to sanity, steered them through adolescence and enabled them to go out into the world, get jobs, marry and have children.

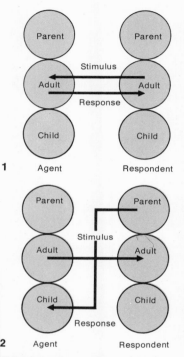

Complementary and crossed transactions
In transactional analysis, Berne gives two kinds of transactions – complementary and crossed. In figure 1, there is a complementary transaction: an adult stimulus receives an adult response – for instance, "Did you call the doctor today?" – "Yes, I made an appointment for Tuesday".
In figure 2, the transaction is crossed: an adult stimulus receives a parental response – "Did you call the doctor today?" – "Why do you expect me to do everything for you? Call the doctor yourself".

Co-counselling

Co-counselling or re-evaluation counselling is a method by which lay people may help each other, without the need, or cost, of professional intervention. The assumption behind it is that illness is often related to a failure to recognize the existence of feelings such as anger, loneliness and inadequacy, locked away in the subconscious. Its aim is to allow such feelings to be released.

Origins

The method originated in the sixties in Seattle – from where it quickly spread, in the process developing breakaway groups that added techniques, such as regression and guided fantasy, providing a transpersonal element to the framework. However, the original emphasis on emotional discharge for psychological health and personal growth, remains. As each person takes an allotted time as client, the peer counsellor's role is to help him or her to recognize those cut-off, hidden emotions, while still allowing the client to remain in charge of the session and what takes place in it. When the allotted time is up, client and counsellor change roles.

Procedure

Each recruit to the counselling network has first to learn the techniques to be used. This involves taking part in a 40-hour training course and studying the manual. "The counsellor is not to comment, or give advice, or sympathize, or share experiences, but only listen . . ." says John Rowan, a London psychotherapist, in his book *Ordinary Ecstasy*. He can, however, repeat "key phrases" used by the client; contradict "self-deprecatory statements"; and use certain other techniques, "but nothing elaborate and nothing mystifying, because the client knows and can use all the same techniques, too. It then becomes crystal clear what is mystified in most other forms of therapy, and may take years to discover – that it is the client who has to do the work. Only the client knows what she is ready to work on and how deep she is ready to go".

The training over, two people can then get together and arrange to meet perhaps once a week for a couple of hours, dividing their time equally between being counsellor and client, for as long as the arrangement is of mutual benefit.

Suitable cases

Co-counselling is especially suitable for those who feel that they have set blocks to their own free emotional expression and want to go back and re-evaluate their reactions to those blocks – and who wish to assist others to do the same.

Bioenergetics/reichian therapy

In the book *Your Body Works*, edited by Gerald Kogan, David Boadella defines bioenergetic therapy as "a system of techniques for mobilizing the energies of people whose forms of expression have become in some way blocked or disturbed. Whereas most existing systems of psychotherapy use primarily verbal techniques for exploring a neurotic problem, in bioenergetic therapy we are concerned with the total expressive behaviour of a person . . . with the quality of bodily movements and the fundamental, rhythmic processes of the body, especially breathing."

Origins

The development of bioenergetics is usually credited to Wilhelm Reich, who joined Sigmund Freud's group of disciples in Vienna at the end of the First World War. Far from shying away from the sexual implications of Freud's theories, Reich had developed the belief that the cause of many disorders is an inability to achieve satisfactory orgasm. This is not just a matter of guilt feelings related to masturbation, he decided; many people who think they experience orgasm are not getting the real thing. It is as if the body *needs* real convulsions, a degree of loss of control, as therapy.

Reich surmised that this need arises because most of us fit ourselves into what he thought of as "armour". As we grow up, we acquire physical characteristics to suit our personality structure, as can be seen in peoples' faces, and their posture. "The organism," as Reich put it in his book *The Sexual Revolution*, "is forced to *armour* itself against the outside world. The armouring of the organism results inevitably in a limitation of the total ability to live". Most people suffer from it, and illness is often a consequence.

The healing power of orgone

Initially, Reich assumed it would be necessary to use analysis to loosen the armour's hold on the body: "If, now, one eliminates the genital inhibitions and genital anxiety, if thus the patient acquires the ability for full orgiastic gratification and has the good fortune to find a suitable sexual partner, one observes a change in the patient's total behaviour, the extent of which is often surprising". Later, Reich began to think in terms of loosening the armour by more direct means such as massage and breathing exercises. Eventually, he moved on to explore the therapeutic use of what he believed to be life energy or what he called "orgone".

Orgone, as Reich regarded it, somewhat resembled Mesmer's theory of animal magnetism (see *Hypnotherapy*, pages 166 to 173), but Reich's experiments, designed to demonstrate both its reality and its healing power, coupled with spasms of paranoia on his part, brought him into conflict with the sceptical United States federal authorities and he died in jail.

❛ The body's life is the life of sensations and emotions. The body feels real hunger, real thirst, real joy in the sun or the snow, real pleasure in the smell of roses or the look of a lilac bush, real anger, real sorrow, real tenderness, real warmth, real passion, real hate, real grief. All the emotions belong to the body and are only recognised by the mind. ❜

D.H. Lawrence,
Sex, Literature and Censorship

One of Reich's disciples, however, while repudiating his later theories, carried on the work on "armour" from where Reich had left off. Muscles, Alexander Lowen argued in *The Language of the Body*, "can become tense when they are consciously holding back an impulse. For example, one can become so angry that the muscles ache from holding back the impulse". They can also become tense, and ache, when the impulse which is being restrained is unconscious, so the process of loosening the armour must take into account the possibility of repressed traumatic events in infancy. This may give a clue to the origins of the armour as well as examining its role in the present, in relation to the patient's relations with family, work and so on.

While rejecting Reich's theory of orgone, Lowen accepted the concept behind it of a life force based on energy; a physical phenomenon, whose identity would eventually be discovered. Its precise nature, he felt, was unimportant: "We work with the hypothesis that there is one fundamental energy in the human body whether it manifests itself in psychic phenomena or in somatic motion. This energy we call bioenergy". "Bioenergetics" has since become the term used to describe the theory and practice of therapy based on this hypothesis.

Procedure

It is hard to give a clear indication of what happens in a bioenergetics' session, other than descriptions by individuals of what actually has happened in their own experience. Sheila Ernst and Lucy Goodison, however, give an interesting example of the way in which a group session develops in *In Our Own Hands*.

The session began with deep breathing in one of the "stress" positions, such as lying on the back with heels reaching to the ceiling. The idea behind this is "that the deep breathing increases the flow of energy to the body and combines with the stress position to stimulate and build up an energy 'charge'".

The group was closely supervised and watched to see if anyone appeared to be emotionally affected, in which case help was sought from the others. On one occasion, June, who had been affected, expressed a wish to kick. She was encouraged to do so, and at the same time to release her feelings. This led her to remember childhood experiences of being held down, kicking and screaming, by her mother. Now, at last, some of the childhood anger, held by June in her muscle blocks, burst out into expression. But this, Ernst and Goodison point out, is only one of many ways in which a similar result might have been achieved. The group "could equally have used deep breathing on its own, or bioenergetic massage applying pressure directly to tense muscles. Or the same experience might have been triggered by a physical experience, like someone in the group holding June down".

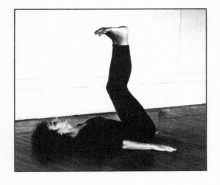

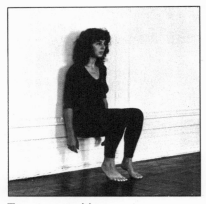

Two stress positions
Bioenergetic "stress" exercises are designed to break down the defensive barriers which cut off any individual from his or her own emotions. During therapy, the patients learn to open up their breathing and then gradually their emotions. Sessions frequently become very emotional – patients may feel pain, anger, terror or sadness which break out violently while they are learning to release.

Different practitioners of bioenergetic therapy have developed their own ideas. One example of this is the "biodynamic psychology" practised by the Norwegian Gerda Boyesen at her London centre. She discovered that parallel to the normal digestive systems, there is an "emotional" digestive system which equates with Reich's concept of the orgasm as a regulator of emotional tension. Attendance at one of her weekend courses has been described by Christopher Macy, a former Manchester *Guardian* staff writer, in *Psychology Today*. There were too many participants for all to benefit from her massage, so they started with exercises resembling ordinary physical training, but conducted with a view to getting them to let bioenergy course through them, and to learn to feel it doing so. "Sure enough, I began to feel the most mysterious tingling all up and down my body, legs and arms, like a gentle electric current".

Sceptics, Macy concluded, would probably have some explanation, but he was impressed ("energy is catching, it seems") and he found its influence pleasurable, not just at the time, but for weeks after. What his account also shows is the cross-fertilization of the developments associated with *Humanistic psychology*.

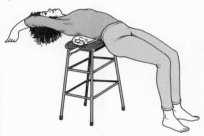

The breathing stool
This is the basic breathing exercise in bioenergetics. The patient bends backwards over a stool with a rolled blanket on top, his arms hanging back behind his head. This is a "stress" position and should only be held for a very short time, during which it is imperative that the patient breathes deeply and calmly.

Suitable cases

Any people with conditions in which there is a suspected underlying psychosomatic element may benefit from bioenergetic therapy in conjunction with a physical therapy such as *Homeopathy* (see pages 66 to 73) or *Acupuncture* (see pages 120 to 133). Generally speaking, those who prefer to work with the body to find release benefit the most.

Polarity therapy

"The principles and practices of polarity therapy", according to Pierre Pannetier in his contribution to Kogan's book *Your Body Works*, "are based on our view of the energy flow in human bodies in the universe. We envision life energy as it flows through the bones, the nerves and all the cells to be like a wireless radio or television. However, it is a more radiant form of energy, which travels everywhere. There are no limits as to the condition of this universal energy".

Polarity therapists use elements from *Nature cure* and *Manipulative*, *Psychological* and *Paranormal* therapies. They believe that by using a variety of techniques, blocks may be removed enabling energy currents to move freely again, circulating from positive to negative poles, creating a harmonious state of neutral.

❝ . . . The polarity system has a holistic approach to health and healing. This means it deals with the whole person: thoughts and attitudes, nutritional needs, special exercises known as 'polarity yoga', and, of course, the polarity session to facilitate the body in healing itself. ❞

Richard Gordon
Your Healing Hands

Origins

The concept of polarity therapy owes its existence to Randolph Stone. Born in Austria, Stone spent his working life in the United States where he made an extensive study of eastern as well as western medicine and trained as an osteopath, chiropractor and naturopath. He then returned to live in India with his spiritual master for the last ten years of his life. Good health, Stone believed, depends on preserving the balance of forces: ill health signifies a block in the energy flow. The basic principle was relatively simple, but a glance at some of the charts mapping the energy flows and wireless circuits in the body, the polarity relationships (positive, negative and neutral) between the different anatomical parts of the body, and the balances between the five centres of the body – those corresponding to the five elements: ether, water, fire, earth and air – reveals some of the complexity of the ideas that Stone was working on and developing during the course of his life.

Procedure

There is an established procedure of case history taking, followed by diagnosis which involves checking reflexes and pressure points throughout the body to establish the energy blocks, and treatment using manipulative techniques, stretching postures, special diets although how the guidelines are followed will depend upon the therapist and the patient's attitude.

Manipulation techniques

A therapist will have a whole repertoire of manipulations to perform which are designed to balance the currents and the five elements, and to release blockages. The hands are used to set up a field between the positive and negative poles in order to apply the correct type of energy for the manipulation. Three types of pressure are used: *neutral* is soothing and balancing and produced by a light touch with the fingertips; *positive* creates movement and involves direct manipulation; *negative* is used to disperse the blockages and involves painful manipulation which goes deep into the tissues.

Stretching postures

The aim of the postures is to help the removal of the energy blocks. Although all the postures help tone up the body generally, some are aimed at specific functions. You are never expected to go beyond your physical capabilities. You will be asked to notice if you feel any physical, emotional or mental changes during the process, and encouraged to express your feelings.

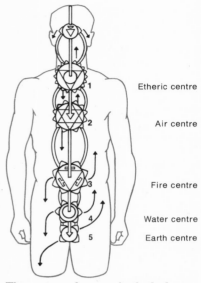

Etheric centre

Air centre

Fire centre

Water centre

Earth centre

The centres of energy in the body
1 Etheric Centre – *governs the voice, hearing and the throat.*
2 Air Centre – *governs the respiration, circulation, lungs and heart.*
3 Fire Centre – *governing digestion, stomach and bowels.*
4 Water Centre – *a generative and emotional force, governing the pelvic and glandular secretions.*
5 Earth Centre – *elimination of solids and liquids, governing the rectum and bladder.*
Polarity therapy requires that all these centres are perfectly balanced in order for energy to flow.

Diet and nutrition

The principles behind polarity suggest following a special diet programme. This may begin with a short "cleansing programme". This may well last for 10 to 14 days – though the length of time depends upon the nature of the disorder – and is intended as a purifier to help the body expel toxins. During this time great emphasis is placed on the consumption of "live foods" – fresh fruit and vegetables – drinking plenty of liquids; and being given the "liver flush" – a drink made from a mixture of lemon juice, olive oil, garlic and ginger root.

This is followed by a longer "health-building diet". Foods are reintroduced gradually and their effects on both body and mind studied by the patient and the therapist. The third stage of the programme is one of maintenance of the state of harmony and balance, most notably by following a vegetarian diet.

Suitable cases

Like the oriental therapies, the emphasis of polarity is not on treating specific symptoms: " We concentrate on balancing the life energy that flows through the body, in order to allow nature to do the healing". But therapists are also keen to point out that any therapeutic work requires commitment and willingness to learn and to change on the part of the patient. As Stone has said: "Effort and diligence is the price of Health and Happiness".

Using polarity therapy

A polarity therapist will begin by balancing the currents and centres of energy in the body using manipulation; he or she will often discuss any problems at the same time. You will then be taught postures the therapist feels will be beneficial to you.

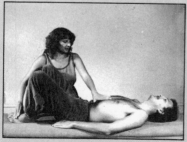

1 *The therapist is manipulating the patient's toes at the same time as pressing into his belly button. This unblocks the fire energy.*

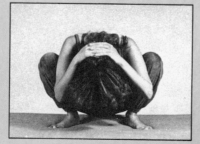

2 *The wide squat or "youth position" opens up the watery centre – the pelvis – and releases gases. Breathe in gently and grunt or groan as you breathe out while rocking gently backwards and forwards.*

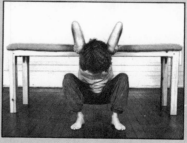

3 *The "Cliffhanger" releases both fire and water energies opening up the lungs, back and pelvis. Breathe deeply during this exercise and yell as you breathe out – this helps expel toxic gases from your lungs.*

Metamorphic technique

According to Gaston St Pierre and Debbie Boater, the practice of prenatal therapy, or the metamorphic technique as it is now called, is based upon the assumption that "it is during the nine months of the gestation period that our physical, mental, emotional and spiritual structures are established. It has been found that by working on the spinal reflex points of the feet, hands and head, they bring the formative period back into focus, and loosen the time structure". This in turn loosens energies blocked off during the prenatal period, "thereby setting free the healing processes of the body, the mind and the spirit".

Origins

The metamorphic technique was first developed in the 1960s by Robert St John. It was originally based on *Reflexology* (see pages 112 to 115) but now the two approaches differ significantly, both in purpose and in method. Metamorphic practitioners do not regard themselves as treating any disorder, but as providing the means whereby the patient may heal himself. Rather than working all over the foot or head, they work on them at points which are considered to correspond with different stages of the nine-month, prenatal period.

Procedure

Practitioners of the technique make no special claims about who can practice. Anyone can learn the technique; the only requirement is the right attitude. The general procedure is to massage each foot for about 30 minutes. No more than an hour's massage per foot, per week, should be given; though with children longer is possible if the massage is spread out over the week. The massage can also include the hands and the head, for these, in their own way, are considered to reflect aspects of a person's state of being that are open to change.

Research

St John's hypothesis that disorders of childhood and adulthood are traceable to experiences in the womb was timely. For example, according to the psychiatrist Myron Hofer of New York's Montefiore Hospital, recent experiments with animals indicate that, contrary to accepted opinion, "prenatal exposure to alcohol, methadone, heroin, major tranquillizers, barbiturates and amphetamines all have been shown to produce long-term effects on the behaviour of offspring, whether juvenile or adult, weeks and months after the intrauterine period of exposure to these substances". The presumption must be that prenatal exposure to such substances could have similar effects on humans, and there is

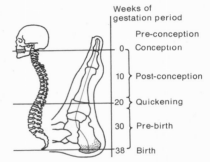

Chart of the prenatal pattern
Devised by Robert St John, the chart correlates the weeks of the prenatal or gestation period with the corresponding areas of the foot, which in turn reflect the spinal vertebrae. The dotted line running laterally down the foot represents the position of the spine reflexes.

Using metamorphic technique

During a typical session, the practitioner sees him or herself as a catalyst using the spinal reflexes of your feet, head and hands as supporting matter for "loosening the prenatal pattern". The aim is not to "massage" these parts of the body but to use them as a focus for the fingers, using probing, vibrating or circular movements, with or without pressure.

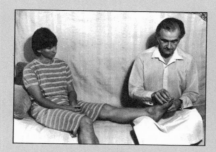

1 *Working on the prenatal pattern, the practitioner starts on the outer side of the big toe and goes down the side of the first and second bones, then on to the foot itself.*

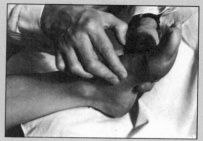

2 *He proceeds on along the side of the bones in the main part of the foot down to below your anklebone.*

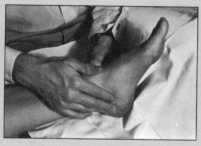

3 *The practitioner will then concentrate on the whole of the side of the heel from the point where the Achilles tendon meets the top of the heel bone.*

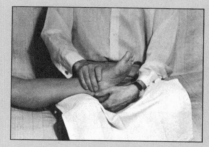

4 *From time to time he works from below the inner side of the anklebone, right across the ankle to a point below the outer side anklebone and back again.*

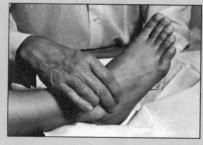

5 *After the ankle, the practitioner goes up and down along the bony ridge on the top of the foot.*

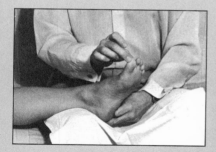

6 *Working on the conceptual pattern involves using vibrating movements or simply holding the top and upper parts of the first phalange or bone of the big toe.*

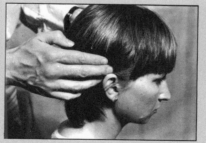

7 *The practitioner stands behind you to work on the head, moving his hands up and down in a straight line from the top down to the base of the skull and along each side towards the ears.*

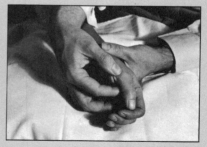

8 *Working on the hands helps release the patient's innate ability to change, started by the work on the feet. The practitioner strokes from the tip of the thumb down its outer edge as far as the wrist.*

now a growing volume of evidence that it does. Metamorphic therapists suspect, however, that it is not just what the mother consumes by way of drugs which can affect the future health of the child, but that her state of mind may also influence it.

Stress and the unborn child

In a recent issue of *Psychology Today*, Charles Spezzano has provided a case history of a healthy 17-year old who gave birth to an apparently healthy baby, which died within 24 hours. The post-mortem revealed the child had three peptic ulcers, and as they are so often stress-related, the doctors surmised that the stress might have been in the mind of the mother. In fact, this young girl's pregnancy had been "extraordinarily stressful. Coerced by her parents into marriage, she had found that her husband was violent, and when she had left him to go back to her parents, he had continued to pester her, eventually throwing a brick through her window, so that the police had to be called in".

This might be coincidental, but Spezzano cites some of the research which has been in progress in this field, including a 20-year study by the psychologist Denis H. Stott in Scotland and in Canada. At the conclusion of his Scottish survey, Stott reported that there was no clear relationship between the children's health and accidents or illnesses of their mothers during pregnancy – or even with severe shocks which the mothers had suffered. "On the other hand, stresses following severe, continual personal tension (in particular marital discord) were closely associated with child morbidity in the form of ill-health, neurological dysfunction, developmental lag and behaviour disturbance".

A great deal more research will need to be done, workers in this area agree, before the picture becomes clear, but it is obvious that the period of development in the womb can no longer be neglected in any search for the causes of unaccountable symptoms.

It is at this point, however, that any corroboration of St John's theories by research ends. For the metamorphic technique claims that there are pre-conceptual and what it calls "non-material" influences (as well as genetic influences) also at work, shaping our futures. Furthermore, the whole *raison d'être* of the technique is that it provides a means of setting right what went awry before birth – the practitioner acting as catalyst for the patient's own power of life to bring about healing. Seen from this view, not even genetic disorders are irreversible.

Suitable cases

Originally designed to help children handicapped from birth, the metamorphic technique has given results which have encouraged its practitioners to extend it "to all persons who are anxious to change themselves for the better".

Primal therapy/rebirthing

The basic assumption of primal therapy is that certain unmet needs of an unborn child or infant cause pain, which if allowed to remain subconsciously festering can give rise to trouble in later life (as repressions of other kinds also can). The aim of primal therapy is to come to terms with and release these pains.

Origins

In his book, *Through Pediatrics to Psycho-analysis*, British pediatrician and psychoanalyst, Donald W. Winnicott, described how, contrary to the strict Freudian principles which he had been conditioned to follow in his training shortly before the First World War, he allowed a patient to act out his feelings. Winnicott observed that the patient behaved in ways which suggested that he was replaying his role at the time of his birth – first going into the fetal position, and then making convulsive movements as if involved in labour. Similar episodes followed with a woman patient who sometimes even fell off the couch, prompting Winnicott to surmise that this represented her unconscious need "to relive the birth process: a performance that she repeated on several occasions". Winnicott realized that the details and even the exact sequence of her birth was being "relived", until eventually the patient worked the experience out of her system as it were, reemerging "with the true self instead of the false self in action".

The significance of this form of acting-out was realized in Britain by Michael Balint, the most influential psychoanalyst in the years following the Second World War; other major contributions to the importance of birth and the effects of pre-birth experiences on healthy development have since been made by a variety of people. R.D. Laing, for example, who was at one time a pupil of Winnicott, introduced the idea of "implantation trauma", that may be experienced by the fertilized ovum as it struggles to secure itself to the wall of the womb. And French obstetrician, Frederick Leboyer, has stressed the importance of those first few minutes outside the womb urging that the new-born should be able to "bond" with the mother, and not be rudely taken away and exposed to a world of noise and bright lights.

Primal therapy as it is practised today therefore involves various techniques and methods devised to deal with the traumas of conception, implantation, birth and infancy. Based on the belief that patterns our lives take are evolved way back in these early days, the aim is to bring patients back to these times to discover and eradicate the root cause of their problems.

Janov and the primal scream

The person, though, whose name is probably the most associated with primal therapy – he really popularized the idea of using

The history of man for the nine months preceding birth would, probably, be far more interesting and contain events of greater moment than all the three score and ten years that follow it.

Samuel Taylor Coleridge
(1772–1834)

cathartic techniques to re-experience infancy and birth traumas – is Arthur Janov, a Los Angeles psychiatrist. Treating a young man for neurosis, Janov persuaded him to shout out "Mommy, Daddy, Mommy, Daddy" repeating the words until he heard something which was to change the course of his life: "an eerie scream welling up from the depths of a young man lying on the floor during a therapy session" which could be likened "only to what one might hear from a person about to be murdered".

Telling this story in the introduction to his formative work, *The Primal Scream*, Janov explained that it had given him the clue to what had been missing in the treatment of neurosis. The scream came from "primal pain" – the pain arising from the "major primal scene", the critical episode in an infant's life when it first realizes that its parents are denying it its basic needs, and frustrating its natural development. Primal therapy consists of helping the patient to relive primal scenes until the "primal pool" ("the inner reservoir of primal pains", as Janov described it in a second book, *The Primal Revolution*) has been systematically emptied out, "dismantling all the patient's defences, leaving only a real self".

After the publication of *The Primal Scream*, groups of Janov's followers began to split from him, and when in 1973 the first meeting of the International Primal Association (IPA) was held in Montreal, it was under the direction of its founder, William Swartley, whose method of primal integration is much broader in its approach and techniques than Janov's.

Re-experiencing birth
This woman had been born two months premature and would have died but for the sudden intervention of two doctors. The rebirthing process helped her to understand the trauma of her birth and overcome her feelings of rage and resentment.

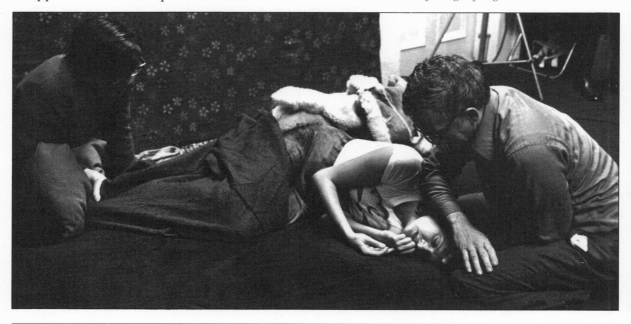

Procedure

In view of the way in which primal therapy has been developing, it is not easy to predict what you can expect if you opt to try it. There are basically four techniques in use to bring you to a primal or rebirthing experience: hypnotic age regression, in which the therapist gradually takes you back in time until you encounter the moments of trauma; psycholitic methods using psychedelics such as LSD (now, of course, on the whole discarded, because illegal); simulation of the birth experience; or breathing. You can expect to spend about 30 hours of therapy spread over six months in individual or group sessions. Most primal work now centres around the birth experience rather than infancy.

Janov's patients have to commit themselves to a full course – usually three weeks of intensive work with a single therapist in order to get back to the "primal scream," which "comes out in shuddering gasps, pushed out by the force of years of suppression and denials of that feeling". This is followed by around 75 group sessions of three hours apiece.

Another and different version of rebirthing focuses on reliving not the birth experience but the first breath taken in the midst of the pain of birth. To Leonard Orr, its originator, rebirthing is healing the breath, learning that breathing (and hence life itself) is not painful but pleasurable. The procedure has been described by Anne Dominique Bindschedler in her contribution to a recent symposium on "birth and rebirth" in the journal *Self and Society*: "The rebirthee lies down and relaxes in the presence of a trained rebirther and works with a simple method of breathing. He is encouraged to keep breathing whatever happens (one wants to stop breathing when some deep feelings arise). In the rebirthing process the rebirthee notices the pain or any other emotion, without 'getting lost in it' . . . but without suppressing it either".

"As the rebirthee relaxes, he experiences physical vibrating sensations (tingling) and the dissolving of the tensions and negative emotions stored in the body. This may last one to three hours". But to actually break the power of the birth trauma may take any number of sessions, from one to one hundred.

Suitable cases

Whilst Janov might claim that primal therapy is *the* cure for neurosis and mental illness, the late Frank Lake, a psychiatrist, has described various diseases whose origins he found could be traced back to perinatal experiences. These include migraine, asthma, depression, claustrophobia, schizophrenia, and hysteria.

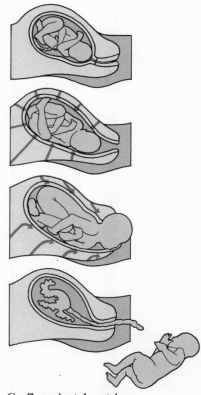

Grof's perinatal matrices
Through work with primal therapy, Stanislav Grof noticed how often life-traumas followed a basic pattern which he found to relate to four stages in our birth and pre-birth experiences. The first stage is associated with the "blissful" pre-birth stage; the second stage, a feeling of a crushing or closing-in, occurs during the initial stages of contraction; the third stage, the struggle for survival is associated with the baby's passage through the birth canal; the final stage is the separation of the baby from the mother – the culmination of the traumatic experience of birth.

TRANSPERSONAL PSYCHOLOGY

Carl Jung used to say that for some people, life's goal is adjustment and normality, but for others, this is boring, and they crave transcendence. These "metaneeds" as Abraham Maslow called them, are catered for in transpersonal psychology, the "fourth force" in modern psychology.

Transpersonal experience has so far eluded attempts to describe it, though Maslow did his best in his book *The Psychology of Being*. The aim of transpersonal psychology is to allow for the development of mystical, spiritual and psychic experience, not as an end in itself, to contribute to the store of human potential.

It follows that many of the disciplines from which transpersonal psychology draws cannot reasonably be regarded as therapies. In *Transpersonal Psychologies*, the massive survey edited by Charles T. Tart, Professor of Psychology at the University of California (Davis), some of the "psychologies" discussed could better be described as faiths or philosophies. These include sufism, buddhism and zen buddhism, along with essays on Gurdjieff's teachings and the arica training, all of which we feel lie outside this book's scope.

The term "transpersonal psychology", even more than is the case with humanistic psychology, can be used to embrace a multitude of groups, and it is even harder to deal with them here, because not many of them actually offer therapy. They come closer to offering new or different approaches to life, the assumption being that if the particular way which is being advocated and taught is properly learned and followed, good health, or at least greatly improved health, will result. These groups may also be only one step (or less) removed from being religious cults, or sects – or simply rackets. Some actually go that way, on occasion with appalling consequences, as in the 1978 Jonestown massacre (in which over 400 black and white Californians, followers of the self-styled Marxist social philosopher, the Reverend Jim Jones, committed ritual suicide in Guyana).

Psychosynthesis

Practitioners of psychosynthesis attempt to harmonize the main aim of western psychology – the creation of a functioning, healthy personality – with the aspiration of eastern philosophies, the exploration of higher levels of consciousness.

Origins

The founding father of psychosynthesis was the Italian psychiatrist Roberto Assagioli, whose doctoral thesis, written before the

First World War had been on psychoanalysis. Having studied under Eugen Bleuler in Zurich, Assagioli returned to Italy, broke with Freudian traditions and began to develop his own ideas, and though he set up an institute in Rome to promote these ideas, the disapproval of the authorities under Mussolini during the Second World War prevented him from disseminating his theories until much later when further institutes were established, for example, in the United States, Greece and England.

Shortly before his death in 1974, Assagioli was interviewed for *Psychology Today* by Sam Keen. He explained how his theory departs from Freud's and resembles Jung's, in that it concentrates less on the morbid symptoms of supposed disorder, and more on remedying temporary malfunctioning in a fundamentally healthy organism. "Nature is always trying to re-establish harmony, and within the psyche the principle of synthesis is dominant", Assagioli claimed. "The task of therapy is to aid the individual in transforming the personality, and integrating apparent contradictions".

The role of the conscious will

In psychosynthesis, however, more attention is paid than in Jungian or other forms of psychotherapy to the role of the conscious will, "the Cinderella of modern psychology", as Assagioli described it, which has been "relegated to the kitchen". One of the unfortunate results of Freud's discoveries about the importance of unconscious motivation was that it had led to a new determinism, whereas Assagioli believed that freedom of the will, and the ability to exercise that freedom, are crucial.

❛ . . . Psychosynthesis . . . aims to build a personality which is free from emotional blocks, has command over all its functions, and a clear awareness of its own centre. On the transpersonal level, it enables the individual to explore those regions full of mystery and wonder, beyond our ordinary awareness, which we call the superconscious, the wellspring of higher intuitions, inspirations, ethical imperatives, and states of illumination. ❜

British Psychosynthesis and Education Trust

1 The Lower Unconscious
2 The Middle Unconscious
3 The Higher Unconscious or Superconscious
4 The Field of Consciousness
5 The Conscious Self or I
6 The Transpersonal Self
7 The Collective Unconscious

Psychosynthesis: the psychic structure
The oval represents the three layers of the unconscious and the circle represents the field of consciousness. Beyond the oval is Jung's "collective unconscious". The broken lines indicate that the sections are not totally self-contained, as movement occurs continually between different parts. Psychosynthesis has central to it the idea that the Conscious Self (5) is directly connected to the Transpersonal Self (6), which is the deeper identity, and that these are simply two aspects of the same entity.

This is not, however, just a matter of will-*power*, in the usual sense. "Strength is a necessary but not sufficient condition of the will", he told Keen. "It is equally important to develop a skilful will and a good will". In particular, psychosynthesis teaches the need to use the "skilful will" in conjunction with, not in opposition to, the imagination. It is no use somebody with an obsession concentrating on getting rid of it by willing it to go away: he or she must use the imagination to find and cultivate a new interest – a different, beneficient, "obsession".

Procedure

Whereas the techniques that you will find used in a psychosynthesis course may not be peculiar to psychosynthesis – they may include painting, working with imagery, self-images, movement and keeping a diary – their employment within a particular treatment framework is. A course in psychosynthesis will aim to guide you through four distinct phases of inner work and development as set out by Assagioli:
● Thorough knowledge of one's personality.
● Control of its various elements.
● Realization of one's true self – the discovery or creation of a unifying centre . . .
● Psychosynthesis: the formation or reconstruction of the personality around the new centre.
And you may expect to find that these phases are realized by focusing the techniques around three main activities: the improvement of the will by stretching the imagination; the development of creativity by the transformation of what are termed "biopsychic energies" (for example, sexual and aggressive energies); and bringing into consciousness, awareness of the superconscious and harnessing its energies.

Suitable cases

While Assagioli's own roots were in psychoanalysis, today's practitioners of psychosynthesis are not, on the whole, trained in this field, and their approach is consequently less oriented towards the treatment of neuroses. Anyone interested in pursuing personal growth – whether spiritual or psychological – can try a course of psychosynthesis; it is also considered to be of particular benefit to those suffering from the problems of modern living, whether in dealing with physical manifestations of stress such as migraine and the like, or with emotional problems arising from relationships. Considerable success has also been reported in the treatment of phobias. Those in the caring professions – doctors, lawyers, teachers, – who want to develop communication skills may also find the courses beneficial.

PARANORMAL THERAPIES

Paranormal therapies assume the existence of psychic or supernatural forces. The usual distinction which is made between these forces is that "supernatural" implies the existence of a being, or beings, capable of overturning or modifying the laws of nature, whereas "psychic" carries the implication that the forces, though they may appear to be contrary to natural laws, are simply unexplained, as yet, and will be found to be natural.

Exploiting extrasensory perception

Some natural therapists accept the existence of extrasensory perception (ESP). The *Silva mind control* method, for example, is one that, to some extent relies on it (see pages 176 to 178). But here we have dealt with the therapies in two main categories. One part of this section deals with a variety of techniques which are based on the belief that there is a healing force or forces which can be tapped for healing purposes. The belief is that this force can be channelled, through individuals who have the ability to tap it, to people in need. Included here, then, is a resumé of the history of healing, from ancient tribal origins, through techniques approved by the established Church, to *Christian Science*, *Spiritualist healing* and *Therapeutic touch*.

In the other main type of therapy, described here as *Radionics and radiesthesia*, a variety of equipment (from the simple, pendulum used in radiesthesia, to sophisticated radionic machinery) is used for exploiting ESP for diagnosis and treatment.

Also included in this paranormal category, though a little apart from the rest, are *Past lives therapy*, which stems from belief in reincarnation, and *Psychic surgery*, which revives shamanist healing methods.

Faith Healing

Before surveying the various types of paranormal therapies, perhaps we should take a look at "faith healing", which is still the common, colloquial term for healing in general. This term is not, however, used by practitioners of healing, who feel it is misleading, because they believe that the healing force may work, and often does, without any faith in it on the part of the patient. This does not mean that they dismiss the possibility of faith as a factor in the healing process. But it cannot be distinguished from the psychological element as displayed in hypnosis and autosuggestion. This point of view was put by Jean-Martin Charcot, the French neurologist who, shortly before his death in 1893, sought to convince the medical profession to accept faith healing, as they had accepted hypnosis.

Charcot argued that cures result from a combination of confidence, credulity and receptivity to suggestion: "the instantaneous cure produced directly by faith healing, which is commonly known in medicine by the name of "miracle" is, as may be shown in the majority of cases, a natural phenomenon which is produced at all times, in the most different levels of civilization, and among the most varied religions".

Charcot, however, went too fast and too far for medical orthodoxy. He believed that faith healing could cure all forms of neurological illness, including multiple sclerosis; he even thought it could cure cancer. The medical profession settled for a compromise: faith healing could successfully be used in the treatment of functional disorders, but not organic ones.

Although "faith healing" remains the common colloquial description of healing in general, it is not practised under this name. Nor is it likely to be, so long as healers repudiate it, and psychologists continue to believe that suggestion, autosuggestion and placebo-effect are an adequate explanation for successful results. Christians may continue to believe in it, on the basis of Jesus's teaching ("thy faith hath made thee whole"), and it can be loosely used to describe what goes on at Lourdes and other such places of pilgrimage, but you are unlikely to find therapists describing themselves as faith healers.

The healing force
Most healers consequently call themselves, simply, healers; some add the qualification "spiritual". Although their methods vary, they have in common a belief in the existence of a healing force which can be channelled through them to patients. Some believe it to be divine, coming from God. Others surmise that it is natural, like magnetism or electricity, but not yet recognized by science, and described it as "psychic", "paranormal" or "paraphysical".

Until very recently healers had little contact with the practitioners of other forms of natural medicine, and even less with the medical profession. There is now, however, a greater (though still grudging) readiness on the part of scientists to admit the possibility of paranormal forces. As Britain's Healing Research Trust recently pointed out, the discoveries of the quantum physicists have made it possible to award healing a measure of scientific respectability. "The ultimate cause of physical illness is seen as arising very often at a paraphysical level and, in order to eliminate it, it is necessary to treat it at that level instead of, or in addition to, providing treatment at the physical level".

The hypothesis is that healers have something in their "energy fields" which is capable of interacting with, and replenishing, the "energy fields" of patients. How this happens remains a mystery, but the admission that it does happen begins to make sense of therapies which have been reported in every era of history.

Tribal origins
Most of the techniques employed by healers today have been described by explorers and anthropologists studying tribal cus-

toms of early civilizations. Almost all the tribes whose customs and beliefs have been studied, have taken for granted the existence of a paraphysical force, a kind of bio-magnetism.

Of the many names for this bio-magnetism, perhaps the most familiar is *mana* of the Pacific islanders. In itself the force is generally held to be neutral, but it can be used for good or ill by the gods and the spirits, and also by certain individuals who in our society would be described as psychics, mediums or sensitives.

Witch doctors, shamans and medicine men

The tribal shaman or medicine man (he was usually male) was ordinarily selected because, in childhood or adolescence, he showed that he had the ability to tap *mana*. He could demonstrate this in two main ways. Firstly, he could display second sight or clairvoyance which among other things, such as telling where game was plentiful, he could use both to diagnose the cause of illness and to prescribe treatment. Secondly, he could exhibit psychokinetic prowess, for example, by levitating or causing objects to materialize or dematerialize.

To exercise his powers, he usually had to enter a trance state in which he appeared to be possessed by a spirit, which would send him into convulsions before taking over and talking through him in a voice not his own. Or he might go off into a dream-like condition from which, when he awoke, he would be able to describe what the spirits had shown or told him, including diagnosis of sickness.

Examining entrails
A witchdoctor in Sumatra employs his powers of second sight as he examines the entrails before a tribal feast.

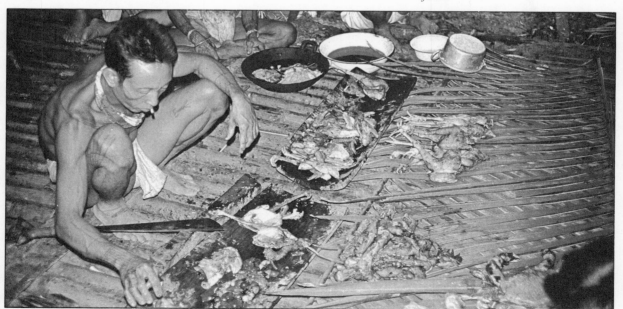

The shaman was expected to function exclusively for the tribe's benefit. Sorcerers or witches were members of the tribe who were suspected of having psychic powers, but of exploiting them for their own selfish, and usually malign, purposes. The tendency consequently was for illness to be attributed either to the spirits or to sorcery. One of the shaman's jobs was to use his powers of second sight (or second smell, Rider Haggard described Gagool "smelling out" witches in *King Solomon's Mines*), to identify sorcerers. He would also, where necessary, use his psychokinetic powers to dematerialize a foreign body which, it was assumed, a sorcerer had caused to materialize in chosen victims.

Religion in tribal communities

The shaman was transformed into the even more powerful prophet with the development of religion in tribal communities. Henceforth he held that his authority came not from the tribe but from the tribal god, as Moses did. Paradoxically this meant that he largely ceased to practise healing. If illness was an indication of divine displeasure, as was assumed by the Greeks in Homer's time and by the Old Testament Israelites, it seemed futile, and indeed wicked, to try to thwart the will of Zeus (or Jehovah) by trying to cure sick people.

It was only when Jesus taught his disciples and showed them, by his example, that people could be restored to the faith by curing their diseases, or restored to health by reviving their faith, that healing was brought back to occupy a central position in the new religion. The Holy Spirit was a form of *mana*, directed by God through Jesus to his disciples for the early Christians, and healing came to be regarded as one of the disciples' most important duties.

Medicine becomes separated from healing

With the introduction in the Middle Ages of a Church with a hierarchy and a priesthood, however, Pentecost-type healing came to be looked upon by the Church authorities with suspicion. In trance states, they feared, the convulsions, the "speaking in tongues" and the healing powers might be a sign that the healer was possessed not by the Holy Spirit but by the Devil, seducing him with such gifts, inflating his pride, and encouraging him to form a breakaway heretical sect. Trances came to be frowned upon. The Holy Spirit was relegated to the role of a shadowy third member of the Trinity. The practice of medicine was handed over to physicians.

The physicians were not healers in the early Christian tradition. They practised medicine from the book – from the texts of Galen and other classical authorities, using bleeding, purging and drugs. "Medicine" and "healing" consequently became two distinct forms of therapy, which rarely overlapped. Physicians came

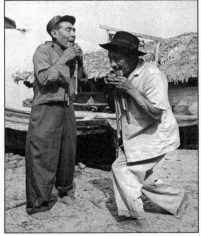

Witch doctors
Tribal shamans or witch doctors still exist in many parts of the world. Here a shaman from Carti Island, one of the San Blas Islands, plays his reed pipe to dispel the spirits.

utterly to reject healing, particularly when it was mixed up with occult practices, astrology and magic, charms and incantations. At a humble level, it continued everywhere, particularly in rural areas, but a healer who became too well-known ran the risk of being hounded in a witch-hunt.

By the Middle Ages, healing as a day-to-day therapeutic method had ceased to be practised by the clergy, and Christians who found they had healing powers were discouraged from using them, at least publicly.

Absent healing

The Christian healing tradition lingered on in ritual: the "laying on of hands" became formalized, and prayers for the sick (also sometimes called absent healing) in churches were introduced. As the name implies, absent healing consists of any form of healing which is undertaken at a distance from the patient. But many healers believe that healing forces can be transmitted without calling upon a divine intermediary.

Formal pleas to God or the saints to intervene, therefore, were substituted for the direct transmission of the Holy Spirit's healing force, through the hands of the healer.

There were, however, a couple of types of healing which were permitted under the Church authorities' watchful eye: visits to healing shrines and exorcism.

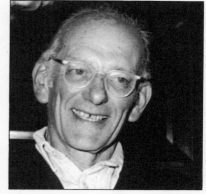

Sir Francis Chichester
When Chichester was diagnosed as having lung cancer in an advanced stage, his wife refused to allow him to have surgery. She took him instead to a nature cure establishment and organized absent healing, rallying people of all faiths to pray for him. The results proved miraculous and less than three years later, Francis Chichester won the first solo transatlantic yacht race.

Healing shrines

If priests, nuns, monks or lay Christians began to earn a massive reputation as miracle workers during their lifetimes, they were held to constitute a risk to the authority of the Church even if of unquestioned holiness; they might, after all, eventually succumb to the sin of pride. As a result, individuals who are said to possess miraculous powers have been subjected to rigid discipline – right down to the celebrated "Padre Pio" in recent times.

As soon as they die, however, it is a very different matter. Whenever reports reach the Vatican of healing miracles occurring at some tomb, the practice is to investigate them and, if the evidence seems clear, to allow the Church connected with the shrine to exploit the reports in order to attract pilgrims. If the healing miracles continue, the traffic is later encouraged, and the dead person, the presumed sponsor of the miracles, is beatified and often later canonized, on the assumption that he or she is out of the Devil's reach.

Though new shrines become popular periodically, there are a few which have been centres for pilgrimages for many generations.

Lourdes, the main healing centre

Easily the best known of these centres is Lourdes, in southern France, where in 1858 the young Bernadette Soubirous had her vision of the Virgin Mary. As usual in such cases, the Vatican initially discouraged what it feared was a dangerous tendency towards hysteria, when stories spread of the healing powers of the water from a hidden spring which Bernadette had discovered in a cave. This official lack of enthusiasm was not surprising as the waters did not benefit Bernadette herself; she remained in chronic ill-health until she died at the age of thirty-five. But with pilgrims arriving in ever-increasing numbers, the pressure became too strong. And the fact that Bernadette herself made no attempt to exploit her fame, preferring the life of a devout nun, calmed Vatican fears. Lourdes quickly became, and has remained, the Church's major healing centre, though there are others –

Pilgrims at Lourdes
In 1858 Saint Bernadette received 18 visions of the Virgin Mary at the Massabielle Rock, Lourdes. Since that time it has become a major Catholic shrine and healing centre. Saint Bernadette was beatified in 1925 and canonized in 1933.

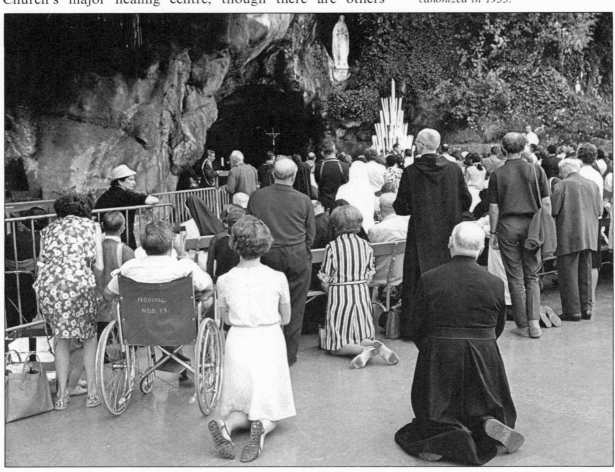

Compostela in Spain, Knock in Ireland – and new ones appear from time-to-time.

Procedure

Most pilgrims visit Lourdes on organized tours, by air, rail or coach, and what happens when they arrive is laid down for them in brochures and by their organizers. They may, however, also express a personal intensity of devotion to the Blessed Virgin in a variety of ways, such as walking barefoot around the Stations of the Cross (the representation of stages in Christ's journey to Calvary). The seriously ill and the crippled are wheeled to baths which have been constructed to contain the flow from the spring Bernadette found. An effort is made to create an atmosphere conducive to acceptance of the possibility of divine miracles, notably by the promenade round the floodlit town at night, with each pilgrim holding a candle. Some visitors, however, find the daytime contrast – all the Bernadette mementoes – unedifying.

The possibility of disappointment

It has often been argued that, as a pilgrimage to Lourdes or any other healing shrine is primarily intended as a religious experience, which may or may not have incidental therapeutic benefits, it ought not to be regarded simply on the basis of its results, measured statistically in terms such as "improvement" or "no change". But as Dr Leslie Weatherhead pointed out in his compassionate *Psychology, Religion and Healing*, as no more than two out of every hundred pilgrims can be expected to report significant benefit, the decision whether or not to encourage patients to go to Lourdes needs to take into consideration the possible consequences of their reaction to disappointment. The effect of losing hope, as he found when he travelled with a group in a train, can be saddening. "On the way down through France they were sure they were going to be better", but as their time in Lourdes ran out, hope began to die. On the journey back, none complained, or grumbled, "but the pathos in the eyes was terrible and the depression hard indeed to overcome. Many patients not only went back home with the last hope gone; it must have been a severe shock to their Christian faith".

Research

One aspect at least of the healing at Lourdes can justifiably be claimed as uncommonly carefully researched. Disturbed at the possibility that false claims would be made of miraculous cures, the Vatican set up a Lourdes International Medical Bureau, which doctors with an interest in the subject (not necessarily Catholics) were invited to join. As members, they were free to examine the records of pilgrims, to investigate individual cases, and submit reports. The records are consequently very detailed and extensive.

There has always been a problem, however: the lack of any agreement on how to distinguish between healing which can be attributed either to coincidence, suggestion and auto-suggestion on the one hand, and healing which can be attributed to actual divine intervention.

Defining miracles

In the eighteenth century, Pope Benedict XIV laid down a set of guidelines (which have since been made more rigorous) which were designed to restrict the use of the term "miraculous" in connection with cures: the disease must be extremely serious; there must be no question of coincidental recovery for other reasons – such as earlier medical treatment beginning to take effect; the recovery must be very sudden, and complete; and there must be no relapse. In addition, any case which is held by doctors to fulfil all these conditions must then be submitted to the scrutiny of a committee of specialists convened for the purpose. But so stringent are the conditions that very few cases qualify for this final vetting, and fewer still pass it – on average, fewer than one every two years.

Whether or nor miraculous cures have taken place at Lourdes has remained a matter for controversy. In his *Eleven Lourdes Miracles*, Dr D.J. West, having examined them, claimed that in none of them was the evidence entirely convincing. Other investigators, looking at the record as a whole, have taken the opposite view. What cannot be disputed is that even if the number of cures which pass the committees' scrutiny is very small, scores of people return from pilgrimages every year convinced that they have greatly benefitted. If their symptoms have disappeared, they may reasonably feel that the issue whether or not the cure was miraculous is academic.

Suitable cases

Most patients attending Lourdes or other shrines have disorders which their doctors have pronounced untreatable, or which have not responded to treatment. The assumption must be that most of them are Catholics, and that they go in hope, if not expectation, of a "miracle", or at least some alleviation. But there have been occasional accounts of sceptics benefitting – including one of a communist who had lost his childhood faith. While watching a badly crippled girl being dipped in the baths, he was moved to pray for her. His prayer had no effect on her, but to his astonishment, the symptoms of an illness from which he himself was suffering disappeared.

Exorcism

The only form of healing in which a living priest has been expected to use methods other than those laid down in the liturgy is in treating cases of what are taken to be diabolic possession, along the lines described in St Mark's gospel, when Jesus cast out an evil spirit which had possessed a boy. "The spirit cried, and rent him sore, and came out of him", leaving the boy as if dead; he quickly recovered. The prayers and rituals are still designed, in the Anglican as well as the Catholic church, for the same purpose.

Trespassing spirits

Writing in the *Journal of the Royal Society of Medicine* recently, Chancellor the Reverend E. Garth Moore has described exorcism as presupposing "the existence of God; the existence of non-material entities, commonly called spirits, and that spirits are sometimes trespassers in a place where they ought not to be." The assumption is that the trespasser is either a "pure" spirit, or the spirit of a deceased person, and that the "trespass" may be either in a place, haunting, or in a person, possession. These trespasses, Moore explains, being contrary to God's will, "can be terminated by the power of God. It is this termination which is called exorcism".

With the decline in belief in diabolic possession after the Renaissance, belief in the value of exorcism also dwindled. But recently it has sprung up again, particularly in the Anglican Church. Dr Coggan (then Archbishop of Canterbury) in the *York Report* laid down that exorcism is permissible because so many people "are so within the grip of the power of evil that they need the aid of the Christian Church in delivering them from it", permissible, that is, so long as it is performed only by clergy licensed by their bishop, working in collaboration with doctors.

This view did not meet with general approval in Anglican circles. Twenty theologians wrote to complain that it was at variance "with the entire history and tradition of the Church of England". Most dioceses, however, now have an exorcist, and many have a number of clergymen who are prepared to investigate cases of apparent possession, and to perform the appropriate rites. The majority of the cases, however, are of haunted houses, rather than of possession of individuals.

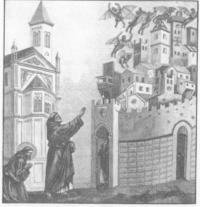

St Francis of Assisi
St Francis of Assisi orders a monk to cast out the devils from Arezzo.

Procedure

The old Christian ritual to drive demons from the afflicted person is still the basis for exorcism. After fasting, prayer and communion, if they are practicable, the ceremony is performed, preferably in a church, according to the rites of that church. What happens in the course of the ceremony is dictated largely by the reaction of the possessed person, or the possessing "demon", which may be violent.

Research

No systematic research has been carried out into the effects of exorcism. Sceptics stress the many examples of its failure, notably in the case of poltergeist hauntings, and also the occasional examples of destructive consequences: for example, a Bavarian girl, suffering from epilepsy, died following exorcism.

Suitable cases

When treating mental illness, some agnostic psychologists are willing to concede that exorcism can work when orthodox methods have failed, in cases where the combination of the ritual and the exorcist's personality are able to make a powerful enough impression. This is not because devils are driven out, they argue, but simply because the occasion administers such a powerful jolt to the patients' imaginations, that they recover – much as a despairing kick sometimes starts up a faulty TV set.

Exorcism at work
Exorcism is based on Jesus' "casting out" of evil spirits. Acting on the old Christian ritual, a vicar is seen here in church, driving out demons from an afflicted girl.

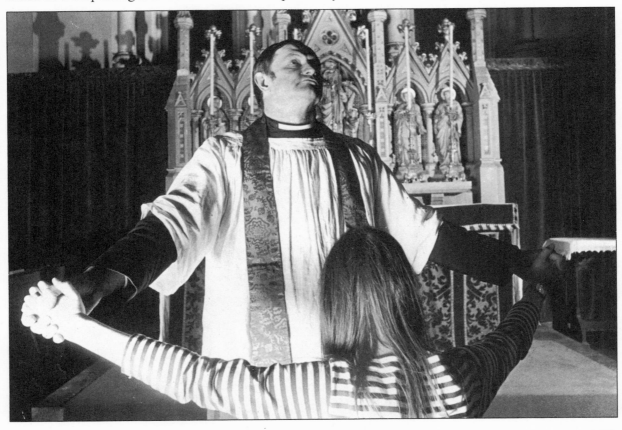

Protestant healing

Most of the Protestant churches have some form of ritual in connection with healing, whether it be prayers for sick people at Sunday services, or a special bedside service for an individual.

Origins

The founders of Protestantism had little inclination to restore healing to the position it had occupied in the early Christian Church, because under Rome it had become identified with the very practices that they were rebelling against – such as the sale of bogus, health-giving relics, and the exploitation of healing shrines. Healing came to be regarded as a deal between the sick person and God. Prayers for the sick and bedside services were designed to bring invalids to God's attention, as it were, in the hope that he would relent and permit them to recover. They were not designed to summon up a healing, Pentecostal-type force – except in some of the small Pentecostal-based sects.

The idea of miraculous healing, in fact, was eventually almost totally rejected by Protestants. By the mid-eighteenth century, the historian W.E.H. Lecky could report that "nearly all educated men receive an account of a miracle taking place in their own day with an absolute and even derisive incredulity that dispenses with all examination of the evidence". Even Protestant bishops and theologians agreed that it must be the renewal of faith of the sick which could bring about their recovery, rather than the holy spirit's healing force.

In the present century, interest in spiritual healing along New Testament lines has revived in the Anglican Church. Initially, this was largely because of irritation at the way in which Christ's healing power was being exploited by the Christian Scientists (see pages 237 to 239). But any chance of the revival spreading throughout the Church was blocked, as it is to this day, by the refusal of the medical establishment to accept healing, coupled with the reluctance of the Anglican establishment to risk a confrontation with the profession on the issue.

The attitude of the medical establishment

Twice, shortly before the First World War, and again shortly after the Second, commissions of inquiry were set up in Britain to look into what, if anything, could be done to facilitate the resumption of "the Church's Healing Mission", as it is commonly known. Both times, the representatives of the British Medical Association politely but firmly squashed the idea that the laying on of hands could have any therapeutic effect, other than through suggestion. This, they insisted, cannot cure organic disease.

As the first of these reports put it, the members of the committee "thankfully recognize that persons suffering from organic disease are greatly comforted and relieved, and even physically benefited, by spiritual ministrations". But healing, "like all treatment by suggestion, can be expected to be permanently effective only in cases of what are generally termed "functional" diseases. The alleged exceptions are so disputable that they cannot be taken into account".

The report following the second investigation, nearly half a century later, followed the same lines as the first, except that by the 1950s the term "functional" (which in effect had meant neurotic or hysterical) had gone out of fashion, and "psychosomatic" had taken its place.

The ministrations of the clergy, it was conceded, might help where the physical symptoms were the result of emotional disturbance. Nevertheless, it concluded, "we have seen no evidence that there is any special type of illness cured solely by spiritual healing which cannot be cured by medical methods which do not involve such claims". Again, the Church's representatives on the committee, though mildly expressing their view that there is more to healing than the report allowed, were not prepared to reject it.

As a result, the Church's organization dedicated to the healing ministry, the Guild of St Raphael, has remained largely impotent. It numbers among it patrons many members of the hierarchy, and states boldly that one of its aims is "to promote the belief that God wills the conquest of disease, as well as sin, through the power of the living Christ". But it reprobates agencies "which make miraculous claims", and emphasizes its full cooperation with the medical profession.

Procedure

As the Church has not dared to assert its independence of the medical profession on this issue, there are only a few members of the clergy who practise healing along the lines of the early Christians – that is to say, working on the assumption that the laying on of hands is not just a ritual, but a way of transmitting the divine healing force supplied by the Holy Spirit. This is usually practised at special healing services. For the most part, clergy think in terms only of performing the appropriate rites, as sanctioned by the Church.

Research

The Church's own investigating committee, The Archibishop's Commission, which was sitting at the same time as the BMA's committee, was clearly a little disgruntled at the latter's verdict. Christian healing, its report insisted, "cannot be completely described in terms of psychological medicine". While it agreed that the kind of scientific testing which the British medical

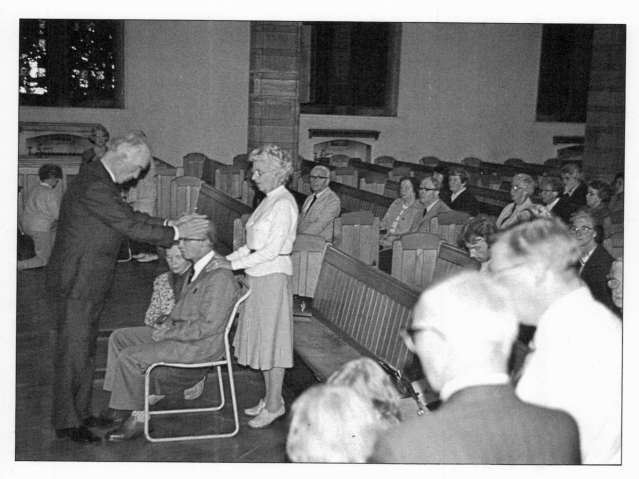

Christian healing
The laying on of hands was a central theme in the healing of the early Christian church and remains so today. The divine healing power is supposed to use the healer as an instrument in reaching the patient.

profession insisted upon could provide a useful corrective for false claims of cures, the report added that it was "idle for the Church, or anyone else, to appeal to science to prove the reality of supernatural power or the truth of theology or metaphysic".

In other words, if God exists, and chooses from time to time to exercise healing power to cure somebody by a miracle, medical science is not qualified either to confirm or deny the miraculous nature of the event. Research of the kind normally undertaken into natural therapies would be considered inappropriate.

Suitable cases

The most that can be said is that those Protestants who feel they are likely to benefit (or have benefitted, on a previous occasion) are the most likely to benefit.

Charismatic healing

A recent development within both Catholic and Protestant churches has been the revival of principles of the kind inculcated by St Paul, and derived from the experience of the disciples at Pentecost, as related in the Bible in "The acts of the apostles".

> *"And suddenly there came a sound from heaven, as of a rushing mighty wind, and it filled all the house where they were sitting.*
> *And there appeared unto them cloven tongues like as of fire, and it sat upon each of them.*
> *And they were all filled with the holy ghost and began to speak in other tongues, as the Spirit gave them utterance".*

Onlookers thought the disciples must be drunk, but St Peter reminded them that they could hardly be, so early in the day. What had happened, he argued, was that the prophecy of the minor Hebrew prophet Joel had been fulfilled: the Holy Spirit had been poured on the faithful, giving them power to prophesy. That is, to speak without conscious thought or control, often in a strange voice or language, as if possessed, and to work miracles, including healing the sick. When a man lame from birth asked for alms as Peter and John were on their way to the temple, Peter made a bold experiment: "Silver and gold I have none", he replied, but "in the name of Jesus Christ of Nazareth stand up and walk". He lifted the man to his feet, "and immediately his feet and ankle bones received strength. And he, leaping up, stood, and walked, and entered with them into the Temple, walking, and leaping, and praising God".

Spirit possession

It is clear from his "Epistles to the Corinthians" that St Paul was a fervent believer in the need for the Holy Spirit to descend on congregations as it had done at Pentecost, and even if the "tongues" might not be easy to understand or interpret, this "spirit possession" was what provided the Christians with their powers of divination and of healing. But caught up as the Christian Church later became in organization, dogma and ritual, Paul's message was later rejected.

From time to time, small sects have harked back to it, as for a while the Society of Friends or Quakers did. But in general, the notion of possession by the Holy Spirit remained out of favour.

The charismatic movement is an attempt to restore the Pentecostal element, at prayer meetings and where permitted in services. The movement is not primarily concerned with healing, so much as with "making whole" but the underlying assumption is that healing forces will be unleashed, and some priests specialize in the healing aspect in ways such as are described by the American Dominican, Francis MacNutt in his books *Healing* and *The Power to Heal*.

Christian science

To its followers, Christian Science is not a therapy but a religion. Today there are over 3,500 Christian Science churches in some 57 countries. However, as Christian Science had its origins in psychic diagnosis as practised by mesmerists (see *Hypnotherapy* pages 166 to 173) and as it can be regarded as a version of *Autosuggestion* (see pages 173 to 176), its implications for natural therapy are worth examining.

Origins

Having seen a mesmerist at work in 1838, Phineas Quimby, a Maine clockmaker, decided to try the technique for himself. He had little success until he encountered a subject who, while in a trance, became clairvoyant and diagnosed that Quimby's back-ache was the result of kidney trouble. The subject then performed the laying on of hands, and Quimby's pain disappeared. Quimby concluded that it must have been his own belief that he was going to be cured that was responsible for the cure, and went on to surmise that his fear that he had serious kidney trouble might have been responsible for his illness. "If I really believed anything", he decided "the effect would follow whether I was thinking it or not".

Putting this principle into practice and convincing people that they could be healed if they believed they could be healed, brought Quimby a big reputation as a healer. In 1861 he successfully treated Mary Patterson, who was to become Mary Baker Eddy, and eventually the founder of Christian Science.

Before she had met him, Mary Baker Eddy had already come to believe that all disease was mind-induced: "If I believe I am sick, I am sick", she had written, "to cure the disease is to correct the error, and as disease is what follows the error, destroy the cause and the effect will cease".

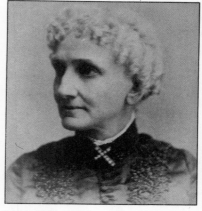

Mary Baker Eddy
Eddy (1821–1910) believed that disease was a consequence of wrong thinking and that by correcting the mind's error a cure would result.

The healing principle

Quimby's healing confirmed Mary Baker Eddy in her belief that it was possible to "correct the error", and cure her own neurasthenia. From this she went on to develop her own theory: that it is not the human mind which cures disease, but the divine mind or God, whom she identified with what she called "the healing principle".

In this belief, Christian Science differs from the traditional Christian attitude to healing. It is not a question of a divine healing force, flowing through the healer's hands. The divine mind is omnipresent, Christian Scientists argue, in and around us all the time. All we need is to have faith in it, tune in to it, and disease will simply disappear. There is no need for a healer, let alone for a doctor, though on occasion a "practitioner" (adviser or counsellor) may be helpful.

Procedure

Christian Science cannot be taken as a therapy in the sense that, say, you can opt for osteopathy or psychosynthesis. The "procedure" is to present yourself at the nearest Church of Christ, Scientist, examine the literature on the subject, and decide whether you would like to become a member.

Research

Christian Scientists have discouraged formal research into the therapeutic benefits of their religion. "Healing physical sickness is the smallest part of Christian Science", Mary Baker Eddy wrote. "The emphatic purpose of Christian Science is the healing of sin". As a current Church manual puts it: "It is a mistake to think of Christian Science as a faith-healing religion. It does not claim to heal sickness, for it claims sickness is an illusion".

Christian Science and longevity

One revealing piece of research, however, was carried out into Christian Science 30 years ago by a sceptical doctor from Seattle, Washington. Irritated by hearing stories of the longevity of its adherents, Dr Gale E. Wilson decided to exploit his post as autopsy surgeon to compare the mortality statistics of Christian Scientists with those of the rest of the community. He was able to do this because, by law, he could investigate the case of anybody who died without a doctor in attendance. He found, as he expected, that the belief that Christian Scientists lived longer was incorrect; there was no significant difference between them and the rest of the population.

Well satisfied with the results of his research, Wilson presented a paper on it to the American Academy of Forensic Sciences in 1956. To his audience, however, his figures came as a disappointment. The period which they covered was the start of the wonder drug era, in which the sulpha drugs, penicillin, and antibiotics had been introduced. If Wilson's sample was representative, it demonstrated that although Christian Scientists had declined to avail themselves of the life-saving new drugs, they had not, in terms of a higher death rate, been any the worse off.

The results of another research project, too, although not directly concerned with Christian Science, clearly have some relevance to it: the investigation of a "denial of illness" reported by Isabelle V. Kendig in the *British Journal of Medical Psychology* in 1963. "Denial of illness" was intended to convey the attitude of people who regard themselves as basically healthy. The results strongly confirmed the hypothesis that such denial, "arising from belief in the integrity of the self and the invulnerability of the body, is associated with the maintenance of health".

Suitable cases

Owing to the Christian Scientists' refusal to divulge information about their membership, it is not easy to find out why people join them. But we were interested to be told by a former member of the Church that in her experience, in Britain at least, "most people who come to Christian Science do so for healing". They do not join for simple reasons of belief, in other words, in the same way they might become a Catholic or a Methodist; they have some form of illness which orthodox medicine (and sometimes also alternative therapy) has been unable to treat effectively. As a result, the role of the "practitioners" has come increasingly to resemble that of a doctor.

Spiritualist healing

One type of Protestantism, though today it is not as a rule described as such, is the Spiritualist movement. Some of its healer members regard themselves as the lineal successors to the early Christians, with their faith in the Holy Spirit as the carrier of the divine healing force. Some of them, however, believe they have a spirit "control" who is their go-between with the spirit of a doctor; the "doctor" provides them with the information they need, for example by clairaudience, and guides their movements.

Healers who accept that their power comes from God, and is mediated by spirits, are variously described as spiritualist healers, spiritual healers or spirit healers.

Origins

From time to time Protestant sects have emerged whose leaders claim that they seek to restore the Pentecostal, spirit-motivated element. The Shakers and the Quakers got their name from the tremors and convulsions they experienced when the Holy Spirit descended upon and possessed them. Healing, however, was usually regarded as a by-product of the Pentecostal manifestations, welcomed when it happened, but not regarded as their mainspring. Although John Wesley believed in the healing power of prayer, he also compiled a book of herbal and other remedies for Methodists.

When spiritualism became a vogue in the middle of the nineteenth century, it was initially a parlour game, with "table-turning" seances in which music played and objects materialized and dematerialized. Later, however, the emphasis switched to communication with the spirits of the departed. Eventually spiritualism acquired a capital "S", as a religious cult, dedicated chiefly to proving that there is an after-life. In the course of their work some mediums, finding that they had healing powers, began to use them – either in healing services in Spiritualist churches, or in their own homes or the homes of friends.

Easily the best-known and most influential healer in Britain in recent times was Harry Edwards, whose career ran from the 1930s to the later 1970s. Asked to give evidence to the Anglican Church's commission in the 1950s he set out his beliefs, and they are still representative of British Spiritualist healers in general – though inevitably individual healers have their own ideas.

The divine healing force

All forms of spiritual healing, Edwards claimed, are the same, coming from God. Healers are obeying Jesus's injunction, also from God, to heal the sick. They do not themselves possess healing powers, but are simply the human instruments through whom the divine plan is carried out with the guidance of God's agents – angels and spirits of the dead – appointed to do his bidding. Healing is *not* "miraculous", in the sense of breaking natural laws. Being God's laws, they "cannot be broken in a favourable discrimination for any person". They take place as part of an ordered procedure, intelligently directed, within the scope of the laws" – spiritual as well as physical.

In the same document, doubtless because Edwards wanted to emphasize the distinction between the Spiritualist point of view and that of the Protestant Church (which in its prayers for the sick appears actually to invite God to intervene in particular cases) he reiterated this belief: "healings do not take place as the result of God's personal intervention on behalf of a favoured individual, over-riding his established laws".

For Spiritualists this point is important. They assume the existence of a divine purpose worked out with, among other things, the help of a divine healing force which can be available to all of us, at any time, through certain human agents. They are chosen much as Jesus's disciples were chosen, because they have the capacity to channel the healing force through themselves into other people. When a healing occurs, therefore, it is not an indication of divine favour; it is simply a further proof that such healing is available to all and sundry, given the individual's desire to be healed.

"Desire", however, is not quite the appropriate term, because it implies consciousness of purpose. This would put Spiritualist healing into the category of psychological healing, through suggestion. Spiritualists believe that there is a latent capacity in people which can be aroused by the divine healing force – even in those who, unaware of the force's existence, scoff at the whole idea of God and spirits.

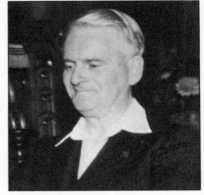

Harry Edwards
The famous British healer Harry Edwards (1893–1976) believed himself to be a medium for healing from the spirit world, with Louis Pasteur and Lord Lister as his spirit guides.

Procedure

Most, though not all, spirit healers go into a trance or altered state of consciousness, but it may be of a kind which is not readily apparent to onlookers, or even to patients. The healers' aim is to make contact with their spirit "guides" – the Spiritualist equivalent of the biblical "guardian angel". The guide may actually possess them, taking over while they are in a trance, so that they do not recall what they have been doing when they come out of it. Or it may simply take over their movements, leaving their minds clear. Or it may give verbal instructions, which the healer picks up by clairaudience and acts upon. Sometimes there is no "guide", no identifiable personality that is manifesting itself to the healer's consciousness. Sometimes the "guide" hands over to another spirit or spirits, who take on the healing function. By analogy, the healer's procedure may be likened to the pilot of an aircraft, either listening to instructions from ground control and putting them into effect, or engaging the automatic pilot, which is itself then operated by ground control – in this instance, spirit control.

Healing services

In many large towns there are Spiritualist meeting places where services are held and people can present themselves for healing. At a service Spiritualist prayers are said, and hymns sung. Instead of a sermon, however, a session with a medium follows, in which members of the congregation are given information about friends and relatives who have passed over. Tea follows, and then those members of the congregation who wish to be treated present themselves to the healer or healers.

Some healers simply place their hands over the patients' heads, or over the affected part of their body. Others employ what looks to be a very gentle form of physiotherapy, as if coaxing arthritic limbs to loosen up. If a healer and patients go into a trance, a Pentecostal atmosphere may be generated.

Spiritual healers constitute by far the largest group of practitioners of natural medicine. The National Federation of Spiritual Healers, which is independent of the Spiritualist movement, has over three thousand members, and there must be thousands more, in other organizations. A great many of the independent practitioners are amateurs, in the sense that they treat only their friends, or people recommended to them by their friends. Because of a tradition that the healing gift will disappear it if is abused for gain, few healers charge a fee, even when the patient is so rich that the temptation to extract money from him or her may be strong. Some will not take money at all; others have the equivalent of a church offertory box, into which grateful patients can put whatever contribution they can afford. Only a few of the well-established healers charge for their time on a pro rata basis.

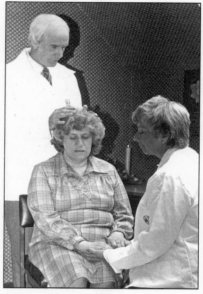

Spiritualist healing
Two practitioners from the National Federation of Spiritualist Healers engaged with their subject at a spiritualist session.

Research

The application of scientific research methods to the investigation of healing was held up for many years by the assumption, common in medical circles, that such success as healers had could be accounted for by either suggestion or coincidence. When Harry Edwards presented evidence of patients who had earlier been diagnosed as having cancer, but who after healing sessions showed no signs of it, he was met by a variety of ingenious explanations. One surgeon explained that what Edwards was claiming as a cure had nothing to do with healing. It must simply be that the piece of tissue removed for biopsy, and found to be cancerous, had coincidentally contained *all* the cancer cells; it was "cure by biopsy"!

The scepticism of the medical profession

Edwards also found, as he complained to the sceptical Dr Louis Rose, author of *Faith Healing*, that whenever a patient had received any medical treatment, his or her recovery, "no matter how remarkable", was attributed to such treatment, and not to spiritual healing. "To satisfy you, the sick person must not have received medical attention at any time" Edwards went on, but, "then you would dispute the healing, because there could not have been a proper diagnosis". It was a case, Edwards complained, of "heads you win, tails I lose".

The only way to impress the medical profession, Edwards realized, would be to set up a trial in which patients diagnosed as having cancer would be offered healing as an alternative to conventional treatment. But this was out of the question, because the General Medical Council's rule that any doctor who recommended patients to have treatment from a healer would be liable to be struck off the Medical Register.

Difficulties in setting up trials

Even a project for a trial of "absent healing" was turned down. The idea was to take a number of cancer patients who were having conventional treatment, divide them into two matched groups, and then give one of the groups treatment by a healer or healers, at a distance. Neither the patients nor the doctors need know about the trial, because conventional treatment would continue. If the healing began to work, presumably in time its effects would be seen; the patients being given the absent healing, though unaware of it, would survive longer than the controls.

Nevertheless, doctors could not be found who would cooperate. Their general assumption was that the whole idea of absent healing was unscientific. But if by any chance it worked, they reminded Edwards, any doctor involved in the trial could be charged with allowing his patients to receive treatment – and, worse, treatment by medically-unqualified practitioners, without their knowledge or consent. Once again, it was a case of "heads you win, tails I lose". When the GMC rescinded its ban in 1977, Edwards was at last able to set up a trial. But he died before the initially promising results could be confirmed (healers have since been involved in tests of a related kind, but these can best be considered in conjunction with research into hand healing).

Suitable cases

Spiritualists are convinced that there are few, if any, *un*suitable cases; even the most hardened sceptics may be converted if their arthritis or asthma disappears. They also emphasize that their ministrations may be of value to patients who are being given orthodox treatment. Because they are in the category of ministers of religion, they are allowed to visit and treat any patient in hospital who asks for them.

Hand healing

There is no clear-cut distinction in practice between "hand healing", as it is coming to be known, and healing through the laying on of hands in the Christian tradition when healing, as distinct from ritual, is involved. To outward appearances a hand healer and a spiritual healer seem to be going through the same motions. The distinction lies in the beliefs of the healer. Hand healers are secular in outlook and they tend to be more pragmatic in their attitudes and methods.

Origins

The first writer to describe hand healing as a natural, rather than a divine, phenomenon was one of the Hippocratic school in Kos in Greece in the fifth century BC. It had often occurred to him, he wrote, that he was able to relieve patients of aches and infirmities "by laying my hands on, or moving them over, the area concerned, as if my hands possessed some strange healing power".

The trend of the mechanistic medicine which the Hippocratic school founded, however, drew it away from healing of this kind, which was practised chiefly by spiritual healers until the Church eventually turned against it. It went underground, to be given only at the risk of prosecution for witchcraft, until the seventeenth century. Then, it saw the light again as "stroking" – moving the hands up and down the body, not necessarily with actual contact.

Strokers and magnetizers

The best-known "stroker" of that era was the Irishman, Valentine Greatrakes or Greatorex, whose social position as a landowner, a magistrate and a friend of some of the most eminent people of his time allowed him to practise and demonstrate "stroking" without the risk of being prosecuted under the still operative witchcraft acts. Some of his friends, notably the founder of modern chemistry, Robert Boyle, testified to Greatrakes' success.

Greatrakes' method was to begin by putting his hands on the patient's head, perhaps gently rubbing it. He then stroked the pain towards the feet, "thrice over from his hip downwards", as he put it, describing the case of a crippled seaman, "until the pain were driven out at his toes' ends". The man then "walked lustily to and fro in the garden, professing his willingness to do so for 10 miles, and carrying the crutches – sometimes in his hand, sometimes triumphantly on his shoulders – which had previously supported him".

The resemblance between the act of stroking for therapeutic purposes and the act of imparting magnetism to a steel bar, led some strokers in the seventeenth and eighteenth centuries to reinforce their treatment by holding magnets in their hands. (It was through watching experiments with magnets in this way that Franz Mesmer developed his healing technique, see *Hypnotherapy*, pages 166 to 173.)

Mesmerism later came to be identified with hypnotism, but some of Mesmer's disciples continued to use "stroking", or, as it was sometimes called, "magnetizing". The notion that actual magnetism played a part fell out of favour during the nineteenth century, but some research towards the end of the century appeared to confirm it, and recent research has provided further evidence that it may be involved. Many hand healers now assume that there is some bio-electromagnetic element in healing.

Whatever the biophysical explanation may turn out to be, the anecdotal evidence for hand healing is so extensive and well attested that it is becoming hard to continue to reject it on the ground that no force has yet been discovered to account for it.

Evidence from the Soviet Union

The most recent testimonial comes from Russia – all the more surprising in that the Soviet authorities have traditionally pursued unbendingly conventional policies and medical unorthodoxy of any kind has been as suspect as political deviation. In 1980, it was reported that President Leonid Brezhnev, no less, had been receiving treatment from a healer.

In the winter of 1979, Brezhnev was obviously a sick man, his speech often slurred, his walk so unsteady that somebody had always to be close to him in case he should stumble. By the spring

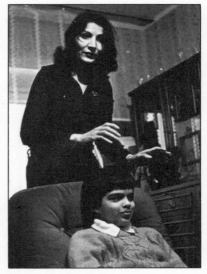

Dzhuna Davitashvili
Three tumours had blinded this young boy and made him increasingly sluggish, with blurred speech. After only one visit to the Russian healer Dzhuna Davitashvili he had regained the sight of one eye and seemed far more cheerful and intelligent. Here he is on his second visit to the healer.

of 1980, however, a marked improvement had clearly taken place, and an article in the *New York Times* by Craig R. Whitney, writing from Moscow, explained why. The miracle had been wrought by a young woman, a former waitress, Dzhuna Davitashvili. Among her other patients had been the Ministers of Planning, and of Public Health, and her Moscow apartment was being besieged by other eminent people wanting appointments, in spite of her charges of around £175 a session.

Dzhuna has since been interviewed by the American writer Henry Gris, co-author of a book on psychical research in the Soviet Union – she apparently uses straightforward hand healing, believing that "bioenergy" streams from her palms.

Procedure

Hand healers often discover their vocation by chance – perhaps a friend has a headache, and when their forehead is stroked, the pain disappears. They then try it out again on other people, and again the pain goes. Then they try it on a child which has fallen down and bruised itself . . . and so on. Because hand healers so often discover their ability in this way, there is no standard method of treatment, but most commonly the hands are placed on, or just above, the patient's head, and then on, or close to the seat of the pain. Some healers make stroking motions; a few actually follow the Greatrakes technique.

The immediate physical effects

Patients' reactions to hand healing vary so greatly as to defy generalization. But there is one very common phenomenon. "When being healed", Dr Alec Forbes, a doctor prominent in the campaign to secure recognition for healing as a valid form of therapy, has written, "a person mostly feels heat, sometimes where the healer's hand are held, sometimes in the disabled area of the body". The heat may be gentle, or it can be so intense that the patient can hardly bear it. Yet, as a rule, there is no actual rise in temperature, of the kind that registers on a thermometer.

Alternatively, Forbes adds, the patient may feel a chill or a sensation of "pins and needles", in the area under the healer's hands; occasionally, "a sensation like an electric shock will run along the limbs to the extremities or along the spine". Or there may be no physical sensation at all. Yet, when the session is over, physical changes may have taken place; for example patients who earlier could hardly bend at all find that they can touch their toes.

In a few well-attested cases, lasting cures have been achieved in a single healing session. Most hand healers, however, warn patients that they may need to return for say, half a dozen sessions – by which time it should be clear whether or not the healing is having a beneficial effect.

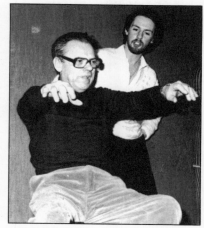

Matthew Manning
This patient could not bend his arms or lift them above this point before consulting Matthew Manning. By the end of the healing session he found himself able to raise both arms above his head.

A new generation of healers

As healers vary so much in their beliefs and techniques, you cannot expect to find an established procedure. What the internationally known British healer Matthew Manning does, however, is representative of at least the younger generation. While still in his twenties, Manning has won an international reputation as a healer, and at the same time he has been conducting research, in collaboration with doctors and scientists, into the healing process.

As a schoolboy, Manning had the unnerving experience of finding himself the storm centre of poltergeist disturbances, at home and at school. Fortunately for him, he had understanding parents and schoolteachers, and eventually he found that he

A hand healing session

Healers differ in their routines. Normally, you will receive treatment lying down though some healers treat patients sitting up. The actual procedure followed during a healing session varies according to your needs. For some of the sessions he or she will work with the hands on your body, but mostly the healer's hands will hover above it.

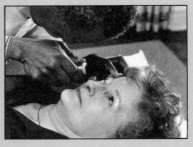

1 *The healer attunes his own energy force with that of the patient, and assesses the energy flow by holding the thumbs, which for him are the focal point of the hands – the body's main outlet of energy.*

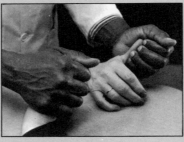

2 *This healer makes use of iridology (see pages 279 to 281) to confirm the diagnosis of the patient's condition that he has already made intuitively.*

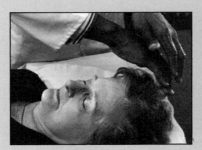

3 *He starts to balance the energy flow through and around the patient's body with his hands above her head. Without touching the body, he will then sweep his hands down to the feet and up again.*

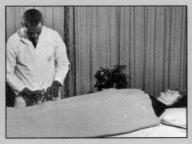

4 *Healing energy is concentrated on the specific area of the body that requires attention. This patient was suffering from rheumatoid arthritis in her knee.*

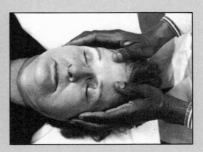

5 *To conclude the session the healer lays his hands on the patient's head and his thumbs on her forehead to "ground" the energy flow from her body.*

could channel the wayward psychic energies into automatic drawing and writing, bringing them under some control.

For a while it appeared as if Manning might follow the trail which Uri Geller had blazed, as he found he had psychokinetic powers. But while still in his early twenties, he decided he would prefer to concentrate his powers on healing. For the past few years he had divided his time between healing sessions, either with individual patients or in demonstrations to audiences, and research projects in different countries – the United States, New Zealand, Japan – in which doctors and scientists have collaborated with him to try to learn more about the healing process.

Matthew Manning's technique

When new patients arrive, Manning talks to each one individually, discussing their problems and hearing about their symptoms, in much the same way as any other natural therapist does. But from the moment he sets to work – he stands behind the patient, initially placing his hands on the patient's shoulders – his hands begin to move as if of their own accord. Sometimes they work together; sometimes there is one hand on each side of the patient's body. They may go to the spot where the pain is, or they may hover over an organ related to the symptoms. In some kinds of eye trouble, he finds that his hands move to either side of the patient's body, in the region of the kidneys, as if they should be considered the real source of the disorder.

Manning's colour codes

Information about a patient is commonly received by Manning in his mind's eye, through what he describes as a colour code: red for pain, yellow for an infection, black for a malignancy. This technique also occasionally enables him to correct an earlier faulty diagnosis, which has led to the patient being given the wrong medical treatment.

Like many healers, Manning finds that the bulk of his patients come with disorders for which orthodox medicine has no effective treatment: backache, arthritis, allergies, cancer, multiple sclerosis. Increasingly, he has found, that people are beginning to go to their doctors for diagnosis – where, for example, they have a pain which they cannot account for – but as soon as they know what is the matter with them, if it is something which orthodox medicine cannot handle effectively, they go to him (though he recommends that they should continue with their orthodox treatment). The same applies when, as so often happens, orthodox tests reveal no "organic" disorder, and a doctor cheerily reassures them that there is nothing the matter.

With diseases such as cancer and multiple sclerosis, Manning makes it clear to patients that he is not in the business of providing miraculous cures. In his experience a high proportion of such cases – up to 90 percent – has been triggered off by some emotionally shattering event, which occurred from 6 to 18 months before the onset of the disease. Simple healing, he points out, cannot work unless the patients come to grips with the painful problems which that stressful event – a messy divorce, the loss of a loved one, or (very common in the early 1980s) redundancy – has caused. It is as if cancer, particularly, is the mechanism by which some people, unable to face life, unconsciously commit hara-kiri. To avoid that fate, Manning says, they must renew their zest for living, and all that healing can do is help start them on their way.

Patients who are being treated occasionally go into a light trance. But ordinarily they are not aware of any effect of the healing – except for those who have the sensation of warmth from his hands – until they realize that their pain is going, or that they can move limbs which had long been made rigid by arthritis. About two out of every three patients, Manning finds, gain relief from the healing session, which usually lasts about 30 minutes.

The will to recover

For some patients, the improvement lasts only a day or two, and it is in this connection that Manning represents what can be regarded as the modern school of healing. He lays particular emphasis on the need for patients to explore self-help. The healing may be no more than an indication that patients *can* recover, but only if they really want to.

If they think of the healer simply as providing an alternative type of tranquillizer or anti-arthritic remedy to the one doctors prescribe, they are unlikely to get more than temporary relief. For those who want to take positive steps to recover their health, he advocates the use of a visualization therapy similar to that developed in the United States by Carl and Stephanie Simonton (see *Meditation* pages 184 to 185), and he has tapes giving his patients guidance in self-healing meditation to bring about pain control and relaxation.

The gradual process of recovery

The occasional "miracle" occurs, as when people who have been stone-deaf for years, or who have lost all sense of smell in an accident suddenly find they can hear or smell once more. Backache, too, may disappear suddenly, and not return. But Manning warns new patients against expecting sudden cures: often they will need to return, from time to time, either for "booster shots" to help to keep their bodies in working order, or as part of a gradual process of recovery, helping the patient's own homeostatic mechanism to recover its lost authority.

From his earlier psychic experiences, Manning is in no doubt about the existence of as yet unexplained paranormal forces which appear to be controlled by some intelligence (not necessarily of a high order – poltergeists are notoriously practical jokers), and he accepts that there may be spirits working on him and through him. But he does not identify them as deceased doctors working through him, as the older generation of healers commonly did (and many still do). His interest lies rather in investigating the healing forces scientifically in the hope of establishing their reality.

Choosing a trustworthy healer

Asked by an interviewer how it is possible to pick out a trustworthy healer, the American investigator of healing, Dr Lawrence LeShan has countered by offering three rules of thumb to identify healers who ought *not* be trusted:

"One is, if a healer promises you results, don't trust him . . . The second is, any healer who doesn't refuse to see you unless you're under a physician's care is a dangerous charlatan . . . The last is, if a healer charges you (or accepts 'love offerings', a polite blackmail for charging) don't trust him".

These are useful warnings, but each needs qualification. There are some honest healers who, on occasion, quite deliberately promise results not out of boastfulness or delusion, but because they feel that certain patients need to be impressed that way – just as other patients are more impressed by modesty. The "under a physician's care" warning was partly the consequence of the law of the land in the United States, where until recently the giving of treatment by anybody but a doctor invited prosecution. In Britain, in any case, with its state welfare scheme and free GP service, the great majority of people who go to a healer do have a doctor as well. Payment by time (as distinct from payment by results) can, in theory at least, be justified. Somebody who finds he or she has healing powers, after all, may be able to use them for the benefit of the community only if he or she can afford to give up regular work.

Matthew Manning is one of the increasing number of healers who charges patients on a time scale – so much per half hour (that being the average time of a session). He is well aware of the long tradition that healers must not seek to profit financially from their gift. But he is also aware that one of the charges commonly levelled against healers by the medical profession is that they do not keep records.

To answer all requests for healing, hundreds every week, and to keep a card index of all patients treated, with details of their disorders and a record of their progress, requires, these days, a formidable outlay on stationery, postage and secretarial assistance. Manning aims to fix his rates to cover his expenses – additional gifts from grateful patients balancing the letting-off of those who cannot afford to pay.

Research

From his research into healing and healers in New York and elsewhere in the 1970s, Dr Lawrence LeShan came to the conclusion that there are two main types of healer.

Some healers move into a condition where they appear to lose their own individuality and become at one with the rest of humanity – a condition which people who have had a mystical experience have often tried to describe, and have usually admitted they cannot put into words. "The 'I' ceases to exist because it has, by a kind of mental osmosis, established communication with, and been dissolved in, the universal pool". Thus wrote Arthur Koestler in the second volume of his autobiography, *The Invisible Writing*, recalling his own experience in a Spanish jail while under sentence of death. "It is this process of dissolution and limitless expansion which is sensed as the 'oceanic feeling', as the draining of all tension, the absolute catharsis, the peace that passeth all understanding".

In this condition, LeShan believes, some people can tune into psychic forces which release healing powers. There is no need, in such circumstances, for the healer to do anything, or even to be with the patient or patients he is trying to heal: the forces at work, whatever they are, transcend space.

Testing healing prayers under lab conditions

An example of research into this category of healing is a "prayer" experiment undertaken with the American healers Ambrose and Olga Worrall. They were asked to see whether they could affect the growth rate of rye grass in a locked-up laboratory in Atlanta, 600 miles from where they lived in Baltimore, the grass's growth rate being monitored on a chart recorder. Precisely at the time they were asked to include the grass in their healing "prayers" (they tried to visualize grass full of energy) the growth rate suddenly began to increase, until it was more than eight times as fast as before.

The other type of healing is more familiar. It is directed specifically at the patient, ordinarily through the healer's hands, and healer and patient are in close proximity. Paradoxically, this makes research into healing powers, as such, more difficult, because if symptoms disappear, suggestion or autosuggestion may be credited. In any case, until the late 1970s, owing to the General Medical Council's ban in Britain and state laws in other countries, such research was blocked.

Healing research using animals

Twenty years ago, however, Dr Bernard Grad, a biochemist at McGill University, Montreal, realized that although research into the effect of healing on humans might still be impracticable, there was no bar to research on the effects of healing on laboratory animals. Dividing a group of mice into three matched groups, he made a small cut in each of them, and invited a well-known healer, Colonel Estebany, a former Polish cavalry officer, to perform the laying on of hands on one of the groups. The second group was subjected to the same "treatment", but not by a healer, and the third group, left to its own devices, acted as the controls.

The wounds of the mice Estebany treated healed significantly faster than those of the other groups, as they did, again, in a further trial – this one carried out "blind"; nobody involved in the experiment knew which were the treated and which the untreated groups until the code identifying them was broken at the end of the test period.

Blind trials with enzymes

Reading about these trials, Sister Justa Smith, a Franciscan who had become a highly qualified biochemist and was Director of Research at the Human Dimensions Institute, Buffalo, New York, decided to find out whether Estebany could produce similar results with enzymes (catalysts formed by living cells which promote chemical changes). When "treated" by Estebany, would a test tube full of enzymes promote changes different from those in test tubes left untreated?

"I approached the possibility of a paranormal healer effecting a cure as a sceptic", Sister Justa Smith has since explained: "No other initial approach is possible for a biochemist". The results startled her. The enzymes were divided into four equal batches. Estebany "treated" one by laying his hands over the glass vessel containing them for 90 minutes at a stretch, an assistant periodically withdrawing some of them to monitor any changes there might be. Of the other batches one was set aside as a control, one was subjected to a high magnetic field, and the fourth exposed to ultraviolet radiation, designed to damage the enzymes, to see whether Estebany could "cure" them. He did, up to a point, but the results with this fourth batch were less striking than with the batch he treated "straight". They resembled the results of the batch subjected to the strong magnetic field – though in Estebany's case, it could not have been straight magnetism, as nothing registered when his hands were metered with a magnetometer.

Sister Justa Smith had another surprise to come: a later trial was a failure. But this, she feels, does not discredit the earlier one. Healers are not automatons, they cannot always produce positive results. In any case, there have been many trials since with other healers which have revealed the influence they can exert, strikingly if not consistently, on a variety of substances.

A typical example is the test in which Olga Worrall, the

American healer, was asked to participate in an experiment designed to discover if she could influence the course of the "Zhabotinsky reaction", in which a chemical "cocktail" changes its colour at regular intervals. Monitored by TV cameras, she made the colours change much more quickly than those of the "cocktail" in the control vessel.

Olga Worrall, who is an ordained minister in the Methodist church, has also been tested informally at a conference of doctors and scientists at Stanford University, Connecticut. According to a report in *Medical Economics*, doctors were invited to bring patients to her who were suffering from disorders for which there was no effective conventional treatment, and 7 out of 10 patients were either cured or showed marked improvement. "A few years ago, reports on the exploits of a faith healer would have drawn little more than snorts of derision from the medical community," the writer commented, "but scores of doctors in the USA and in foreign countries have gone to Olga Worrall for treatment of their

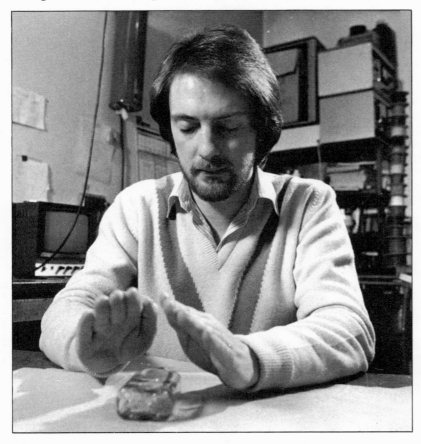

An experiment with cancer cells
Matthew Manning has recently demonstrated that he can influence the life of cancer cells in a flask – even from several rooms away. He reported that he would imagine the cells surrounded with white light and mentally tell them to go elsewhere.

own ailments, and many more have unofficially referred 'hope-less' patients to this faith healer''.

Influencing cancer cells

Matthew Manning has worked with scientists on a variety of research projects, ranging from trials to discover whether he can influence cells in test tubes, to a pilot study at a London hospital designed to discover whether there were any healing effects with patients.

That he can, and does, influence cell growth in laboratory conditions has been demonstrated on many occasions, including one on television. The series on the paranormal which Dr Kit Pedler presented on Thames TV showed a controlled trial in which Manning succeeded in making significant biochemical changes in the contents of a flask, while the "control" flasks, one being "treated" by Pedler and the other left alone, showed no change. So far, however, Manning has not produced consistent results in such trials – hardly surprising in itself as, like all healers, he is keenly aware of the extent to which his mood can influence healing's course.

The trials at the London hospital, though on too small a scale to allow of any positive conclusions, confirmed the desirability of rapport – that is, a deeply sceptical patient who brings no expectations to a healing session is less likely to feel benefit from it than somebody who accepts healing.

Evidence of healing in the Soviet Union

The Russian healer, Dzhuna Davitashvili, has also been involved in some trials of "bioenergy", as Soviet healers describe it, and one of them was reported in the official trade union newspaper, *Trud*. In his report, a member of the Soviet Academy of Sciences described how Davitashvili was asked to treat an ulcer. The effects of her hand healing were to speed up immensely the normally gradual "drying out" process. It was completed in a quarter of an hour and "in the five minutes after that, a light pink film appeared, evidencing the formation of skin cells".

The need for further research

Research into healing is still in its infancy. It can expect to continue to encounter the same apathy from within the medical establishment, and also sniping from the "rationalists" and humanists, in their eccentric alliance, fighting a last-ditch campaign against what they feel is a return to obscurantism and miracle-worship. But the evidence of trials, small-scale though they have been, leaves little room for doubt that some healing force must be at work. Further trials now in progress should make it possible for us to achieve a better understanding of it.

Therapeutic touch

"In our adulation of things mechanical, synthetic and, frequently, anti-human", the laying on of hands has come to be "all but forgotten in this scientific age".

This statement is the opinion of Dr Dolores Krieger, Professor of Nursing at New York University. She has therefore sought to restore it by a procedure she describes as "therapeutic touch". This technique, she points out, "has recaptured this simple but elegant mode of healing, and mated it with the rigor and power of modern science".

Origins

Dissatisfied with the way in which present-day nursing has become rationalized into soullessness, Dolores Krieger's interest was aroused when she read about Dr Bernard Grad's experiments with mice and hand healing at McGill University, Montreal. She then went to watch the healer, Colonel Estebany (see also page 251) at work and conducted a trial herself, in which she set him to see if he could influence hemoglobin, the oxygen-carrying red blood cells or corpuscles. If his healing powers worked, she reckoned, the cells ought to be in better condition after it than they were before.

Encouraged by the results, Krieger began to train nurses in a secular version of the laying on of hands, in effect, a version of hand healing. The form it takes can vary much as hand healing does; some people use stroking techniques, others simply place the hands above or on the afflicted part of the patient's body to bring relief.

Procedure

Therapeutic touch does not require a trained practitioner, Krieger maintains, so any two people can try it out on each other, one acting as the "sender" the other as the "receiver". The sender tries to achieve a relaxed state, to allow the healing force to work through the receiver. "Stroking" is used to "unruffle the field", to open up the receiver to accept the healing force, which is transmitted by hand healing. When it works, its effects can be detected by a number of indications: the voice of the receiver becomes quieter; respiration slows down and deepens; there is a general relaxation, often gratefully expressed by the receiver; the skin gradually takes on a pinker hue, starting with the face and spreading through the body.

Working on a patient's energy field

That a healer or psychic is not essential to the therapy does not mean, Krieger insists, that it is "all psychological". Communication between sender and receiver may be through extrasensory

Learning therapeutic touch

Dolores Kreiger believes that hand healing is a gift that any can use. However, she emphasizes the need to be clear about your interest in, and attraction to, the art of healing, because a very close interaction is set up between the "healer" and the "patient"

which can wreak psychological havoc if not handled correctly. Being a healer requires self-knowledge, correct motivation, and an understanding of the "dynamics" of healing: ultimately the patient heals him or herself, the healer merely sets the process in motion.

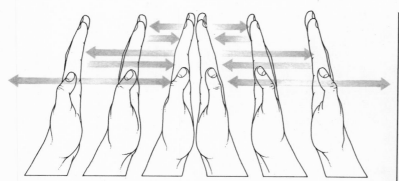

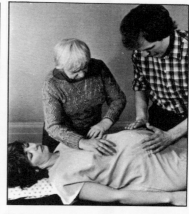

Learning to feel the hand energy
Hold your hands away from your body and bring the palms as close as possible without actually touching. Separate your hands by about 5 cm (2 in) and very slowly bring them back to the original position. Separate your hands again, this time by about 10 cm (4 in) and slowly return them to the original position. Repeat separating your

hands by about 15 cm (6 in) and returning your hands slowly to the original position; notice if you feel a build up of pressure or any significant sensation. Finally separate your hands by about 20 cm (8 in) and bring your hands back together slowly and steadily stopping every 5 cm (2 in) to experience the "pressure field". If at any stage you go wrong, start again.

Helping pregnancy and childbirth
Teaching a father how to feel the difference between the energy fields of the mother and of his baby, gives him a sense of contact and involvement with his unborn child. Therapeutic touch can also be used to help reduce pain in childbirth.

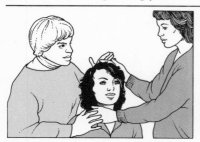

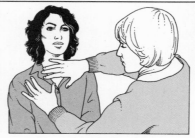

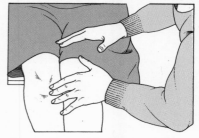

If you are learning therapeutic touch one of the first exercises you should practise is scanning a person's head. Hold your hands 5 to 6 cm (2 to 3 in) away from the head and feel for changes in temperature.

To assess the person's energy field, run your hands down each side of the body, feeling for signs of congestion or imbalance, which you will experience as heat, cold, tingling, pressure, slight electric shocks or pulsations.

You must get rid of areas of congestion by unruffling the field, before directing energy to particular parts of the body that require it by holding your hands over the trouble spots.

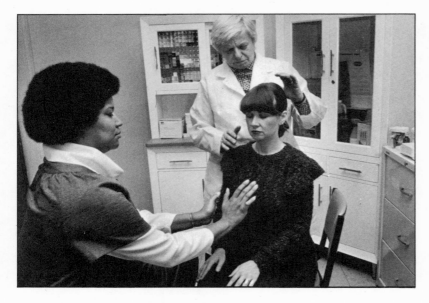

Therapeutic touch technique
Dr Dolores Krieger (standing), Professor of Nursing at New York University's School of Nursing demonstrates her technique of therapeutic touch to two of her graduate nursing students.

perception. The "unruffling", stroking process is based on the assumption that the body's real boundaries extend outside the physical body, in the form of an energy field. The field can be detected by dowsing instruments, but as science has not yet accepted it, it remains in the paranormal category.

Research

The initial pilot experiment with Estebany was set up with 28 patients, nine of them acting as the controls. The hemoglobin of the 19 who received the healing responded to it significantly. A further experiment with 76 patients produced a similar result.

This encouraged Krieger to begin trials to find out whether the ability to heal requires special powers on the part of the healer. Sixteen registered nurses each used therapeutic touch on two patients, while another 16 nurses gave ordinary care, also each to two patients (the two sets of patients were matched as closely as possible for age, severity of illness, and so on). As in the earlier trials, there was no difference in the hemoglobin of the control group, but the treated group's had significantly improved.

Suitable cases

The chief value of therapeutic touch, Krieger feels, is that it can be used in any and all cases of illness as an adjunct to whatever form of treatment has been decided upon. She has also found that it provides great relief for women in the painful stages of childbirth.

Radionics and radiesthesia

As well as those who have regarded psychic or occult forces as divine or diabolic, there have long been scientists and savants who prefer to think of them as neutral. By analogy, the waves that bring sounds on the radio, or pictures on the television screen, are not perceptible to us, unless and until the set is switched on. The theory is that we need to be switched on to receive psychic transmissions, and their effect on us will depend to some extent on the programme-maker. Some men and women have the capacity to transmit a steady flow of healing; others, the sorcerers, on occasion transmit harm. Most of us have the ability (if we can find how to exercise it) to switch on to receive healing, and occasionally to provide it.

Radionics and radiesthesia are methods of recapturing and exploiting these largely dormant powers. The two are distinguishable, in theory, in that radiesthesia is the application of the principles and techniques of dowsing (see page 257) to medicine, whereas radionics also involves the use of some instrumentation. In practice, however, it must be said that radionic practitioners will be found to vary in their use of instruments – from none to a range of up-to-date equipment.

' Radionics is a method of healing at a distance using specially designed instruments in conjunction with the radiesthesthetic faculty . . . In radionic therapy, any disharmonies or distortions in these energy patterns can be identified and measured so that the trained practitioner using the instrument for analysis builds up a holistic 'blueprint' of the patient which incorporates mental, emotional and physical levels. '

Radionic Association

Origins

The use of aids for healing purposes can be traced back to shamanism. When a shaman experienced difficulty in entering into communication with the spirits, or when the spirit messages were garbled in transmission, he might use a stick – the original of the magician's wand. Or he would employ a primitive form of pendulum, a pebble hung on a thread, and ask it questions. The way it moved, whether back and forth or sideways, or clockwise or anti-clockwise, provided him with the answers.

Water divining

A variety of such devices has been employed for divination ever since, the best known being the forked hazel twig commonly used by dowsers (water diviners). Dowsing, however, is not only used to locate water, but other "hidden" things, such as oil, archaeological objects, lost articles and even missing persons.

Some dowsers have preferred to use a pendulum. Early this century, a French priest, the Abbé Mermet, conceived the idea that if with the help of a pendulum he could diagnose the condition of an underground stream, he might also be able to use it to diagnose the condition of a patient's blood stream. He found that he could. In the 1920s, he began to give demonstrations in hospitals to which, as a member of a religious order, he had access. He would ask the doctors to select a batch of patients, the nature of whose illness he would then use his pendulum to diagnose. It was not necessary, he explained, that he should see

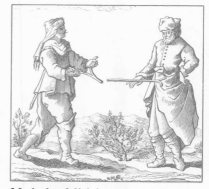

Methods of divining
This drawing from a seventeenth-century treatise on "occult physics", shows two ways of holding a divining rod. The man on the left clasps the forks of a branch in both hands, while the one on the right balances the rod on the back of his out-stretched hand.

the patients. Even if they were covered with sheets, his pendulum would still spell out what was the matter with them – often sufficiently accurately to surprise onlookers, and mortify sceptics.

Mermet's concept of radiesthesia

On the strength of his discoveries, Mermet wrote his *Principles and Practice of Radiesthesia*, the term he coined to describe dowsing for medical purposes. All substances, he claimed, emit radiations. The human body is capable of acting as a receiver, if it is tuned into them by means of some ordinarily imperceptible current which flows through the hands. If a rod or a pendulum is held, its movements can be understood to indicate where the radiations are coming from, and provide a measure of their strength. When the book was published in 1935, however, medical science was not prepared to accept such a theory. The idea of anybody thinking he could diagnose disease by holding a pendulum over the patients seemed simply ludicrous – the more so if he were an abbé.

Abrams' theory of "biocurrents"

By this time, however, there had been another, totally unexpected, development in this field of research. Investigating the phenomenon of percussion, whereby a doctor taps the body of a patient in order to elicit information about the condition of the internal organs, the American neurologist Albert Abrams had noted that if a patient was facing due west, the sound varied according to the area percussed and the disease that he was suffering from. Following this up, out of curiosity, he found that if he tapped the body of a healthy patient who was holding a piece of diseased tissue, the tapping would produce the characteristic sound of the diseased tissue, rather than of the healthy body. The explanation, he reasoned, must be the existence of what he called a "biocurrent", not far removed from Mesmer's theory of "animal magnetism" (see *Hypnotherapy*, pages 166 to 173). If this biocurrent existed, Abrams surmised, there might be no need for patients to be present for diagnostic purposes. Might not a drop of their blood be sufficient? He found that it was.

Although Abrams does not appear to have been aware of it, through his research he was providing a clue to the understanding of one of the mysteries of ancient magic: the use by tribal shamans and sorcerers, of portions of an individual's clothing, hair or fingernail parings over which to weave spells, for healing or harm.

At this point, however, Abrams made what in retrospect was a dangerous mistake. By nature and temperament he was as dedicated a materialist as his fellow-neurologist and contemporary, Sigmund Freud. Abrams longed to win scientific sanction for his discovery. For this, he realized, he must be able to demonstrate it had objective validity. Assuming that some electromagnetic force must be involved, he began to experiment further, and found that his assistant did not actually need to hold the diseased tissue: he could be connected to it by a length of wire. By placing the equivalent of electrical resistances on the wire, therefore, and by watching the effect on the biocurrent, he could distinguish more clearly between different diseases than had been possible by simple percussion.

The Abrams box

It proved relatively easy to design the diagnostic instrument which became known as "the box"; but here Abrams made a further mistake – manufacturing it and selling it himself. This was less for the profit (he was a wealthy man) than to keep his invention in his own hands. Inevitably it aroused suspicion, particularly as the box looked as if it were intended to operate through electricity, which it did not use. And although for some purchasers the boxes worked well, for others they gave unreliable results; some users could get no response at all.

Abrams had not allowed for the possibility that his bioenergy might be influenced by the people involved in operating the equipment, as well as the equipment itself. If so, they would have to be "tuned in", as well as the box. When Abrams died in 1924, the device was apparently discredited. Some of his disciples in the United States carried on his work, but the better their results were, the more they were tempted to prove that orthodox science had been wrong to dismiss Abrams as a charlatan. This was not simply out of professional pride, it was also because in many states of the Union they could be prosecuted and jailed for using the box. But in the attempt to demonstrate that it could provide consistent results they made the same mistake as Abrams, as Ruth Drown, an American chiropractor, found to her cost.

The Ruth Drown débâcle

Drown's box worked differently. A very similar principle had, in fact, been discovered by anthropologists who reported that some African witch doctors rubbed two pieces of wood together, obtaining answers to their questions according to whether they moved smoothly over each other, grated, or stuck. Ruth Drown used stretched rubber skeins instead of pieces of wood; the point at which they became "tacky" to the touch could be used for diagnosis. But her box also incorporated a means of treating patients, which, taken together with the diagnostic procedures she was using smelled highly of quackery to the medical establishment. The Food and Drug Administration (FDA) was the first to bring proceedings against her, which amounted to a heavy fine. Then at the age of 72, she was accused of fraud, jailed, and her papers and equipment were destroyed. Tragically, before her trial she suffered a stroke and died.

The de la Warr case

In England, George de la Warr, an engineer who had set out to investigate radionics (as the use of gadgets to tune into bioenergy for therapeutic purposes had now come to be called), was lucky to escape a similar fate. He, too, believed that he could convince scientists that his boxes – including his "camera" which responded to blood spots placed inside it by producing negatives of the organs of the person or animal from which it was obtained, though there was no lens – could be shown to work objectively. He, too, often failed in test conditions, and he, too, was prosecuted by someone who bought one of his boxes. The jury, however, was not called upon to give an opinion on the merits of the de la Warr box, only on whether he genuinely believed in it or was selling it under false pretences. As they decided that he believed in it, de la Warr was found not guilty.

Towards the end of his life, he realized, and admitted, that he had made a mistake in thinking he could demonstrate his devices in ways which would convince orthodox scientists, and there has since been more readiness among radionic practitioners to concentrate upon employing the pendulum, or the box and pendulum, for therapy without worrying about proving they are "scientific", in orthodoxy's sense. They hope empirical evidence can be accumulated which will eventually carry conviction, as it has done with acupuncture, even without a satisfactory explanation of how it works.

Procedure

Techniques in radionic practice have tended to change over the years. Most practitioners have now moved from the use of the "stick pad", as Ruth Drown's means of obtaining contact with the patient was called, to the use of the pendulum. Otherwise it will be found that emphases vary from interpretation of the movements of a pendulum, to treatments generated by specially constructed geometric charts, and to readings and treatments

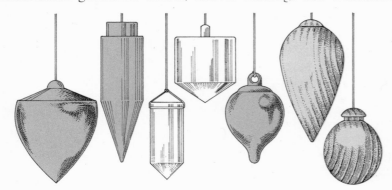

Pendulums used in radiesthesia
Radiesthesia is a development of the ancient art of dowsing and the "Divining rod" (or Virgula Divina) became the pendulum. Here are just some of the many different types of pendulum, each of which has its own specific use in radiesthesia.

from various "boxes" which may be of simple construction, or bristling with dials.

Regarding diagnosis, some practitioners may find that they work best using the pendulum alone – really just practising radiesthesia – obtaining sufficient guidance from its movements (by perhaps swinging clockwise for yes, anti-clockwise for no) to answer their questions; some employ charts with the names of symptoms and remedies round them. A number of practitioners – herbalists, homeopaths, aromatherapists, among others – may use this method or a variant to confirm decisions they have made regarding diagnosis and treatment, or to help them make a final choice if a number of therapies could, theoretically be used with equal effect (see *Aromatherapy*, pages 58 to 62). Most radionic

Consulting a practitioner

Radionics may be used both to diagnose and treat illness even without your meeting the therapist. Most practitioners, however, prefer to have at least one meeting. On initial contact you will be given a questionnaire, asking for details of your medical history. A radionic practitioner will always dowse to find out if he or she can help you.

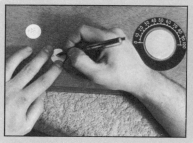

1 *You will be required to provide a "witness" – a drop of blood on a piece of blotting paper, for example, or a lock of hair – that can be used both to diagnose and treat your condition.*

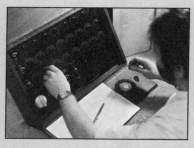

2 *To analyse your state of health, the practitioner must focus his mind on you. He may do this by placing your witness on a "diagnostic" machine and, holding a pendulum over it, proceed with a series of questions.*

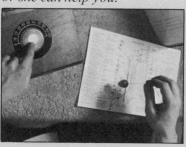

3 *Alternatively, he may dowse over anatomical and physiological diagrams of the body, allowing the pendulum to indicate which part or parts of the body require particular investigation.*

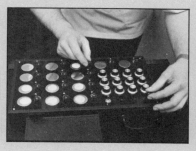

4 *Treatment depends on the diagnosis and on the variety of instruments the practitioner possesses. This instrument pulses out treatment for 2.2 minutes each time it is tuned in to a particular patient.*

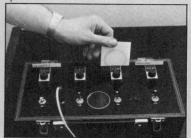

5 *Sometimes dowsing will indicate the need for another therapy in addition to or instead of radionic treatment. This specially constructed machine simulates the manufacture of homeopathic remedies.*

practitioners, however, will use some kind of instrument for treatment, even if this is only to simulate a remedy that the patient may take in pill form; though some find that they work better practising a form of absent healing – no box, no charts, no medicine, but simply the projection of psychic or spiritual energy for the healing of the patient.

There is a sense, however, in which the method the practitioner adopts is of little concern to the patient who, after all, is interested primarily in the results. Radionic therapy provides the easiest of all options for patients, in that they do not necessarily need to visit the practitioner (although some do like to meet their patients to talk to them about the treatment).

Radionic diagnosis

All that is required of you, if you wish a diagnosis, is that you should contact the radionic practitioner to obtain a questionnaire to fill in. This will then provide a general case history of past illnesses and injuries and how they have been treated, and general details of any symptoms causing you pain or worry. For the protection of the practitioner, you will also be asked if you are quite clear what radionics entails, to ensure you realize it is not a therapy endorsed by orthodoxy. When you return the completed questionnaire, you send with it either a drop of your blood on some lint or litmus paper, or a lock of your hair.

That is all. You take no further active part, as the diagnosis and the healing process is done in the radionic practitioner's own time. Subsequently the practitioner keeps you informed about what, if anything, you are expected to do; you, of course, keep him or her informed of any changes in your condition, and settle your bill.

Until recently, radionic practitioners often tended to diagnose and treat symptoms along what, in one sense, were orthodox lines: they would pick up "asthma" or "indigestion", and project "bioenergy" with a view to removing them. Now they, too, are being converted to holism. They even avoid the term "diagnosis" both in their questionnaire, and in their own questions to pendulum or box, they put emphasis on the patients' general condition, rather than on particular symptoms. They are also more willing to recognize their own limitations, and admit that about a quarter of the people who try radionic therapy for the first time find it does not give satisfactory results.

Some practitioners do not rely solely on projecting bioenergy back to the patient; they may write, recommending herbal or homeopathic remedies or exercise, or psychotherapy.

Research

Humiliating though the results were of the efforts of Abrams, Drown and de la Warr to convince scientists of the existence of bioenergy and of its potential therapeutic usefulness, there has been one very striking vindication of the validity of both the theory and the practice of the radionic box, under strict controlled conditions. In the early 1920s, some members of the medical profession in Britain, alerted by the controversy over the Abrams box in the United States decided that one way to vindicate orthodox scientific methods, and at the same time to discredit the box before it caught on in Britain, would be to set up a high-powered committee of investigation – the only investigation of its kind of an unconventional therapy to take place between the wars.

The Horder report

Headed by Sir Thomas (later Lord) Horder, and containing a number of well-known scientists, the committee examined a British variant of the Abrams box, the emanometer, operated by W.E. Boyd, a homeopathic doctor from Scotland. In two separate trials, Boyd was asked to identify substances and chemicals with the help of the box. In conditions where there was no possibility of his finding out what they were, his results were almost 100 percent correct. The odds against his having guessed them by chance, Horder told an audience which had come to the Royal Society of Medicine to hear the committee's report, were millions to one against.

Another striking feature of the trials, so far as Horder himself was concerned, was that when he and another investigator, acting in the capacity of assistants to Boyd, held each successive specimen, not merely did they hear a change in tone registered by the emanometer but they could also, on occasion, feel an alteration in their own stomach muscles. It was as if they, too, were registering the symptoms which the system was designed to detect. The investigation had therefore confirmed Boyd's claim, the report admitted, "beyond any reasonable doubt". It had also, up to a point, vindicated Abrams, but he had died shortly before the report appeared.

Radionics in the United States

Such research as has been conducted since that time has been carried out by individual practitioners, and their anecdotal findings have not been acceptable. Nevertheless, some of the evidence confirms that of the Horder enquiry. In Florida, for example, Frances Farrelly has for many years been offering a radionic diagnostic service to doctors (by law, she is not allowed to treat patients herself).

The doctors send her blood samples from their patients. Farrelly focusses her attention on each individual sample until a diagnosis comes into her mind, and she then reports it to the doctor concerned. She may never know, in other words, whether

her diagnosis in any particular case is correct, or even what proportion of the diagnoses in general are correct. But one clear indication that her method works, is that she has been diagnosing cases for nearly 100 doctors, some for many years.

Suitable cases

Initially most cases presented to radionic practitioners are for diagnosis: "suitability", therefore is often decided negatively by the fact that the symptoms have eluded diagnosis conducted along orthodox lines. Similarly, suitable cases for radionic treatment are commonly those which have not responded to other therapies. According to the Radionic Association "Many long standing cases of asthma, hay fever and other allergic diseases have been helped by radionics. Mental illness, hypersensitivity and psychological states often respond well, although not necessarily quickly".

Past lives therapy

If we have souls which survive death, or if reincarnation exists, it would not be surprising if traces of our past lives should periodically filter down into a present life, causing mental or emotional disturbance. Past lives therapy is based on the assumption that some disorders arise because of past lives burrowing their way, as it were, into an individual's subconscious, and that these psychic intrusions may need to be brought to the surface, on the same principle that Freud introduced psychoanalysis to bring up repressed traumas.

Origins

When psychical researchers began to explore mediumship towards the end of the nineteenth century, some of them encountered mediums who while in their trance would appear to be "possessed" by the spirit of some historical character.

Sometimes, though not always, this was a recognizable person, often convincingly "in period". A critical but sympathetic investigation of one such medium by the Swiss psychologist Théodore Flournoy revealed that in her case the past lives were largely fantasy, but she had not consciously invented the characters. She was indeed "possessed".

Since then there have been a few cases where the evidence for actual reincarnation has been stronger. In a series of books the psychiatrist Dr Arthur Guirdham has described in considerable

❛ Patients recreate scenes in past lives for the purpose of understanding certain problems they have in the present; it would be pointless to question the veracity of the material they are reporting. Past lives therapy does not depend on the 'truth of reincarnation', but on putting aside the question of 'truth' in order to work toward curing the patient's behavioural problem.❜

Morris Netherton
Past lives therapist

detail what he believes to be a group reincarnation, involving eight people, all of whom had a previous experience as Cathars (an ascetic Christian religious sect) in the thirteenth century, in the Languedoc area of France, and all of whom have lived in or around Bristol in England in the twentieth century. Their past lives have been traced in the records of the Inquisition, each of them being an identifiable character. One of the strange indications of the links between past and present has been that their thirteenth-century experiences have tended to impinge on their present lives, causing nightmares and even physical illness.

How past lives influence the present

"The next step in our evolution as doctors is to recognize more the influence of the psyche imprisoned in matter", Dr Guirdham urges in his book *We are one another.* "Its recollections of experience in past lives are related to present symptoms". As it happens, independently of Guirdham's work, a therapy based on the assumption that symptoms which resist orthodox diagnosis and treatment may be the consequence of the impact of a past life on the present one has been introduced in the United States and is beginning to spread across the Atlantic.

How it works has been described by the Los Angeles psychologist Morris Netherton, founder of the Institute for Past Lives Awareness, and his co-author Nancy Schiffrin, in their book *Past Lives Therapy.* Netherton is naturally aware that his belief in the unconscious mind's ability not just to pick up events from past lives, but to be affected by them to the point of being seriously ill, will leave many people incredulous. Reincarnation, he is often told by sceptical patients, has yet to be established as a proven fact. This he does not dispute; he doubts if reincarnation *can* ever be proven. It is merely a convenient hypothesis, he explains, to account for the way in which certain people in a state of trance appear to become a different person, talking as though they were living in a different century, and providing supporting evidence that they really were. Similarly, there is no need to prove the truth of a past lives experience, because what really matters is whether it works as a device to cure a patient's behavioral problems.

The Bloxham tapes

Perhaps the best-known example of a past life experience was a case of regression under hypnosis carried out by Arnall Bloxham, a hypnotherapist who practised in Cardiff. Under hypnosis, twentieth-century Jane Evans became Rebecca, a Jewess who had lived in York in the twelfth century and had been one of the victims of the pogrom of 1189.

The case was unusual in that one of the scenes which she "relived" was in a church crypt, the existence of which was not known until after the TV programme had been put out, so that there could be no question of Jane Evans knowing about it. Bloxham recorded Evans' experience and the tapes were featured on a BBC television programme and formed the basis for Jeffrey Iverson's *More Lives Than One?*

Past lives therapists, however, reiterate that from their point of view, it is immaterial whether or not Jane Evans' terror, as displayed while she was under hypnosis, was the result of a playback of a past life. Equally, it could have arisen out of some fantasy, such as a nightmare she had dreamed which had stuck in her unconscious mind. The therapists argue that such buried material, whatever its source, if not brought to the surface is capable of disrupting our lives.

Morris Netherton cites cases (as Guirdham had also done) where weals, or what appear to be burns, appear on the flesh of patients in response to the playback of the past lives "memories". Sometimes a plausible historical link can be established, as in the case of Guirdham's Cathars, who met their cruel fate at the hands of the Inquisition. More often, the symptoms relate to some specific episode such as the maltreatment of a slave by his master, which is unlikely to be traceable in any records. But this is beside the point in past lives therapy, in which the memory needs to be brought up to the level of consciousness, where it can be dealt with. This is like nightmares, for example, which are terrifying at the time they are being experienced, but cease to alarm us when we are fully awake.

It does not matter, therefore, if the reality of the events remembered cannot be established. It does not even matter if investigation proves conclusively that the past life was not in fact lived, that the person whom the patient appears to become in the course of treatment did not historically exist, or that the events described never took place. Something is bothering the patient and presenting itself in this way, much as it can in a dream. The object of the therapy is to make patients aware of it, and to help them to come to terms with it.

Procedure

Some past lives therapists use a method not unlike psychoanalysis, the subject remaining conscious while, together with the therapist, he or she reaches for the buried material. Others prefer to use hypnosis as a means of helping the subjects to go back in time to find whether some past life comes up, with traumatic episodes which can be linked with the subject's present life problems, or symptoms. As Sue Hinton, who has attended a past lives weekend at a London workshop has said, "the techniques for getting into your past life are much the same as for *Primal therapy* (see pages 217 to 219) or *Psychodrama* (see pages 205 to 222). You take a problem, a focal point, a memory or anything that can be used as a catalyst, and work on it with the therapist and the rest of the group to really get to the point where, although you start off acting, it suddenly becomes real, and you feel that what you are acting has become re-living".

While some therapists run workshops where a number of people are encouraged to interact together, often over a weekend, others prefer to see patients on a one-to-one basis over an extended period of time.

Research

The point Netherton has made about the unimportance of validating past lives experiences is important, because most of the research which has been undertaken recently examining ancient records to try to find whether there is evidence containing the possibility of reincarnation, has been designed to try to discover whether the past events described actually happened, and, if so, whether there was any way in which the individuals who remembered them could have learned about them by, say, hearing tales about them when too young to remember, and then storing them away in the unconscious.

Some investigators, notably Professor Ian Stevenson of the University of Virginia, have meticulously checked a great number of cases, and found evidence that supports the idea that certain individuals can describe past events accurately, without having had any such access to information about them. As Stevenson has been careful to insist, this does not prove the reality of reincarnation, but it does demonstrate that some individuals appear to have "memories" which cannot be accounted for by straightforward remembering, whether conscious or unconscious.

These individuals do not just "see" the past; they may also experience it, and the experiences they "relive" during therapy can be terrifying. This has frequently been demonstrated in the course of regression under hypnosis, when subjects are asked to go back not just to their childhood – a method some therapists commonly use to try to track down episodes which may be linked to neurotic symptoms – but also beyond, to the distant past.

Suitable cases

Those people who have tried other forms of psychotherapy for unexplained symptoms, particularly emotional problems – worry, anxiety, "nerves" – which cannot be traced to any obvious cause may find past live therapy particularly helpful. Tracking down some ancient trauma does not necessarily remove the symptoms, Guirdham has found, but it does remove the fear that they come from some organic disease or are a warning of incipient mental illness.

Psychic surgery

Psychic surgery is widely practised in several parts of the world, notably Brazil and the Philippines, but has only a few practitioners in North America and Europe. It has aroused more interest and controversy, however, than many more commonly encountered therapies and there have been several articles and several TV documentaries on the subject. We include it not because it is a kind of therapy which is much practised here (nor is it likely to be in the foreseeable future), but because its implications for the future of medicine, if the phenomena associated with it should turn out to be genuine and capable of being satisfactorily demonstrated, would be of profound importance.

There are two main types of psychic surgery. In one, widespread throughout Brazil, the "surgeon" uses a knife to open up the patient's body, but diagnosis and action appear to be guided (as he believes) by spirits, and the wound left by the knife seals itself up at the close of the operation. In the other, as practised in the Philippines, no instrument is used. The body appears to open up as if in response to the surgeon's fingers, and close up again, leaving no scar.

Origins

Of the two most widely accepted causes of illness in tribal communities – loss of the soul, which has been "spirited" away, and the introduction into the sick person's body of a pathogenic object or substance – dealing with the second has commonly been explained to onlookers from the West, explorers, and anthropologists, as imitation or ritual surgery. The shaman or witch doctor extracts the object with the help of his psychic powers, drawing it from the patient's body by motions of his hands or by "suction".

Psychic surgery in tribal communities

Watching shamans at work, anthropologists found two different types of "surgery" being practised in tribal communities. In one, the shaman sought to dematerialize the object placed by sorcery in the patient's body, and rematerialize it to demonstrate that he had been successful. In the other, though he went through the same motions, he would hold an object or fetish in his hand (or in his mouth) into which he would draw the sorcerer's magic, thereby rendering the sorcery impotent.

Some anthropologists have jumped to the conclusion that in the second of these methods the shaman, required by his tribe to be able to work magic, is pretending to extract the object, while in fact using sleight-of-hand. This, the eminent historian of medicine, Henry Sigerist, pointed out, is a misconception. It is because the pathogenic object has been introduced by a sorcerer "not physically but magically, on the strength of certain rites", that it has to be removed in the same way. The shaman puts his fetish in his mouth before he begins the treatment: "By performing the rites, of which sucking is one, he expects his object to attract the foreign body from the patient's parts so that the two become one magically. Thus he can produce the object in all sincerity".

Professor Mircea Eliade, the world's leading authority on shamanism, has since made the same point. No deception is involved: the tribesmen know that the shaman has the fetish objects in his mouth all the time. As one of them replied to an investigator, when questioned on the subject, "he draws the sickness into them, he uses them to catch the poison, otherwise how could he catch it?"

In modern times, these two strands of psychic surgery have become intertwined with nineteenth-century spiritualist beliefs and practices, and a great deal of confusion has been caused because some investigators (notably journalists looking for an easy "exposure") have attempted to separate these strands. They have confused the use of magic to materialize and dematerialize objects, and the use of ritual to obtain the same results without any attempt to produce psychokinetic effects, with sleight-of-hand.

The Brazilian "surgeons"

Here at least, there is no question of sleight-of-hand. The operations by the Brazilian "surgeons" are real, performed with a kitchen knife or scissors or whatever is to hand. The most famous exponent in recent times has been José de Freitas, better known as Arigo, who was clairaudient. For healing, he allowed himself to be "possessed" by the spirit of a deceased German doctor, Dr Fritz, who gave him instant diagnoses of patients' ills, and sometimes recommended appropriate drugs. When Dr Fritz advised an operation, Arigo took up a blunt knife, made the incision, removed the troublesome organ, and rejoined the skin simply by pressing it together. "This is one of the great mysteries of psychic surgery", Guy Lyon Playfair, who investigated the subject in Brazil, has written, "yet I have seen it happen both on film and in the flesh (mine included). The flesh simply comes together leaving a faint red line, which subsequently disappears altogether, where the incision was made".

Patients operated on by Arigo felt little pain. There was no sterilization, yet nobody died of blood poisoning. If anybody had, Playfair points out, "the story would have been over all of the country overnight, and Arigo would have been jailed for life". Arigo was jailed on one occasion for practising medicine without a licence, but his reputation as a healer remained untouched by any scandal until 1971, when he was killed in a road accident. He had been investigated scores of times, often by doctors who could not believe what they had been told about him. He welcomed investigation, and gave them every facility to watch him at work.

Whatever their opinion of his methods, his investigators could detect no sign of fakery.

Psychic surgery in the Philippines

It is less easy to investigate the activities of the Philippino surgeons. Some use the ritual method, drawing the poison out of the body by magic into the object they are holding – which Western sceptics have often assumed to be evidence that they are cheating. Some doubtless do cheat; the droves of rich Americans looking for miracle cures provide a tempting target. But others are doing what the shamans do – producing the object (perhaps obtained at the local butcher's shop) as part of the ritual. People who scoff at this are apt to forget that it is standard practice in those Christian churches where the wafer and the wine are presented for consumption as the body and blood of Christ.

Procedure

British healers who use the technique of psychic surgery have a modified version, which they call spirit healing or spirit surgery. They go into a trance, and perform what looks like a surgical operation, going through motions similar to those which a surgeon could be expected to make while removing, say, an appendix, but performing them *above* the patient's body. The theory is that they are operating on the patient's etheric or astral body, and that this will have the same effect as a surgical operation on the physical body: toxic substances will disappear, tumours will dematerialize. Many healers of this type are spiritualists, using "guides" who were themselves qualified doctors or medical specialists of some kind when they were alive (see also *Spiritualist healing* pages 239 to 243).

Research

A fair amount of research has been carried out by individual investigators in Brazil and in the Philippines, and although there have been some exposures of fraud, there have also been reports which suggest that fraud alone is an inadequate explanation of the techniques used. A number of observers have described watching Juan Blance of Pasig "make real incisions in the bodies of his patients", as Lyall Watson has recalled in *The Romeo Error*, "without a knife and from a distance. He simply points his finger at the skin and a cut appears instantaneously!" To test him, Watson interposed a sheet of plastic foil between him and the patient: the cut still appeared. There can be no question of its being imaginary. Watson insists; patients feel it, and the subcutaneous tissue is clearly visible. Yet afterwards, the skin comes together again, and only a faint scar line remains.

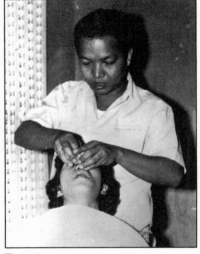

Tony Agpaoa
This Philippine healer has performed a number of remarkable "operations". During tests in Tokyo, it was found that several physiological changes occurred while Agpaoa was healing, including an increase in galvanic skin response and a predominance of alpha waves.

In 1973, nine scientists from the United States and Europe went to the Philippines, bringing 50 selected patients who had volunteered to test healers. The factual existence and daily practice of several types of psychoenergetic phenomena by several native healers was clearly established, as George W. Meek, who led the team, subsequently reported. These included "the practice of materializing and dematerializing human blood, tissue and organs as well as non-human objects".

All nine members of the team testified to the fact that the healing they had watched had been carried out without fraud. And although orthodox precautions such as sterilization had not been taken, none of the patients had been adversely affected. After they had returned home, some of the patients were reported by their own doctors to have made complete recoveries from illnesses which had been diagnosed as hopeless before they left. A biochemist with a brain tumour had been told it was inoperable: after a couple of sessions with Tony Agpaoa, the best known of the Philippine healers, the tumour had disappeared.

Suitable cases

Most of the patients who opt for psychic or spirit surgery undergo the British form where the "operation" is carried out on the etheric body. This, as a rule, means they are spiritualists who have been impressed by the reputation of the practitioner, and who suffer from inoperable tumours or less serious disorders which orthodox treatment has failed to treat effectively. If one of the Philippine healers is brought over for a few weeks, the patients who present themselves for treatment are also mostly spiritualists.

Inevitably, there are charges of fraud on such occasions, but if sleight-of-hand is involved, at least patients are likely to suffer only in their bank balances – and not by any worrying amount. Surgery which does not involve opening up the body may be a futile waste of time, but it can hardly do much harm beyond the inevitable disappointment if it does not work.

PARANORMAL DIAGNOSIS

There are some forms of diagnosis which have either yet to be explained or have yet to become acceptable to orthodoxy. For convenience they can be described as "paranormal", though some of their practitioners jib at the use of the term in connection with what they feel are scientific procedures which orthodox science has blindly ignored or rejected. In this section, therefore, we have included *Psychic diagnosis, Kirlian photography, Palmistry, Iridology, Biorhythms* and *Astrology*.

Psychic diagnosis

Most natural therapists, and not a few doctors, are aware that from time to time they realize what is the matter with a patient in a flash of what can be described either as intuition or extrasensory perception (ESP). Often there is no way of deciding which is responsible. Nobody has, as yet, been able to quantify intuition in such a way as would enable it to be distinguished from ESP. Whether a hunch or clairvoyance is responsible, some healers rely upon it, and others welcome it as a bonus when it comes to them spontaneously.

The development of psychic diagnosis

Throughout the world, psychic diagnosis was once standard practice in most tribal communities, and it has remained a feature of all forms of psychic healing. Occasionally the "divining" faculty has been so well-developed in individuals that they have styled themselves "psychic diagnosticians", as the Kentucky-born Edgar Cayce, the best-known of them all, used to do. From the turn of the century until his death in 1945, Cayce gave "readings" – information he had acquired about patients while he was under hypnosis. In his case, intuition could be ruled out as he did not even see the patients, and often knew nothing about them. He was perfectly willing to allow his readings to be checked by the medical profession, and as even those sceptics who investigated him were compelled to admit, they were astonishingly accurate.

Today, you are unlikely to come across anybody calling himself or herself a "psychic diagnostician", in the way Cayce did, partly to protect himself or herself from prosecution as an unlicensed practitioner of medicine. (Cayce was himself, in fact, once prosecuted in New York State for fortune-telling, but was acquitted of the charge). However, psychic diagnosis is practised in some groups, such as the Inner Light Consciousness, which is based in Virginia Beach, by some healers, and by all *Radionic* practitioners (see pages 257 to 263).

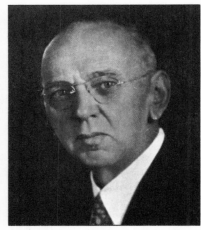

Edgar Cayce
Known as "the sleeping prophet", Cayce (1877–1945) became famous for the accuracy of his diagnoses while in the trance state.

Kirlian photography

Kirlian photography is a technique of high-frequency photography named after its inventors, Semyon and Valentina Kirlian. The belief is that the display of patterns and colours produced using this technique can be used as a diagnostic tool for detecting both psychological disorders and physical illness before the onset of visible symptoms.

Origins

Throughout history there have been reports of "auras", luminous areas surrounding people, much as phosphorescence appears with sea creatures. The circumstances in which auras have been seen often appear to preclude the possibility that they are physical, in the ordinary sense of the word. Could they, then, be regarded as etheric, visible only in certain circumstances, and perhaps only to certain people – people with psychic powers? Eileen Garrett, who made an impressive contribution to research into mediumship before and after the Second World War, claimed that for her, living things were always "encircled by a misty surround", and their colours and brightness varied.

When *Psi: Psychic Discoveries Behind the Iron Curtain* was published in 1970, its authors, Sheila Ostrander and Lynn Schroeder, made much of the fact that Semyon Kirlian, an electrician from Krasnador in the Kuban, and his wife Valentina, appeared to have found a way to photograph the aura. Very spectacular the results could be, with striking colours emerging from a finger, or even a leaf from a tree. The colours, they found, dimmed as the leaf withered, fading away altogether when it was "dead". When their discovery was tested by a representative of a Soviet research institute, it was found that their method actually detected "sickness" in a leaf which had been contaminated with a plant disease, though there appeared to be nothing wrong with it.

The implications were startling, particularly if they proved to be true of pictures of humans. Semyon Kirlian duly found that when he was ill, pictures of his hands became blurred and cloudy, while those of Valentina, who was well, remained clear and bright. This set off research in the Soviet Union, the satellite countries, and – in the 1970s – in the West, to see if the method could be used to provide reliable diagnoses.

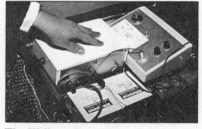

The Kirlian effect
This machine for photographing the Kirlian effect consists of a high-frequency field delivered to an aluminium plate. On top of this is a glass plate, then a film and finally a piece of protective plastic to protect the film from the salt in the skin. There is also a pressure gauge to ensure consistency of hand pressure.

Procedure

This is much the same as for *Palmistry* (see pages 276 to 278), except that the hand print is obtained by means of photography, and the interpretation based on the patterns and colours which show up on the Kirlian photograph. Tendencies may be identified and a therapist may recommend homeopathy, acupuncture, or psychotherapy, depending on what the photograph shows.

Research

It has to be said that although some of the research results have lent confirmation to the belief that Kirlian photography could eventually become a standard diagnostic tool, the problems of interpreting the pictures have often proved formidable. As Professor Arthur Ellison of the City University, London, has pointed out in a critique, objective assessment is hampered by the fact that there are so many variables, any one of which may affect the outcome.

Factors affecting Kirlian photographs

Most important of all the variables affecting interpretation, obviously, is the degree of pressure of the fingertip on the photographic apparatus, which can drastically alter the picture. But "other factors are clearly of importance, too, such as the temperature, the humidity of the air, the voltage wave-form and consistency, the duration of the discharge (along with its frequency) and the consistency of the film."

Using the photographs for diagnosis

Leonard W. Konikiewicz of the Polyclinic Medical Centre, Harrisburg, Pennsylvania, has shown that it is possible, under strictly controlled conditions, to use Kirlian photography successfully for diagnosis of certain disorders. But he has also shown how unreliable the results can be if the conditions are *not* strictly controlled, and few practitioners have the required facilities.

Menstrual cycle photographs
A range of photographs of the finger pads taken throughout a normal menstrual cycle. It is now thought that it is possible, by using this technique, to determine the time of ovulation. In this case the "aura" can be seen to be most prominent on the twelfth and thirteenth days of the cycle.

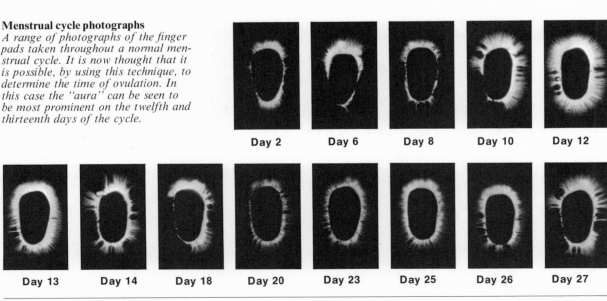

| Day 2 | Day 6 | Day 8 | Day 10 | Day 12 |

| Day 13 | Day 14 | Day 18 | Day 20 | Day 23 | Day 25 | Day 26 | Day 27 |

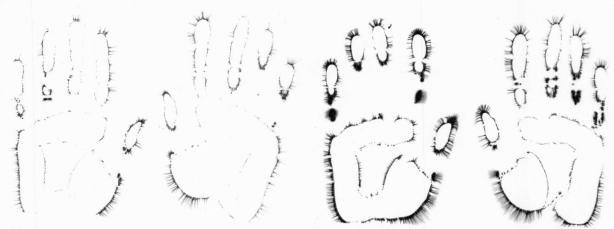

Although not unsympathetic to the paranormal (he was President of the Society for Psychical Research in 1982, its jubilee year), Professor Ellison is convinced that the information which a Kirlian photograph provides "is very much of *this* world, and no other". In other words, the aura can be accounted for by the fact that the body is surrounded by electromagnetic and thermal fields, not to mention the effects of sweat (as exploited in *Biofeedback*, see pages 188 to 193, and "lie-detector" machines).

The possibility remains, however, that a paranormal element may be mixed up with the observation of these physical surrounds of the body, which would account for the experience of Eileen Garrett, and other mediums who have claimed they have seen auras, and can judge from them whether an individual is, or is not, in good health.

Unfortunately, the Kirlian enthusiasts have tended to make much of the value of the method for the detection of cancer in its early stages. In view of the absence of any certainty that early detection of cancer is a reliable indication that the disease is going to progress, and also the fact that the method does not indicate the site of the cancer, this diagnosis may do nothing but give cause for alarm.

The effects of yoga on the aura
The two hands on the left have been photographed by Kirlian technique. After 15 minutes of yoga, the hands were rephotographed (right) and show a more relaxed, "complete" aura – the result of the gentle, energizing postures of yoga. Interestingly, the experiment was repeated with the same person doing standard gymnastics – this time there was no change.

Suitable cases

In some cases, Kirlian photography has given apparently useful diagnostic indications where other methods have failed; it cannot yet be relied upon, however. Brian Snellgrove, one of the pioneers of Kirlian photography in Britain, believes this photographic technique could have hundreds of applications, from "measuring the life force in seeds and plants" to "investigating the residual toxic effects of drug addiction", evaluating "the effect of parental conflict on children", assessing "the psychological compatibility between two people" and "evaluating the ability of a therapist to activate the self-healing process in a patient".

Palmistry

In *Modern Guide to Palmistry*, Beryl Hutchinson says "there are three distinct approaches to hand interpretations which have to be appreciated separately, then woven into a pattern of cause and effect to obtain a true map of the personality."

One approach is through *chirognomy*, the study of the shape of the hand, including such characteristics as its flexibility, colour, and texture, and even the way the hands are used. A second, which is what the public tends to equate with palmistry, is *chiromancy*, the interpretation of the lines of the hand. The third, *dermatoglyphics*, relates to the skin patterns – of the kind, for example, that are displayed in fingerprinting. There is another element in palmistry, however, which some of its practitioners consider the most important of all. After studying the hand for its physical characteristics, they try to "tune in" by intuition or clairvoyance to the individual. For diagnostic purposes, either the physiological evidence alone can be assessed, or it can be combined with the information obtained intuitively.

Origins

One of the first scientists to devote attention to the subject was the British scientist and explorer Sir Francis Galton, whose work on fingerprints at the turn of the century helped to establish them as a standard method of detecting criminals. But the medical profession was slow to pursue research along the lines he had pioneered, and palmistry remained as a rather frivolous fairground or church-fête activity until an American anatomist, Professor Harold Cummins took it up between the wars, and demonstrated that there is a more serious side to it. Later, a German-born researcher, Dr Charlotte Wolff, provided detailed evidence to prove that there are links between the condition of the hand and illnesses. It was not just a matter of reading the lines, Wolff insisted, temperature, humidity, colour and flexibility all count, "and their significance is as much psychological as indicative of physical health".

Procedure

Inevitably, much depends upon the particular preconceptions and interests of the therapist. If you go to an established palmist, he or she may "read" your hand immediately or palm prints may be taken with the help of a piece of glass, a sheet of paper, ink and a roller. The prints are then studied at leisure by the palmist, and a diagnosis provided. As with *Astrology* (see pages 286 to 291), the diagnosis (except where it is intuitive or clairvoyant) is rarely specific. Rather it is chiefly concerned with a predisposition to certain types of disorder which, as research has confirmed, can be gauged from reading the hand.

6 . . . the findings and knowledge are of essential importance for psychologists, doctors and educationists. It is a valuable contribution to a character research in its widest application. 9

Carl Gustav Jung

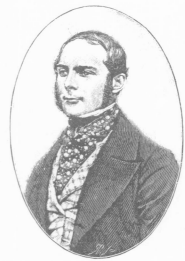

Sir Francis Galton
The scientist Galton (1822–1911) did pioneering work on fingerprints, classifying them according to three patterns – loops, arches, and whorls.

Research

The fairground image of palmistry was so strong that research into palmistry in connection with disease made little impression until, in the late 1950s, work at the Galton Laboratory showed that Down's syndrome or mongolism, which is the consequence of a chromosomal abnormality, is accompanied in three cases out of four by a line across the top of the palm, which is known as "the simian crease". Then, in 1966, two pediatricians at the State University of New York, Ruth Achs and Rita Harper, investigating a group of babies with abnormal handprints, found that they had all been born during a German measles epidemic, suggesting that the abnormalities had some link with the epidemic. The following year, a report of research at Japan's Osaka Hospital claimed that the doctors there, simply by examining palm prints, could accurately estimate patients' susceptibility to diseases.

Research along these lines may eventually provide clues that will be valuable in preventive medicine. For example, if a link were to be found between certain characteristics of the hand and heart disease, it could be added to the growing list of "risk factors", and perhaps give advance warning to those who have those characteristics that they must be careful to avoid such risks as are avoidable, such as smoking. For the present, however, the intuitive/clairvoyant type of palmistry is more likely to give useful warnings of this kind.

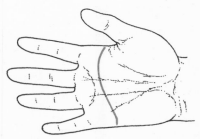

The simian crease
The simian crease is a line across the top of the palm which replaces both the lines of the head and the heart (see overleaf), commonly found on an ape's hand. It has also been shown to be present in three out of four cases of mongolism.

Consulting a palmist

Many practitioners of palmistry use their art as a form of counselling or psychotherapy. You can always expect a full character analysis, working either from prints or directly from your hands. A personal consultation generally lasts about half an hour.

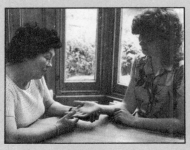

1 *The palmist pinches the client's fingertips to find out whether they are hard or soft. Hard fingertips indicate a self-willed personality, softer ones denote nervousness.*

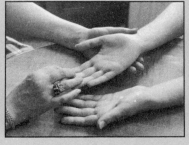

2 *Reading from both palms, she interprets the lines and other characteristics and gives the client her "diagnosis".*

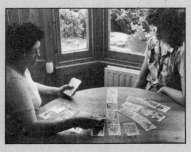

3 *Some palmists use Tarot cards as an adjunct to their main work, to "tune in" to the client and predict future trends.*

Suitable cases

Suitability is largely determined by curiosity. Most people who go to a palmist are hoping for a glimpse into the future. If the glimpse they are given turns out, in time, to be accurate, they may well consider returning to the palmist for information about the health aspect of their lives.

Dr Charlotte Wolff, who over the years has made extensive studies of hands from the point of view of psychological diagnosis, is of the opinion that "the hand is the visible part of the brain". Given that this is the case, we *all* carry maps of our own lives in the palms of our hands. The essential value of palmistry, then, is to help us to learn more about ourselves.

Self-help

In his book *Palmistry*, Fred Gettings gave instructions on how best you can read your own, or other peoples' palm prints. "Try, in the first instance, to look at the prints 'emotionally', resisting any attempt to make an intellectual analysis", he advised; "do not force anything, but simply register what your emotions tell you about the hand prints". To do this you should be sitting comfortably, relaxed, and breathing deeply, then "when you feel emotionally alert, look at the print".

For a time, Gettings warned, all sorts of ideas will come crowding into your mind. "Let it chatter on in its own way, and make some attempt to register what you feel about the hand. After only a little practice you will be astonished to find that you have a very useful tool for investigating the world which you have probably not used at all until now".

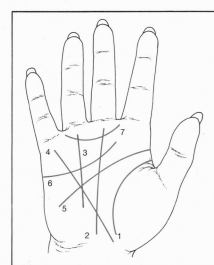

The lines of the hand

1 The line of life *does not foretell the length of your life – it is related rather to your vitality. Breaks can indicate illness, or equally, a major change.*

2 The line of fate *does not tell our fate – it shows certain things which may come to bear on us, though not what our reactions to them will be.*

3 The line of the sun *suggests artistic inclinations. If in harmony with all the other lines, it promises a successful life.*

4 The line of health *is not present on all hands. If it is, you should take extra care of your health.*

5 The line of head *is linked with intelligence and the mentality generally. The palmist sees its significance in conjunction with the life line.*

6 The line of heart *should, in turn, be read against the head line and governs your emotional and sexual life.*

7 The girdle of Venus *denotes restlessness – someone constantly searching for new experiences or with a moody, changeable personality.*

Iridology

The assumption behind iridology is that the condition of the eyes, and in particular, the iris, provides indications which can be used in the diagnosis of mental and physical disorders. Iridologists believe that examination of the iris can reveal not merely what is the matter with you, but what has been the matter with you in the past, as well as giving advance warning of what may be the matter with you in the future.

"The eye is where the nervous system comes to the surface and the iris reflects, via the nervous system, all parts of the body, and hence the mind and spirit, too", John Morley of Iridology Research explains. "The lines, flecks and pigments of the iris thus give a detailed, on-line picture of the status of the whole of the system, including past history and future tendencies".

The beauty of the iris diagnosis is that it reveals tendencies that may not yet have begun to express themselves as actual symptoms. This makes it possible to plan our lifestyle, including appropriate treatment, according to our natural strengths and weaknesses, likes and dislikes.

John Morley
Iridology Research, London

Origins

The eye has been examined for diagnostic purposes for centuries. There are a number of references to the significance of bloodshot eyes in the Hippocratic writings, for instance, and the general colour and brightness of the eyes has always been taken into account in orthodox examinations of sick patients.

The theory that the iris can give more precise information about disease was first independently propounded by a Hungarian, Ignatz von Peczely, and a Swede, Nils Liljequist, about a century ago.

In the United States, Dr Bernard Jensen was the pioneer of the science of iridology and has developed a comprehensive iris chart which shows the location of the organs as they reflect in the iris.

In iridology, the iris is "mapped", divided up like a clock face into segments, each of which represents an organ or function. Where a segment is flecked, or has an unusual colour or marking, it is presumed to be a pointer to a disorder.

In surveying the iris, according to Bernard Jensen, author of *The Science and Practice of Iridology*, "attention is given to the purity or brightness of the colouring. In a state of good health, the colors are bright and clear; in ill health, or a toxic condition, the colors are defiled and dull". The texture of the iris, which can resemble "the fineness of woven silk or the coarseness of burlap", provides further information.

Procedure

Many therapists, including osteopaths, acupuncturists, herbalists and homeopaths, use iridology as an aid to diagnosis alongside their other physical tests. These people often only use a magnifying glass and torch to examine the iris.

Up-to-date specialist practitioners of iridology, however, use purpose-built equipment to enable a photograph of the eyes to be taken, from which slides are made. These are then projected onto a screen and a diagnosis can be made at leisure, in consultation with the patient. An iridologist who is also an acupuncturist or a naturopath, for instance, will then suggest which type of treatment, if any, is most suitable for the condition which has been diagnosed. Alternatively, natural therapists who, perhaps, want a second opinion are increasingly sending their clients for iridology diagnosis. The patients then return to their practitioner for treatment. Either way, more photographs may be taken at intervals later on so checks can be made on the effectiveness of the treatment which the patient has undertaken.

Consulting an iridologist

As a diagnostic tool, iridology has several obvious advantages over other systems. Merely by studying the two irises, the therapist can obtain information about all parts of your body simultaneously. And he or she can deduce not only your present state of health but also predict potential trouble spots. In addition, iridology is completely safe, painless, and extremely quick.

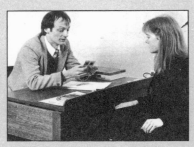

1 *This therapist begins by explaining that he will be taking a slide of each eye in order to find out if there are any irregular markings or colours in the iris that signify possible disorders.*

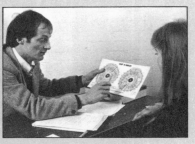

2 *He shows the patient the diagnostic charts (see opposite) which he will use in conjunction with the slides to pinpoint exactly which part of the body is malfunctioning.*

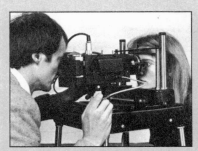

3 *A special camera is needed to photograph the irises. It is mounted so that it can move across three planes – up/down, left/right, and in/out. Fibre-optic side-lighting ensures the eye's contours are well-lit.*

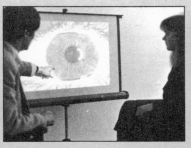

4 *At the second appointment, the therapist projects the patient's slides and explains how he has reached his diagnosis. He suggests a course of treatment and directs the patient to a suitable practitioner.*

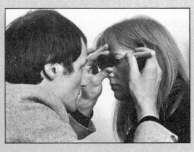

5 *The therapist may also use a magnifying glass and penlight to confirm his diagnosis or, at a later date, to check the success of his recommended treatment.*

Suitable cases

Iris diagnosis can in theory be used in conjunction with any therapy in which the therapist has doubts about diagnosis. It is even applicable, on occasion, where there are no doubts, but the therapist welcomes supplementary information about what course to pursue.

People who are squeamish about submitting to blood tests or who prefer not to have X-rays may feel that they prefer to opt for iridology as a painless diagnostic procedure.

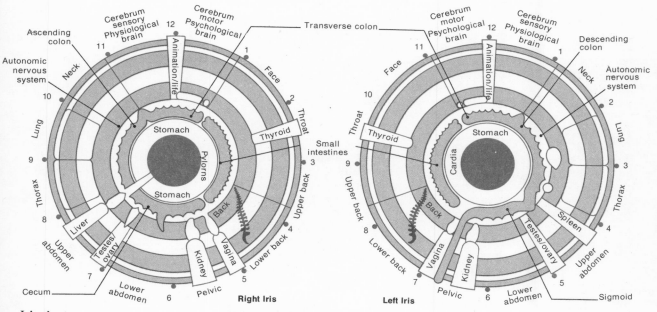

Right Iris　　　**Left Iris**

Iris chart

Developed by Dr Bernard Jensen, the iris chart shows where the various parts of the body reflex in the eyes. The left iris corresponds to the left side of the body, the right iris to the right side. At the top of each iris, the brain and organs of the head are to be found, whilst the feet are at the bottom. From pupil to outer rim, the irises are divided concentrically into 3 zones. Organs of digestion and absorption are contained in the innermost zone, organs of transport, utilization, and elimination through the kidneys in the middle zone, and organs of structure and elimination, including the skeletal system and the skin in the outermost zone.

Using the chart

This is a photograph of the left eye of a woman aged 27 who had a lump in her left breast and a history of digestive problems, headaches, depression, and bladder infections. The eye indicates: severe gastro-intestinal toxicity and congestion, resulting in irritation in the bladder and lower back; a tendency to lymphatic stagnation and weakness in the lymphatic cleansing system; underactivity in the ovaries and uterus; spasticity throughout the large intestine; sinus headaches; and depression.

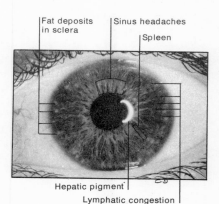

Fat deposits in sclera　Sinus headaches　Spleen

Hepatic pigment

Lymphatic congestion

Biorhythms

The theory of biorhythms, Bernard Gittleson, a New York exponent of the subject, has written, "holds that when a person is born, the trauma of leaving the safe and warm confines of the mother's womb sets in motion a series of three cycles which will continue to reoccur at regular intervals until death".

The three cycles

There is a physical cycle of 23 days, an emotional cycle of 28 days, and an intellectual cycle of 33 days. Each cycle, if charted on a graph, forms a wave pattern. "It is while crossing the middle of each cycle, either from high to low or from low to high, that the individual experiences an unstable or 'critical period' " – which is more significant if the "critical" periods of two or three cycles happen to coincide on the same day. It is during these critical periods that the individual is more accident- or illness-prone, so knowledge of one's own cycle may be useful in making decisions about what to do, or what not to do – for example, in knowing when to take care to avoid stressful occasions.

Origins

The founder of the biorhythm theory was Sigmund Freud's sometime friend (like most of Freud's friends, they eventually quarrelled), Dr Wilhelm Fliess, a German physican fascinated by the patterns of the menstrual cycle. Fliess developed the idea that men, as well as women have a bisexual, sex-linked cycle from birth to death – usually 28 days for women, and 23 for men – which determines stages in growth and the dates upon which people fall ill. The research on which he based this finding looked impressive, accurately predicting the onset of illness. But as Freud was later to tell his biographer Ernest Jones, Fliess was an expert with figures, "and by multiplying 23 and 28 by the difference between them and adding or subtracting the results, or by even more complicated arithmetic, he would always arrive at the number he wanted".

One of Freud's former pupils, however, Professor Herman Swoboda, an Austrian psychologist, had by that time taken up the idea, and had produced more convincing evidence for the periodicity of certain disorders. Swoboda's theory has continued to attract attention. Recently this has extended to the study of "circadian" rhythms, to take in evidence of *daily* cycles. Lyall Watson's book *Supernature*, published in 1973, alerted the public for the first time to the possibility that what had been dismissed as occult fancy, might soon have to be recognized as scientific fact.

Procedure

Computers have now rendered elaborate mathematical calculations unnecessary, and it is possible to consult any of the

❛When the moon is full, people with problems such as ulcers should be especially sure to take their medicine, a University of Illinois researcher says. Ralph Morris said he studied more than 100 patients over five years, and found that bleeding ulcers and chest pains became more frequent in two-thirds of the patients at times of a full moon.❜

Associated Press release
The Guardian, 8 Jan 1982

reputable agencies which advertise in the press. They will require your name and date of birth, and in return for a small fee you will be sent a personalized print-out. This will display information about your cycles and will enable you to see which days during the coming three or four weeks are going to be critical for you, to help you to tell how your body will react to certain situations – which are good days for making decisions, for instance, and on which days to avoid emotional confrontations.

Research

The evidence for biorhythms is still mainly empirical, based on observation more than on experience: "even at this stage there is still no definitive proof that biorhythms exist", Gittleson admits. But he adds that "it is clearly beyond the hypothetical stage, for thousands of well-documented cases already support the theory", and he cites the work of Harold R. Willis, a Professor of Psychology at Southern State College in America. Examining the records of patients who had died during 1973 in a local hospital, Willis found that over half had died on what for them would have been critical days, in biorhythm terms. The following year, a follow-up study of over 100 cases showed the same pattern. Even more significantly, in terms of potential usefulness of biorhythms for accident prevention, when the pharmaceutical company Pfizer introduced a staff safety programme which was partially based on biorhythm principles, they found that the accident rate was halved.

Not all research projects, however, have produced such clear-cut results; some findings have been negative. An examination of the biorhythms of drivers involved in accidents, undertaken by the British Transport and Road Research Laboratory, provided no evidence of a correlation between accidents and critical days. A more sophisticated approach is to accept that there is evidence for biorhythms, but to qualify it by the assumption that individuals react in their individual ways to critical periods. On this theory, somebody who is prone to stress disorders may succumb to them, but somebody else who thrives on adversity may be on top of their form.

More research will be required, therefore, before the role of biorhythms in health and disease can be established. In the meantime, if you are interested in them, you can conduct your own research. See how well the critical days tally with personal experience, and, if they do indeed appear to indicate proneness to illness or accidents, work out how best to avoid them.

Our internal "clocks"

Among the examples of research into circadian rhythms, those daily cycles which Lyall Watson cited, was one which may have implications for humans, even though the objects of research were cockroaches. In the 1956 Journal of Experimental Biology, Janet Harker described how she had changed the internal "clocks" of cockroaches by the use of artificial light during the night, and artificial darkness during the daylight hours (their active time). When she transplanted the "clock" of one of them into a cockroach which lived normal hours, the outcome was unnerving. As Lyall Watson put it, "having two time-keepers sending out two completely different signals, the poor insect was thrown into turmoil. Its behaviour became completely disorganized and it soon developed acute stress symptoms such as malignant tumours in the gut, and died".

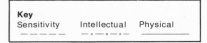

Key
Sensitivity   Intellectual   Physical

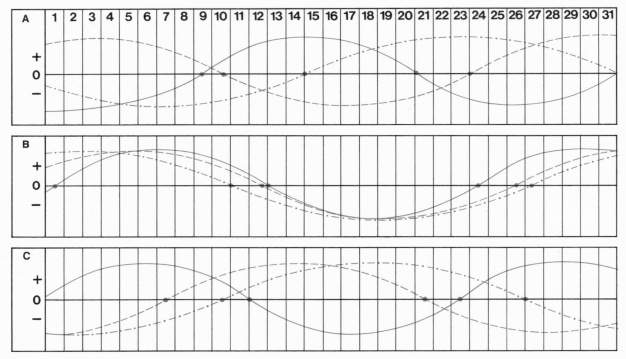

How to read a biorhythm chart
A biorhythm chart is made up from three cycles: these are the physical, the sensitivity and the intellectual. The physical cycles takes 23 days and governs strength, endurance, confidence, sex drive and immunity to and recovery from illness. The sensitivity cycle is 28 days long and governs moods, emotions, nervous reactions and creative abilities. The intellectual cycle is 33 days long,

governing reasoning, decision making, memory and the ability to absorb new facts. When your chart is drawn on to a monthly plan, these cycles are known as "sine curves". Through the centre of each chart runs a horizontal line, the caution line. Above this line, the cycle is positive and its attributes are enhanced; below, it is negative and the cycle is passing through a recuperative phase, gathering energy for the next positive stage. When a

curve passes through the caution line, the subject is most vulnerable in that particular cycle. On caution days, subjects can become accident-prone or aggressive or absent-minded. On double or triple caution days (when two or three cycles pass through the caution line) these problems are exacerbated. It can be seen for example, that the second subject will go through a bad period around the 10 to 12 of the month.

If disruptions of our internal "clocks" can similarly lead to stress disorders, this may well be of concern, for example to airline crews jetting from one continent to another and back. The time has come for more research into human biorhythms, and the results of one project have recently been reported in the *IRCS Journal of Medical Science*.

A seven-man team from Boston and New York, knowing that people show considerable physiological variations according to the time of day (blood pressure, for example, can vary in some patients by as much as 25 percent), decided to monitor patients coming into two coronary care units following heart attacks to find at what time of day their attacks had come on. Their vague expectation was that some link might be found to stressful periods of the day. What they actually found was that the onset of the attacks was fairly evenly distributed throughout the day and night, except for two peak periods, between eight and ten o'clock in the morning, and between eight and ten o'clock in the evening: half the attacks had begun in these two periods.

No plausible history has yet been put forward to account for this phenomenon, but it suggests that there are diurnal fluctuations in levels of health, or of resistance to ill-health, which, if they could be properly mapped (and eventually explained) would be of importance in our understanding of disease, and would enable us to prevent it.

Suitable cases

As with *Palmistry* and *Astrology* (see pages 276 to 278 and 286 to 287), curiosity provides the main reason for exploring the possibility that a knowledge of your biorhythms will help you stay healthy. There can now be little doubt that some of us are subject to periodicity in our illnesses, and it can be useful to know our "critical" days, if experience shows that they tend to be significantly related to illness or accident. It might also be useful for all of us to have more information about our internal clocks or circadian rhythms, though this will be very much harder to translate into active, preventive measures.

Self-help

As soon as your biorhythm periodicity has been established, you can take on the monitoring process yourself. Most suppliers of biorhythm charts provide the information on a 6- or 12-month basis, and it is a very simple process to have it updated as required. Alternatively, you can buy a book devoted to the subject and work out your own biorhythm cycles according to the charts provided; some shops sell specially-programmed calculators from which you can work out your cycle.

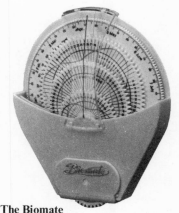

The Biomate
The Biomate is a new device for computing your biorhythms. You key in your own birthdate and it works out all three cycles and your critical days thereafter.

Astrology

Astrology, when it is concerned with health, derives from the belief that there is a correspondence between the positions of the sun, moon and planets in the twelve zodiac signs and physical, mental, spiritual and emotional well-being. At the moment of birth, astrologers believe, the planetary positions establish a pattern, which is unique to individuals throughout their lifetimes. By ascertaining what the map of the heavens was like at a person's birth, it should be possible for the astrologer to gauge the prospects for good health, or proneness to illness, enabling steps to be taken to preserve the former and avoid the latter.

These days, few practitioners are solely medical astrologers, but all admit that health, whether physical or psychological, is an integral part of the reading and interpretation of a birth chart.

Origins

In most early civilizations the importance of astronomy and astrology in relation to health was taken for granted. A good physician, the ancient Greek author of the Hippocratic treatise *Airs, Waters and Places* claimed, should pay attention to climatic conditions, and must also be "familiar with the progress of the seasons and the dates of the rising and the setting of the stars", if he or she wanted to enjoy good health and have a successful medical practice. "If it should be thought that this is more the business of the meteorologist, then learn that astronomy plays a very important part in medicine since the changes of the seasons produce changes in diseases".

Although belief in cosmic forces as a factor in physical diseases tended to die away after the Renaissance, it did retain a hold in connection with mental disorders. In Britain, for instance, the mentally ill were divided into two categories: the insane, who were chronically disturbed; and the lunatic, who became disturbed only at the time of a full moon.

Procedure

Not all astrologers are prepared to advise on medical issues, and only a very few specialize in them. Ordinarily they work on an appointment system, and as a preliminary they will require your name, date, place, and time of birth.

Casting the horoscope

The first step is something which anybody can do, given the necessary information, the ability to cope with astronomical tables, and a sufficient knowledge of mathematics. A horoscope is, in effect, a map of the solar system at the time of birth, as seen from the birthplace. This is done by drawing a circle and dividing it into 12 segments or "houses", each of which represents aspects

'A doctor, too, emerged as we proceeded;
No one alive could talk as well as he did
On points of medicine and of surgery,
For, being grounded in astronomy,
He watched his patient's favourable star
And, by his Natural Magic, knew what are
The lucky hours and planetary degrees
For making charms and magic effigies.'

Chaucer
The Canterbury Tales

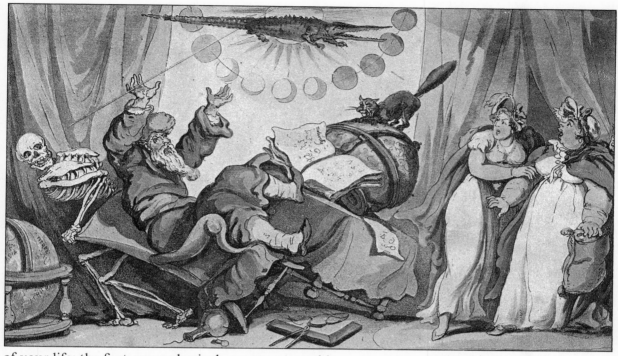

The fortune teller
In 1815, the artist Rowlandson portrayed the contemporary, and rather alarming, view of a visit to a fortune teller.

of your life: the first, your physical appearance and how you see the world about you; the second, your resources; the third, your intellect – and so on. On to this is mapped your horoscope. It is at this point that medical astrology becomes a matter of interpretation. The relationships of the sun, moon and planets all need to be taken into consideration, along with further complexities.

There are several loose generalizations that can be made: for example, if your sun sign is Cancer, you are said to be prone to stomach disorders; if Sagittarius, to trouble with the hips and thighs; if Leo, to heart disease, and so on. But medical astrologers tend to regard these as superficial indicators. To find what disorders to look out for needs a more detailed inspection of your horoscope, and a better knowledge of you an an individual, than can be obtained simply from knowing the sun sign under which you were born.

Research

One of the most notable of the recent investigations into the effect of the moon on personality was reported by the American Institute of Medical Climatology. This showed that certain crimes (among them arson, kleptomania and dangerous driving) are more common during the period of the full moon.

Planetary positions and the moment of birth

It is not discoveries of this kind, however, which brought astrology back into contention, so much as the researches of Michel Gauquelin and his wife. Until Gauquelin's *The Cosmic Clocks* was published in 1969, most scientists had assumed astrology was a debased superstition traded upon by the writers of popular astrology columns in newspapers and magazines. Gauquelin, a psychologist and statistician at the Psychophysiological Laboratory in Strasbourg, had thought of an ingenious but simple way of finding out whether horoscopes are accurate in one of the ways they are traditionally supposed to be. If the moment of birth influences the type of career a person is going to follow, he reasoned, it should show up in the statistics. And using as his sample the birth dates of some 600 members of the French Academy of Medicine, Gauquelin found that a significantly high proportion of them had been born when Mars and Saturn occupied particular positions on a person's horoscope.

As this might have been a chance finding, Gauquelin took a further sample of 500 eminent doctors, and got a similar result. Certain planetary positions, further investigation showed, linked with a significantly high proportion of famous athletes, politicians and military leaders. A further test along the same lines in

Consulting an astrologer

Astrology is potentially such a vast source of information that an astrologer will often ask you for a detailed brief of your particular requirements, as well as the date, place and time of your birth. When you meet the astrologer, you will receive the birthchart, an hour or more of explanation and, often, a cassette recording of the session.

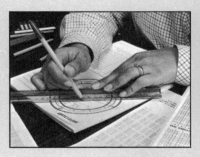

1 *The astrologer draws in the client's "aspects" – the relationships between the planetary positions at birth. Some aspects are stressful, others harmonious; together they will make up the life-pattern.*

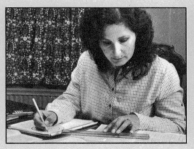

2 *The current planetary positions are noted, for if they are close to sensitive points on the chart, they may stimulate or block certain traits in the subject's nature, producing trends in the life-pattern.*

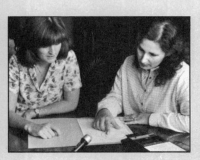

3 *During the consultation, the astrologer will explain the client's astrological make-up and help her explore any unsuspected qualities which may emerge and accept any conflicts in her character.*

the United States, carried out by sceptics, has since confirmed Gauquelin's result, much to their embarrassment – they even tried, unsuccessfully, to hush their findings up. Gauquelin's work has also been evaluated, and recognized as valid, by Professor Hans Eysenck – a testimonial worth having.

Horoscopes and diagnosis

The findings have been leading a few formerly sceptical people to investigate the value of horoscopes as an aid to diagnosis and treatment. Their use in this way was, in fact, pioneered by Carl Jung, the Swiss psychiatrist, who placed considerable reliance on them. The renewed interest in astrology, however, has led to a growing realization that interpretation of a horoscope requires a much more sophisticated approach than had earlier been considered necessary.

One contemporary astrologer, Liz Greene, has explained that confusion about astrology has arisen because of a tendency to think of it in fatalistic terms, as it has occasionally been, in the Far East. But as the astronomer Johann Kepler pointed out several centuries ago, if we are influenced by the heavens, it is in much the same way as a pumpkin is influenced by the bindings which a farmer uses on it: "they do not make the pumpkin grow, but they determine its shape".

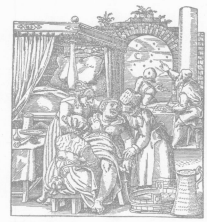

The birthchart
This sixteenth-century German engraving shows astrologers plotting the positions of sun, moon, and planets in order to cast the natal horoscope of the baby of a labouring mother.

Our astrological "programmes"

Liz Greene, however, would allow the heavens rather more of a role. Astrology, she feels "can offer psychology a blueprint of the individual's potential, which not only determines what kind of seed, but what timing and what patterns of growth, must be considered". We tend to be programmed by convention and the necessity of earning a living. But many of us, because we are programmed differently in astrological terms, really need to break convention's mould. If we are not aware of this need, ill-health can be one of the consequences of the stresses set up. The progression of the planets does not make things happen; rather it is, "in a sense, like the bell indicating coffee is ready".

Medical astrology, in other words, is invaluable as an aid to diagnosis, but it does not provide any firm prognostications. Unluckily, many members of the public believe it does. Some become "childishly dependent upon astrologers, incapable of making decisions for themselves"; others may be frightened off, for fear of hearing that they are "fated" in some unwelcome way. The value of a horoscope, Liz Greene insists, should lie not in predicting some actual occurrence, but in prompting recognition of some inner need, the "integration of some dormant quality into conscious awareness".

In Kaslof's *Wholistic Dimensions of Healing*, Dr Mario Jones makes a similar point. In medical astrology, psychology is

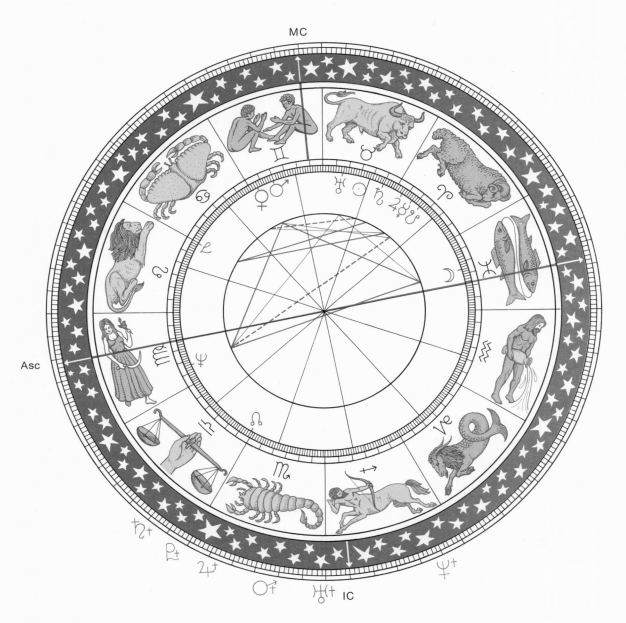

The birthchart

The astrological birthchart is an accurate astronomical map of the solar system at the time and place of the subject's birth. It shows the rising and culminating degrees of the ecliptic, as well as the symbols of the planets in their exact degrees of zodiacal longitude. Each planet represents a basic drive – for example, Mars stands for physical energy and will; Mercury for mental and nervous energy; and the Moon for emotional response, especially the need to nurture or be nurtured. Calculating a chart takes about 2 hours, unless a calculator or computer is used. Many more hours are required to analyze and synthesize its meaning.

essential, he argues: "Astrology shows how psychological and somatic considerations in disease go hand in hand. A psychological definition is necessary to know how the disease is going to affect the total life of the patient and to find appropriate therapeutic means". As he goes on to observe, however, "if to the many different astrological approaches we add the diverse psychological systems, we end up with a distinct approach for every astrologer, a state of confusion that can lead to a number of valid approaches to the patient's problem, but not to a systematic study". There is the further complication of environmental influences, because any astrological reading needs to take into account the client's lifestyle, and life problems.

Suitable cases

Mario Jones suggests five ways in which medical astrology can help. First, it gives a quick overall view of the individual. Second, it may provide indications of what to look out for in the way of disorders, which can be a help where orthodox diagnosis has failed to establish what is the matter. Third, it can help to establish what is the most promising form of treatment. Fourth, it can give a clear prognosis ("here, astrology reigns supreme", Jones claims; "it can define with amazing accuracy a crisis during an illness, and the long-term possibility of a recurrence"). And fifth, it can enable us to plan our lives, to make decisions about diet, activities, precautions and so on.

What this amounts to is that there are no particular types of disorder for which medical astrology is pre-eminently suitable. Its value lies chiefly in the assistance it can give to people who feel the need to reassess their lifestyle and habits, to secure better health, or who are suffering from disorders, especially from psychological and psychosomatic disorders, for which other types of therapy have not brought relief. But to obtain full benefit it is necessary to avoid the fatalistic approach, and to think of the diagnosis and prognosis as an aid, rather than as an instruction, in deciding what to do.

CONCLUSIONS

We have tried to keep this survey of unconventional therapies simple and coherent, but we must reiterate that in practice, they are in a state of flux. Not merely are they proliferating, with new therapies and variations on established ones emerging every year; they are cross-fertilizing, so that the distinctions between them are breaking down.

As we have emphasized, this means that there can be no easy way to select the "right therapy", let alone the "right therapist", to suit your particular needs. It means that you have to shop around. It means, too, that you will be taking on a greater responsibility for your own health than, in all probability, you have done in the past – particularly if you have believed that your doctor will have the appropriate prescription for whatever your symptoms may be.

Self-management of health

In one sense, this is not so much of a revolution as it may sound. Research projects in the last few years have been showing the extent to which people have already come to rely on self-management to keep themselves well; to diagnose what is the matter with themselves if they feel ill; and to prescribe for themselves, often on the advice of relations, friends, or the local chemist. One research team found that over a two week period, three out of four women and six out of ten men took some medicine which they themselves had prescribed.

Natural therapists, however, feel that most self-management of this kind, particularly when it leads to endless self-medication, is unnecessary – and in the long run, dangerous. There is a sense, in fact, in which the more effective self-medication seems to be, the greater the long-term risk, because people who continually use sedatives, painkillers, purges and indigestion cures are not merely masking their symptoms, rather than finding the cause and dealing with it, but are also running the risk of undermining their bodies' self-protective mechanism, which can easily lose its resilience.

The holistic principle

The most valuable contribution that the practitioners of alternative therapies have made, in fact, is not the technique they practise, but their insistence upon the holistic principle: the principle that it is *you* who is being considered, not just your symptoms. But this in turn requires a willingness on your part to abandon entrenched attitudes and habits, largely derived from the assumption that specific symptoms have to be treated by specific drugs. Any one of a score of different therapies may be capable of banishing your headaches or indigestion, not by acting on your forehead or your gut, but by removing the stresses, physical and psychological, that give rise to these symptoms.

What of the future? The course events are likely to take is hard to predict, in view of the extensive monopoly powers still wielded by the medical profession and the reluctance of governments to contemplate changes which will not merely offend the profession, but may require the raising of additional revenue, at least for a time. But there are many indications that the monopoly is everywhere being eroded. The World Health Organization (WHO) has been pressing for a change of attitude to primary health care, shifting it away from professional doctors to paramedicals and to lay care and natural therapists.

Delays in legal acceptance of alternative medicine

In Europe, the WHO now has programmes of research into what is being called "supportive health education" – ways in which through self-help, self-care and "mutual aid" people can be encouraged to play an active role in pursuit of their own health. In the Netherlands, pressure from the public and a recommendation for a change in the laws governing who should be allowed to practice medicine led in 1977 to the formation by the government of a Committee on Alternative Medicine. Three years later, it presented its findings and recommendations, and although these called for more research and for supervision of present training courses – all very cautious, first steps towards including alternative therapies within the Dutch system of health care – the report itself has produced its inevitable criticisms and counter-attacks from the medical profession. For the time being, then, it seems there is no forward movement to gaining official, legal acceptance of alternative medicine.

The singer not the song

What governments do, however, is likely to be of less importance in the immediate future than what the public chooses to do. All the indications are that the demand for the services of practitioners of what have hitherto been regarded as unconventional forms of therapy will continue to increase. This has its dangers, as some of the practitioners are bound to be unscrupulous, and some will be corrupted by adulation and new-found wealth, just as doctors sometimes are. But the existence of this risk only reinforces the need to think in terms of finding *the right therapist*, and not just the right therapy: the singer, not the song.

FINDING THE RIGHT THERAPIST

"Should I place myself in the hands of someone who may not have medical qualifications? How do I choose the right type of therapist? How do I know they will be any good? How long will it take? How much will I have to pay?" These are the sort of questions which naturally arise when you decide you want to try an alternative to orthodox medical treatment. If you have made the decision but you are not sure how (or indeed whether) to go about it, here are some questions and answers which should help reassure you over any misgivings you might have.

Q *Is it really safe for me to go to a practitioner without medical qualifications?*

A It is tempting, here, to suggest that you ask yourself instead the question. "How safe is it to go to my doctor?" Today's drugs are so powerful that if anything goes wrong, you may find the effects of the remedy worse than the disease. On balance, natural medicine is safer simply because it places less reliance on drugs.

Your own doctor may assure you that he has come across cases where a medically unqualified practitioner has failed to diagnose, say, cancer. But as most natural therapists' cases come to them *after* they have been medically diagnosed, and patients have been told either that there is nothing the matter with them or that if there is, nothing can be done about it, responsibility for the failure to make a diagnosis commonly rests first with the GP or hospital.

Similarly, many orthopedic surgeons have scare stories about patients crippled by an osteopath or chiropractor. But then, most osteopaths and chiropractors have similar stories about patients crippled by a slipped disc operation.

You need to remember that each side sees the other side's failures and rejects. They may well be resentful after what has happened, and because of this willing to spread around the worse interpretation.

Q *Are you suggesting that I should give up going to my doctor?*

A No. In one respect – diagnosis – your doctor is likely to be better qualified than the great majority of practitioners of natural medicine. Your doctor's diagnostic skill is most required, admittedly, in connection with relatively rare diseases, but on those occasions it may be vital.

Q *If I go to a natural therapist who is not medically qualified, should I tell my doctor?*

A This depends upon your doctor. Some are happy to let patients go to a local osteopath, acupuncturist or healer whom they have learned to trust. It relieves them of the worry of having to keep on trying to treat patients who do not respond to any drug. If your GP feels this way, there is nothing to stop you from continuing to go to him or her, if you feel the need to keep on the safe side, while trying alternative forms of treatment.

In practice, however, some doctors still feel mortified, or even outraged (like a Roman Catholic priest on hearing one of his parishioners has been going to a Protestant pastor – or vice-versa) when they hear that a patient of theirs has sought alternative treatment. But such sticklers for orthodoxy are becoming increasingly rare. It is sensible, if you can, to keep your doctor informed, as he or she is supposed to keep an eye on you while you are being treated elsewhere. If unhappy about the results, the doctor will tell you. If you are happy about them, you can tell the doctor and perhaps help further to break down the barriers between orthodoxy and the fringe.

Q *Some doctors take a course in acupuncture, say, or osteopathy, and offer it to their patients. Would it not be sensible to go to one of them, if possible, rather than to a practitioner without medical qualifications?*

A Yes – and no. Yes, if the doctor is one of the relatively small number who have recognized that a natural therapy is of real value in its own right, and who have qualified in it the hard way, not just by taking some short course of instruction and then gaining experience at patients' expense. Medical qualifications do not in themselves make anybody a better therapist than somebody who has not done the standard medical training. Rather the reverse, in fact, as the standard training is only too likely to condition medical students into accepting ideas and attitudes inimical to the practice of natural medicine.

Q *If I decide, with or without the agreement of my own doctor, to try natural therapy, how should I choose which type?*

A That is not easy to answer. This book can take you part of the way, but it can only give you general guidance; it cannot cater for all your needs.

Obviously if your problem is backache, you are more likely to opt for an osteopath or chiropractor than a herbalist. But should your backache turn out to be psychosomatic, you may have to think again.

If you have an intuitive "feel" for some particular type of therapy, it is not a bad idea to test it out, in the hope that your hunch will pay off. Should you have friends who have tried a natural therapy, their advice may be helpful, so long as they are people you feel you can trust.

Again, a useful rule of thumb is that, other things being equal, the choice of a therapist is often more important than choosing the type of therapy. This is not just because an experienced, skilled chiropractor, say, is likely to be more successful than an inexperienced osteopath, or vice-versa. It is not simply a matter of experience, or even skill, but also of rapport between patient and therapist (just as it is in conventional medicine – though owing to their desire for what they regard as a more scientific approach, doctors have tended to play down, even to snigger at, "bedside manner").

There are some organizations which can give guidance about natural therapies. It looks, too, as if a system which originated in the United States will shortly become widespread elsewhere: a house is taken in which practitioners of different natural therapies can rent consulting rooms. In these health centres there is ordinarily somebody who gives advice to prospective patients who are uncertain which type of therapist will best suit their needs.

Q *If I have decided on a therapy, how can I tell whether the particular therapist I am thinking of consulting is any good?*

A Chiefly by word of mouth, though even that is not always to be relied upon. Some charlatans have done very well for themselves, as, indeed, they have in the medical profession.

But you *can* find out whether a practitioner has qualified at any standard school or training course. Under British law absolutely anybody can put up a plate or advertise their services as a therapist. It is only if these people pretend to have qualifications when they do not, that they fall foul of the law. Most practitioners who have qualifications put the appropriate letters after their names on their plates or in the telephone books, and this at least indicates that they have graduated from a course which has led to their qualification.

Again, the duration and intensity of the training do not, necessarily, make for more accomplished practitioners. But they do provide a measure of security for the patient; the more so in that the longer it takes for students to qualify, the most likely it is that the organization which they then join will have some influence over those who display its initials.

Practitioners without medical qualifications, too, rely heavily on word of mouth to bring in patients. Those who begin to earn a reputation as extortioners will quickly cease to get patients.

Q *If the disciplinary bodies of the natural medicine organizations do not have legally enforceable sanctions, does this not leave me open to being injured or conned, without redress?*

A No. Paradoxically it is easier, or has been in the past, for you to recover damages for incompetent or hazardous treatment from somebody who is not medically qualified than from a doctor.

The medical profession has shown itself remarkably skilled at preventing actions from reaching the courts by what amount to cover-ups – colleagues declining to provide evidence against each other. Where cases do reach the courts, proof of incompetence or negligence have rarely been sufficient to secure a verdict in a patient's favour. The doctor needs to have done something positively dangerous, like prescribing a lethal dose or amputating the wrong limb, for a case to go against him or her.

Natural therapists have not been able to rely on well-disposed judges and juries. Nevertheless cases where practitioners of medicine who lack medical qualifications have been prosecuted or sued have been very rare – with one curious exception. There have been a number of cases in the past few years of individuals practising as doctors, obtaining hospital appointments, and carrying out their functions, who have eventually been found never to have qualified, nor even to have attended medical schools.

Q *What is the law on the subject? Could going to a natural therapist land me in legal difficulties?*

A No. In Britain, adults are entitled to receive treatment from anybody, be they your clergyman, your dustman or your MP. In other countries the situation may be different.

The law does, however, place some restrictions on medically unqualified practitioners in this country. They must not claim qualifications which they do not possess, or prescribe drugs which may only be dispensed by a chemist with a doctor's signature; they are not permitted to attend to women in childbirth, or treat certain specific diseases. There are also restrictions on the advertising of nostrums. It seems likely that there will soon be other regulations, designed to bring British law into line with the laws of the European Economic Community. Plans are under consideration to give local authorities in Britain more powers to regulate therapists and these will be of concern to the therapists.

Q *Are not some fringe ideas crazy? Massaging or rubbing the sole of a patient's foot to treat headache, or "operating" on someone without the use of surgery can't really be effective surely?*

A Firstly, what could sound crazier than the idea of sticking a needle or two into patients to enable them to have pain-free major operations? In the past, acupuncture was, in fact, often singled out as an example of how long a primitive superstition could survive, in spite of being so obviously spurious. Yet today . . .

Secondly, research into the effects of suggestion under hypnosis show that it can sometimes have therapeutic effects so dramatic that they appear miraculous. Allowances should always be made for the possibility that some such process may be at work to make *any* therapy, however eccentric, effective for some people, in some circumstances.

The last point to make is that many of the world's most eminent physicists are now convinced that paranormal forces, and in particular the action of mind over matter, can no longer be ruled out (as used to be assumed) by the "laws of nature". Some physicists have gone on record as saying that in quantum theory, paranormal action is not merely possible but predictable. And if mind can act on matter, then a great many cases of healing which in the past have been inexplicable except in terms of miracles, or fraud, may be explained.

Difficult though it is for many of us to accept that, say, a tumour may be "de-materialized" by a psychic healer, the evidence becoming available through research into psychokinesis suggests that it is no longer sensible to reject such a possibility out of hand.

Q *Is it not deplorable that people with, say, terminal cancer should be deceived into wasting their money in what must often be a vain search for a cure?*

A Again, yes – but the operative work is "vain". There have been some well-attested cases where people with cancer who have been told their case is hopeless have survived far longer than expected, or ceased to suffer pain, following treatment by a healer, or after a course of visualization therapy; in a few cases the cancer has actually regressed or disappeared altogether. Rare though such cases are, they encourage the belief that in certain circumstances, the diagnosis of terminal cancer need not be taken to be a death sentence.

Undoubtedly there have been, and will contdue to be, harpies preying on the gullible, or dedicated cranks who genuinely believe in their bogus remedies. Many spiritual and psychic healers, however, make no charge for their services, and to learn some of the therapies involving meditation often costs nothing. Such treatments may promote hopes which turn out to be false, but is that worse than leaving people with no hope?

Q *Is it correct that few, if any, of the therapies in this book have proven scientific support?*

A Yes. In part, however, this is because medical scientists have declined to test them. Indeed, in some cases they have been unable to test them owing to the regulation that once existed in Britain which meant that any doctor who collaborated with a medically unqualified therapist could be struck off the Medical Register – as was the fate of the anesthetist who worked for the celebrated bonesetter, Sir Herbert Barker, earlier this century. Harry Edwards, the best known healer in Britain in recent years, made repeated attempts to persuade the medical profession to set up a controlled trial of his work, but his proposals were always turned down, using this as an excuse.

Since the GMC rescinded this rule, the main problem has been that few of those researchers who are willing to enter this still suspect area have been able to attract financial support. The Medical Research Council has shown little interest, the charitable foundations which raise money for research into particular illnesses have shied away from it, and the most substantial source of revenue for research purposes, the pharmaceutical industry, has understandably shown interest only in those branches of natural medicine which, like herbalism, offer the prospect of providing new drugs.

There is also the problem that controlled trials of the kind that have developed to test drugs are inappropriate to most forms of natural therapy. The aim of a drug trial is, as far as possible, to eliminate the subjective element and ensure that the effect of the drug is evaluated on the basis of chemical actions and reactions in a patient. This effect should be unaffected by the patient's own hopes and expectations, or those of the doctor who prescribed it. But where the rapport between patient and therapy – or patient and therapists – is integral to the success of the method, such objective analysis becomes difficult.

To take an obvious example: with manipulative therapy, it may be desirable for a patient to achieve a state of relaxation which they can only reach if they have full confidence in the manipulator, or his or her method, or both. In any case, it would be almost as difficult to make an objective assessment of a manipulator as of a pianist: success, for both of them, depends not just on whether the right spot is found but also on delicacy, or where necessary, forcefulness, of touch.

Q *Can I obtain natural therapy on the National Health Service?*

A Not unless you are lucky. Your best chance is if your doctor happens to have taken a course in one of the natural therapies, as GPs are doing in increasing numbers. But his or her speciality may not happen to be the particular therapy which you need and your doctor may not, therefore, be sufficiently acquainted with the other alternatives to make a proper recommendation.

Q *If I cannot get it under the state system, how much is natural therapy, if I try it, likely to cost me?*

A Impossible to say, because the cost is determined largely by market forces – the operation of the law of supply and demand. Recently the natural therapists have been enjoying a massive increase in the demand for their services, and a favoured few have been able to raise their fees until they are now the envy of some doctors in private practice.

Most natural therapists remain modest in their charges, however. According to a recent survey, therapists (apart from healers) charge an average of £6 to £15 for a first consultation and £6 to £10 thereafter. The cost of X-rays or blood or other tests, if needed, is usually extra. Healers quite often do not charge at all, believing that, as their gift comes from God, they ought not to exploit it for gain. As a rule, however, they have the equivalent of a church offertory box, into which patients are expected to put donations which will defray the healer's costs.

Q *Why can't these therapies, or some of them, be made available under the provisions of the National Health Service?*

A In theory, they could be, but in practice there are serious problems to be solved first.

The obvious step would be to incorporate them in the Professions Supplementary to Medicine, along with physiotherapists, chiropodists and the rest, which have become established within the NHS by a series of accidents of socio-economic history.

When the medical profession was given statutory recognition in the middle of the nineteenth century, the equivalent of an officer class was created in the form of physicians and surgeons who virtually controlled medicine through their control of the royal colleges and of the teaching hospitals. The apothecaries, who were to become the general practitioners, then occupied a status roughly equivalent to that of army warrant officers. The "other ranks" were the nurses, with their own equivalent of sergeant majors, corporals, and privates.

There were a few anomalies. Dentists, for example, managed to secure independent status, so that patients could go to them directly to have their teeth attended to. But they were the exception. The General Medical Council's ruling that doctors were not permitted to refer patients to medically unqualified practitioners, other than those licensed to work as auxiliaries, led to the development of a heterogeneous collection of licensees whose status was not settled until 1960, when they were given statutory recognition as "professions supplementary to medicine": physiotherapists, medical laboratory scientific officers, radiographers, occupational therapists, chiropodists, dieticians, orthoptists and remedial gymnasts. By 1980 there were more than 50,000 of them, in all.

Most of these are likely to remain content with their auxiliary role; they would not have much of a prospect outside the NHS. There have been some grumblings among physiotherapists, who feel that all too often specialists neither know nor care which patients are suitable for their treatment, but none of the organisations either wish to leave the safe haven of the NHS or relish the prospect of having it invaded by osteopaths, acupuncturists, and the like.

Natural therapists, for their part, are ambivalent. Some would like to be within the NHS, but all fear that in order to obtain admission, they might be called upon to lose some of the independence they have enjoyed up to now. In particular, they would not wish to agree to accept only such patients as would be referred to them by a member of the medical profession. In addition, owing to the recent boom in the demand for their services they have become accustomed to "payment per item of service", which means that they earn more in one hour's session than a GP receives per patient per *year* and often their annual income is far higher than they could hope to receive as one of the Professions Supplementary to Medicine.

For the present, in any case, this is a non-issue. Not merely would the Department of Health not care to tackle so thorny a problem; it has no likelihood of raising the funds to provide the newcomers, if they came in, with their salaries or fees. All natural therapists are convinced that if they were in the NHS, the cost of the service to the taxpayer would eventually plummet, because their treatment, they believe, would be far cheaper and more effective. But this would take a little time and meanwhile the initial expense of incorporating them would horrify the Treasury Department.

The
DISORDERS

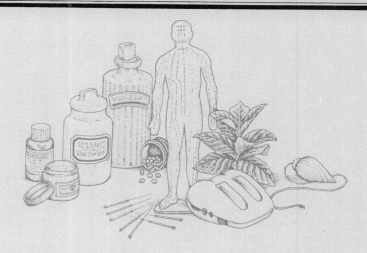

Introduction

In theory, it might appear to be a simple matter to list disorders and symptoms alphabetically, so that you could look up anything, say, "acne" or "xanthogranulomatosis" in the index, turn to the relevant page, see which form of therapy is appropriate, and find a description of the treatment. But the natural therapists do not work this way. One of conventional medicine's most serious mistakes, they feel, has been to pay far too much attention to the treatment of symptoms.

However, it remains true that most people making an appointment with a natural therapist for the first time do so because they have some symptom or syndrome (a constellation of symptoms) which they want to have cured, and if possible, prevented from recurring. Accordingly symptoms and syndromes may be split by therapists into sections according to the type or site of the disorders.

Before we examine those disorders which are related to some part of the anatomy, however, we survey ways of looking at all of them – wherever they may be located: the concept of illness as *Psychosocial* which includes *psychosomatic* or *stress-induced* illness. Following these, we have included four types of illness which straddle the usually accepted diagnostic frontiers – *Just being sick*, *Pain*, *Allergy* and *Addiction* – before moving on to heart disease, cancer and the rest.

Orthodox medicine versus Alternative medicine
Introducing each section, we draw attention to some of the limitations and defects of orthodox medicine, to explain why people have been drifting away from it. This is followed by details of the alternative therapies which have been most successful in the treatment of each disorder.

This means that in one respect, the picture is unbalanced, because we are not concerned here with those services which the medical profession can and does provide, and provides well. We do not for example, deal with the treatment of accidents because if the consequences of an accident are too serious for self-treatment, your GP or local hospital, is better-equipped to deal with them than any practitioner of alternative medicine is likely to be. Similarly where diagnosis is crucial and can best be provided by some instrument you are unlikely to find it outside the medical profession (though some alternative practitioners do use X-rays).

We have set out this part of the book on the assumption that you have already tried conventional medicine and found it wanting. The notion that therapists who do not have medical qualifications are unable to detect where conventional treatment would be, or could be, effective is a myth. They gain experience of which cases they can and cannot treat – just as orthodox practitioners do.

Children's Disorders
What to do about sick children represents a special problem. Adults who take the decision not to go to a doctor, but instead to try a medically unqualified practitioner, know that they do so at their own risk. To subject a child to such an experiment is more worrying – even apart from the fear of what family and friends will think, and perhaps even say, if something does go wrong.

With children the important issue is trust. Where parents have a practitioner of some natural therapy they have come to rely upon for themselves, they can observe how the children react, and how the therapist reacts to them. Some *Naturopaths*, *Homeopaths*, and practitioners of other therapies become accomplished family "doctors", and in this capacity they have one distinct advantage over most GPs in that they tend to give more time and are more willing *not* to intervene with some powerful drug, but they will leave a minor illness to run its natural course.

Where a disorder is of a kind which orthodox medicine cannot treat, or fails to treat effectively, natural therapists can sometimes offer new hope. Even more important, natural therapists feel, is their role in preventive medicine. Naturopaths and homeopaths point out that their methods are designed to work *with* the body's homeostatic mechanism, not to supplant it or override it, as conventional drugs do. Manipulative therapists claim that they can achieve the best results on young, still supple bodies. And psychological disorders of later life can be averted if the "blocks" created in infancy and childhood can be recognized and removed in time.

PSYCHOSOCIAL DISORDERS

The term "psychosocial" has been coming into use to encompass both psychosomatic and stress disorders, and also to bring in other elements of a person's lifestyle, such as air pollution, faulty diet, lack of exercise, smoking and drinking, which may have a role in promoting or precipitating illness. Recognition of the importance of psychosocial disorders has been largely the result of research into the relationship of social habits to proneness to heart disease. And although there is endless dispute over whether smoking, an unbalanced diet and lack of exercise should be regarded as actual *causes* of disease, nobody can now seriously dispute that they are associated with heart attacks and many other diseases.

Psychosocial medicine

Natural therapists make it one of their claims for greater recognition that while the medical profession is still concentrating on the treatment of disease by drugs and surgery, they are practising what, in effect, is psychosocial medicine. Their emphasis is on the importance of a balanced diet, avoidance of cigarettes (and of alcohol in excess), adequate exercise, and freedom from emotional stress for prevention of disease and maintenance of health.

Eminent members of the medical profession quite often claim that the psychosocial element in disease is now given due weight, but this is not the experience of natural therapists. Many of their patients come to them because their doctors are apparently helpless to do anything for them except prescribe drugs. Although some GPs emphasize the importance of stopping smoking and taking some exercise, very few examine a patient for background "psychosocial" information as a matter of course. It is to this failure to recognize the pervasive importance of the psychosocial element that natural therapists owe much of their present custom.

Psychosomatic illness

One of the perennial limitations of the medical profession is an unwillingness to regard illness as essentially psychosomatic, and recognize the need to take the mind as well as the body into consideration both in the treatment and in the prevention of illness.

"Psyche", in a loose sense, can be taken to mean the mind, including not just thought and emotion, but also all the quirks which add up to make a personality structure. It also includes "spirit" (even "the spirits", for people who believe in an after-life). "Soma", of course, stands for the physical aspect. "Psyche" and "soma", in other words, *interact* in the process by which we stay well, or fall ill.

The key word here is "interact". Thanks to the conditioning process to which the public has long been subjected by the medical profession, people still tend to think of illness in either/or terms: *either* caused by a bug, *or* psychologically induced. However, "psychosomatic" implies, or should carry the implication that the disorder is a combined operation in which physical, psychological, spiritual, genetic, constitutional and environmental influences all may have some say in when and how we fall ill.

Colloquially, however, the term is commonly used to convey one of two allied impressions, both derogatory. Often it is employed as the equivalent of "all in the mind". A psychosomatic illness, the implication is, represents the belief of patients that they are ill when there is really nothing the matter with them. The term is more commonly used, however, to convey the impression that although the patients are ill, the source of their symptoms is emotional, or, to put it bluntly, that they are being hysterical or neurotic.

Stress disorders

No clear-cut distinction is ordinarily made between psychosomatic symptoms and stress-related symptoms, but they can be differentiated for the purpose of better understanding of the various processes involved.

The stress theory of disease is related more to the effect of specific *events* on people – not necessarily emotional events, as stress can be the consequence of, say, fatigue. Although its importance had been recognized earlier by the psychosomatic researchers, it was not put on the map as a theory in its own right until Hans Selye's book, *The Stress of Life*, appeared in 1956.

There is some confusion of terminology here in view of the fact that the term "stress" is commonly used in conversation to describe something which imposes a strain on people, as well as the strain imposed – cause as well as effect.

Technically, the term "stressor" should be used for the cause and stress for the effect. As Hans Selye demonstrated in his book, stressors do not necessarily cause disease, in fact they may promote health. The risk of ill-health arises when the stressors impose excessive and prolonged strain.

In *Mind as Healer, Mind as Slayer*, Kenneth Pelletier, director of the Psychosomatic Medicine Center in Berkeley, California, has outlined the stages by which stress and personality type combine to cause illness. First, "a base-line level of tolerable stress is escalated to a level of excessive stress". If that level is not reduced, and is prolonged, "it produces alterations in neuro-physiological functioning, which can create the preconditions for the development of a disorder". At this point, the disorder may be precipitated either by a high concentration of stressful events, such as a bereavement and the loss of a job, or by a single, persistent cause of stress, such as the impending break-up of a marriage.

The form the disorder takes may be dictated by the presence of some pathogen at the critical time ("the bug that's going around"), or it may be related to the individual. The nature of the symptoms, in other words, may be determined by the proneness of the individual to arthritis, or asthma, or whatever disorder he or she is programmed to have, genetically, constitutionally and by personality.

Sleeplessness as a disease
Although the term "stress disorder" needs to be used sparingly, because stress can be a component in any illness, there is one ailment from which almost everybody suffers from time to time and which nobody disputes is stress-linked: insomnia.

In itself, sleeplessness is not an illness. Deprivation of sleep over a protracted period can cause neurosis and eventually hallucinations – hence its use in interrogations to break down victims' resistance. But ordinarily, the amount of sleep we need is far less than the amount we take (or hope to take). What is unhealthy is the common reaction to insomnia – tossing and turning and fretting.

There is some evidence that sleep is not, as most of us have tended to regard it, basically a means of recuperation, of recharging the batteries. The possibility remains that as the human mind has evolved, it has begun to exploit sleep for its own creative purposes.

There are many tales of the way in which people have "slept on a problem", waking up to find the solution in their minds, and many of dreams or daydreams which have provided useful and sometimes valuable information to the dreamer. The atomic scientist, Niels Bohr, saw the model of the atom on which atomic physics was to be based in a dream. It was in a dream, too, that the nineteenth-century German chemist Friedrich Kekulé von Stradonitz discovered the benzene formula, which was to revolutionize organic chemistry. Many musicians have composed in their sleep: "I heard and wrote what I heard", Igor Stravinsky recalled, "I am the vessel through which *The Rite of Spring* passed".

Freud's *Interpretation of Dreams* and subsequent works by his disciples have since added further evidence of the way in which dreaming can help us, even if sleep may not be necessary. Even people who do not remember their dreams (and everyone dreams, every night) may be benefitting from them. In any case, as convention keeps most of us in bed for most of the night, sleep is surely preferable to the boredom of lying awake.

Orthodox treatment

There has recently been a greater willingness in orthodox circles to accept the role of stress as, in the words of a recent *Lancet* editorial, "a major contributor to illness". Coronary heart disease, hypertension, cancer, ulcerative colitis "and other diseases commonly labelled psychosomatic", the editorial goes on, "can all be influenced by stress".

It cannot be said, however, that the medical profession in general has got the message. In any case the advance of specialization has made it more difficult for consultants, removed as they usually are from any knowledge of their patients' stressors, to estimate the degree to which stress is a factor in an individual case. The *Lancet* editorial itself provided a convenient rationalization for leaving stress out of clinical calculations. Although the theories are plausible, it argued, "none predicts disease in advance or specifies what way it will become manifest. Until there is progress in this sphere doctors cannot be accused of being found wanting if they fail to act on the psychologists' suggestions, still less delegate responsibility for illness to the psychologists".

This is not merely incorrect – it *is* possible to predict those individuals who are prone to heart attack (the work of Lawrence LeShan and others has also made it possible to predict the cancer-prone individuals, see pages 313 to 314) – it is also misleading. It gives the impression that the stress theory threatens doctors with the prospect of ultimately being compelled to hand over their patients to psychologists. The alternative, that doctors should themselves be trained as psychologists, has clearly not been grasped. Stress can be a component of any disorder: it should be looked out for in diagnosis even where there appear to be clear-cut physical causes.

Standard remedies for insomnia
"Hypnotics" or sleep-inducing drugs such as the barbiturates have long been orthodox medicine's answer to insomnia. In recent years, an attempt has been made within the medical profession to reduce the quantity prescribed: CURB, the Campaign on the Use and Restriction of Barbiturates, has had some effect – but not much. Most effective hypnotics are highly addictive, and they also breed tolerance, so that addicts have to increase the dose if it is going to continue to work.

Cases of self-poisoning – whether deliberate or accidental – are alarmingly common, running into tens of thousands annually. There is some evidence, too, that the sleep these drugs induce is of an unrewarding kind.

Alternative treatment

Owing to the holistic premise of natural medicine, its practitioners are more predisposed to look for possible psychological causes and precipitants of illness. Unlike members of the medical profession, they have never unconsciously divided up symptoms into "organic" on the one hand and "functional" or "psychosomatic" on the other. Almost all illnesses, they assume, have some psychosomatic element among their causes, and a substantial psychosomatic element must be included in the processes by which they are cured.

Most natural therapists believe that people must be considered as whole persons, and those who are diseased must be studied by both physical and psychological methods. In some diseases, admittedly, the physical aspect can be of greater importance than the psychological, but the therapist is not tempted to conclude from this that there are physical diseases and psychological diseases.

The essential point about psychosomatic diseases, in other words, is that they do *not* constitute a separate category.

Natural therapists are generally agreed that the primary cause of insomnia is unresolved tension. In his *History of the Second World War*, Winston Churchill described how, following what for most people would have been a nerve-racking day (the Wehrmacht had moved into the Low Countries, Chamberlain had resigned, and he himself had become Prime Minister), he was conscious only of a profound sense of relief, and slept soundly. As he now had the supreme authority, his tensions had been resolved.

Nature cure

Of course there can be other elements apart from tension involved in sleeplessness – diet, for one. Anybody who suffers from indigestion is unlikely to sleep well, so eating a heavy meal soon before retiring is to be avoided. (See *Nature cure*, pages 16 to 43.)

Psychological therapies

If there is no reason to attribute sleeping badly to any particular cause, the prescription most natural therapists give is that you should try to find whatever it is that is promoting the tension – perhaps with the help of one of the *Psychological therapies* (see pages 162 to 222) – and find ways to release it. Practitioners of *Hypnotherapy*, in particular, have reported considerable success with insomniacs (see pages 166 to 173).

Self-help

There are many relaxation exercises which can be tried by those who find it difficult to go to sleep. Some are based on a principle derived from observing that people about to go to bed traditonally stretch when they yawn. In bed, as soon as you are ready to sleep, first stretch and relax your fingers, one by one. Then do the same with your arms and legs, the idea being that the relaxation following the tension is transmitted in this way throughout the body. Learning techniques of relaxation as taught by practitioners of *Yoga* (see pages 138 to 144), *Meditation* (see pages 182 to 188) or *Autogenic training* (see pages 178 to 181) can also be of considerable help to insomniacs.

JUST BEING SICK

In his book *The Stress of Life*, Hans Selye recalled that when he was a medical student in Prague seeing hospital patients for the first time, he noticed that there were certain symptoms common to most of them: they "looked and felt ill, had a coated tongue, complained of more or less diffuse aches and pains in the joints and of intestinal disturbances and loss of appetite. Most of them also had fever (sometimes with mental confusion), an enlarged spleen or liver, inflamed tonsils, a skin rash and so forth". Selye found that his teachers ignored these symptoms, and this was hard for him to understand. If it were important to find remedies for specific disorders, he believed it should also be important to learn something about the mechanism of being sick and the means of treating this "general syndrome of sickness which is apparently superimposed upon all individual diseases".

Orthodox treatment

The syndrome of "just being sick" remains a very common form of illness, yet to this day it has not attracted much attention from the medical profession. Generally speaking, the syndrome is not even regarded as a medical problem – not, at least, one which should concern doctors. The chances are that anybody seeing a doctor with the symptoms Selye described and with no specific disease, will be seen as a hypochondriac or a nuisance.

Alternative treatment

Natural therapists, by contrast, regard the syndrome of "just being sick" as important, for a number of reasons. The main one is that it is an indicator of what is the matter with a patient. While it does not indicate a "cause", in the sense of a germ, or virus, it does provide clues of the kind which will help to answer the questions the Scots physician J.L. Halliday asked in his book *Psychosocial Medicine* nearly fifty years ago: "Why did this person become ill in the manner he did? What kind of person is he, that he should have this type of illness? And why did he become ill when he did?" For it is only by finding the answers to these and related questions that effective preventive measures can be decided upon.

Whether a natural therapist will pursue the Halliday line depends on many variables: the amount of interest he or she has in preventive measures (and in particular, those which allow for stress in the home or at work); the amount of time available to spend with patients; and what type of therapy he or she practices.

The general rule, in dealing with this syndrome, is "let nature take its course". If we fall ill, it is because for some reason we need to be ill; the prescription is rest, a balanced diet, and the banishment, as far as possible, of worries.

Nature cure

To natural therapists, the symptoms are not regarded as nuisances to be suppressed, so much as signs that the body's homeostatic mechanism is in working order, and doing its job of fighting off illness.

Naturopaths, for example, can be relied upon to emphasize the need for a well-balanced diet, avoidance of cigarettes, and regular exercise, (some add getting rid of stress, but others pay relatively little attention to patient's emotional problems, which they feel is outside their territory).

Palliatives may be prescribed by

naturopaths to ease pain or irritation, but not to try to suppress a cough, to stop diarrhea, or to clear up a rash: the prescribing of powerful drugs such as antibiotics or steroids as symptom-removers is regarded with abhorrence.

Systems of medicine

Homeopathic remedies (see pages 66 to 74) on the other hand, are favourably regarded in the treatment of the syndrome of "just being sick" because they are held to work in alliance with the body's own homeostatic system rather than to override it.

PAIN

Pain of one kind or another is easily the commonest form of illness. Each week nearly a million people in the United Kingdom go to a doctor for pain relief. Yet it is only in the last few years that pain has come to be regarded as a disorder in its own right.

Of the many types of pain which the human race can suffer, two stand out because they are so common at all ages: headache and toothache. No effective ways have been found to prevent either of them by an conventional means, nor any effective treatment.

Orthodox treatment

The mechanist assumption, when it established itself in orthodox medicine in the nineteenth century, was that pain must represent something wrong with the part of the body in which it was felt. Arthritis, for example, was attributed to a loss of free movement in the joint affected. And there was "referred" pain, sometimes traceable to a different part of the body from that in which the pain was felt. This could be plausibly attributed to a fault or anomaly in the body's communications system, comparable to crossed lines on a telephone. The doctor's job was simply to find the cause of the pain, and deal with it in the best way possible.

Drugs and surgery

Pain used to be seen as a warning signal and there was a tendency in the medical profession to regard its removal with the use of drugs as dangerous; it could cite the disastrous effects of addiction to the painkilling opiates, as chronicled by Thomas de Quincey in his book *Confessions of an Opium-eater*.

There was also a quite widespread belief that suffering was good for the soul. With children, in particular, doctors were inclined to think that it was character-building.

With adults, however, it was not so easy for the doctor to refuse to prescribe painkillers such as the opiates, despite the risk of addiction. Ironically, heroin was initially introduced and widely prescribed because it was believed to carry no addiction risk.

Where no straightforward explanation of the pain, such as an injury or an abscess, could be found, doctors commonly resorted to surgery. The idea was to cut off the channels by which pain signals are transmitted to the conscious mind.

New theories of pain

As, until the 1970s, it was taken for granted that pain must be transmitted by the equivalent of a telegraph system, the logical inference was that pain could be stopped simply by cutting the wires. Sometimes this worked, but all too often it did not and the pain would continue. With the enforced recognition in the early 1970s of the painkilling properties of acupuncture, the basis upon which medical students had been instructed about pain was undermined. There were no "wires" to account for it. Worse was to follow, with the discovery in the mid-1970s of the enkephalins and endorphins, often described as the body's homemade opiates. The human mind, this discovery revealed, has the capacity to treat the human body with drugs which the body itself manufactures, and which our minds can prescribe.

"Chronic pain is now recognized as a disease state", the *British Medical Journal* proclaimed in a recent editorial, "and its treatment and management are now receiving increasing attention". However, it is proving very difficult for doctors (and indeed, for most patients) to come to terms with the chief implication of recent discoveries: *that pain is not necessarily related to any specific physical cause.*

The assumption in the past has been that the pain is roughly proportionate to the severity of the illness, or injury, or the after-effects of surgery, and in hospitals painkillers have often been doled out on that rule of thumb. As a result, patients who protested that the pain-killing effects of the drug were inadequate, or had worn off too soon, were often given to understand that they were not telling the truth.

Now it is realized that the intensity of a pain cannot be equated with the severity of an injury; it is likely to be related to the reaction of the patient, which itself may be influenced by many factors. Some people have a notoriously low pain threshold, others a high one.

Alternative treatment

The risk of drug addiction in cases of chronic pain, has prompted the *British Medical Journal* to admit in its editorial that conventional methods of pain relief have proved inadequate, and to offer a list of alternatives which, it feels, could profitably be tried. Significantly, the alternatives it gave had all been developed outside orthodox medicine, either by natural therapists or by clinical psychologists: in particular acupuncture with or without electrical stimulation, biofeedback with relaxation, and counselling.

Psychotherapies

Almost all the natural therapies claim to offer a measure of relief from pain, either directly or indirectly. But the most immediately effective did not appear in the *British Medical Journal's* list: suggestion under hypnosis. For those who are susceptible to it, hypnotism can not merely remove pain almost instantaneously, but it can prevent them from feeling pain for a few hours – which is why it is used increasingly by dentists (see *Hypnotherapy*, pages 166 to 173).

The simplest way of proving to yourself that the mind can relieve pain is to observe the effects of distraction. This will be obvious to anybody who has had his or her attention deflected from pain by the need to perform some task which requires concentration. One of the pioneers of *Biofeedback* (see pages 188 to 193), Elmer Green, elected to do his doctoral thesis on pain perception in humans under conditions of sensory barrage – noise, vibration, flashing lights and so on. He found that the focus of attention is in the perception of pain: "When attention is directed away from pain, pain is not felt".

He and his wife Alyce went on to investigate the powers of the mind in altered states of consciousness, such as those displayed by yogis. A variety of techniques such as *Autosuggestion* (see pages 173 to 176), *Autogenic training* (see pages 178 to 181), *Meditation* (see pages 182 to 188), and others, could help, they found, to control pain. A few individuals who acted as guinea-pigs in their research showed they were able to switch pain off at will, by entering the appropriate altered state of consciousness.

Oriental therapies

Many people have found that, with practice, it is possible to learn a measure of pain control. For those of us who lack this ability, however, there is *Acupuncture* (see pages 120 to 133), whose painkilling properties have been so strikingly demonstrated in the films taken in Chinese hospitals showing patients undergoing major operations with no anesthetic, and chatting and laughing throughout.

Various gadgets designed to remove pain by giving small electric shocks (transcutaneous electrical nerve stimulation or TNS) have arrived on the market and appear to work on much the same principle as acupuncture. One

theory is that in some as yet unexplained way, the shocks switch off the communication of pain; another theory is that they stimulate the body's own painkillers, goading them into action. Perhaps the shocks perform both services. Whatever the reason, some patients who have used them find them more satisfactory than drugs; provided the machine which gives the shocks is safe, there is no risk and no known side-effects.

Manipulative therapies

Osteopathy and *chiropractic* (see pages 80 to 95) also often afford pain relief, not just in cases of backache, but also where the pain is "referred" to other parts of the body. *The Alexander principle* (see pages 104 to 108) offers the prospect of eventually getting rid of pain if this has resulted from bad postural habits.

It needs to be said that although the idea that our lives may be ennobled by suffering no longer has many advocates, some natural therapists do actually commend pain, in certain circumstances and for certain purposes. With *Rolfing* (see pages 101 to 104) for example, pain is virtually inevitable, as the aim is to loosen up the bone and muscle system by controlled violence. Some practitioners of *Shiatsu* (see pages 133 to 137) and *Reflexology* (see pages 112 to 116) commend some degree of pain as part of the treatment, demonstrating as they treat patients where an area of weakness lies. During *Massage* (see pages 95 to 100) pain is often experienced when the therapist is working on areas of muscle tension, but patients and practitioners alike think of this in terms of "grateful" pain.

Nature cure

One of the most promising, as well as one of the simplest, forms of treatment for headache which has developed recently is the use of "negative ions" (see *Air ionization*

therapy, pages 38 to 39). In 1980 the London *Times* reported the results of "double-blind" tests conducted in offices: they showed that "in a negatively-ionized office, the incidence of headaches fell from a quarter of those surveyed to about 5 percent".

Herbal medicine & Homeopathy

Homeopathy (see pages 66 to 73) has had a certain amount of success in dealing with migraine headache. Recently, however, the supporters of *Herbalism* (see pages 45 to 57) have been delighted at the news that one of their remedies has demonstrated its value.

Writing in a recent issue of the British Migraine Association's *Newsletter*, Dr William A.R. Thomson remarked that addicts of the herb feverfew would be interested to hear "that their faith in this old herbal remedy is being confirmed by those clever back-room boys who claim to know all – or at least more than most of us". A report in the *Lancet* from the research department of a drug company had shown that feverfew has an action very like aspirin's, in that it inhibits the production in the body of prostaglandin, "the substance responsible for many of the aches and pains to which man (and woman) is heir". This discovery, the company thought, would justify the plant's earlier reputation in herbals, dating since the time of the Anglo-Saxon domination of Britain. "So now we know", Dr Thomson concluded, "and those who swear by feverfew have the consolation of knowing that this benefit is not a figment of their imagination, but has a sound scientific basis. Thus do we – and the back-room boys – live and learn".

Self-help

The great majority of cases of pain are treated by self-medication, with drugs such as aspirin. Valuable though this has proved, it can have unwelcome and sometimes serious

305

gastro-intestinal side-effects.

The chief aim of self-help should be to make recourse to drugs of any kind unnecessary. For a start, it is worth looking at Norman Cousins' list in *Anatomy of an Illness* of the abuses of modern society which can lead to pain, and, where possible, taking his advice. You can eradicate the abuses, "by finding ways to eliminate boredom or frustration, by taking more exercise and less drink, or making whatever changes you think most appropriate in your lifestyle". Only if such measures fail will it be necessary for you to try one or other of the natural therapies, beginning with those which are designed primarily to provide you with both mental and physical relaxation.

The reasonably recent discovery that we are capable of manufacturing our own opiates is obviously of great importance – if we can find out how to do it. Unluckily further research has tended to confuse, rather than clarify, the role of these agents. Inevitably, instead of concentrating on finding out how the mind sets them to work, and how that process can be simplified, researchers have tended to concentrate on the potentially more lucrative business of finding ways to manufacture artificial enkephalins or endorphins, so that they can be marketed as drugs.

Still, now that we know the mind has its messengers to the body, we can explore for ourselves all the different methods which have been used to increase the range of the mind's control over pain.

ADDICTION

It is possible to look up "addiction" in medical encyclopedias, only to find that it does not even rate an entry. Yet it is demonstrably one of the most widespread and destructive of the disorders of our civilization, both in its effects, which range from obesity to lung cancer, and in its side-effects, in particular, the appalling toll of death and injury which result from drunken driving.

The term is ordinarily used in connection with mood-altering drugs – some socially acceptable, such as alcohol, caffeine and tobacco (though tobacco is being slowly squeezed out of respectability), and some illegal, such as cannabis, LSD and heroin. Gambling is also known to be addictive. But the commonest addictions of all are to everyday foods such as sugar and salt, both of which have come under fire recently as potential risk factors in promoting ill health. The heavy consumption of salt in particular, has been implicated in relation to high blood pressure and heart attacks.

Obesity

It is only recently that fat people came to be regarded as being anything other than figures of fun. Research projects have been revealing, however, that the more overweight people are, the shorter their life expectation – particularly in the 30–40 age group. Most doctors agree that if you are 10 percent over your ideal weight you are overweight; if you are 20 percent over you are obese (see page 36). By this token 50 percent of the British and American populations are overweight, and half of those are obese. Obesity is often linked to diabetes and to heart disease, it can exacerbate arthritis, and it is a danger in childbearing.

The causes of obesity

There is a genetic element in obesity, it can be the result of endocrine or neurological complications and it can be caused by drugs. Most people who are overweight, however, have reached that condition because of ill-advised eating and drinking habits. These are commonly the consequence of addiction to particular foods, or to incorrect eating patterns.

The chief culprit is junk food. Here, the problem appears to be that the balance between nourishment and calorie intake is disturbed. It is as if the body's metabolism is overwhelmed by the sheer quantity of useless food that it is required to deal with, so that it ceases to be capable of making effective use of the beneficial elements, vitamins and minerals, even if they are present in the food or added as supplements.

Cigarette smoking

Although cigarette smoking has yet to be shown to *cause* lung cancer or heart attacks it has firmly established itself as a "risk factor" in both – that is, the statistical chances of a heavy smoker contracting either disease are very much higher than those of people who do not smoke, and the risk is roughly proportionate to the number of cigarettes smoked. Its links with respiratory disorders are also well established.

Alcoholism

Apart from the fact that alcoholism can culminate in cirrhosis of the liver or delirium tremens, the social consequences are so grave that it presents western countries (and also, apparently the Russians and the eastern bloc) with one of their most intractable problems.

Medical drugs

Addiction to medical drugs has been increasing rapidly since the introduction of the tranquillizers such as librium and valium. Originally thought not to be addictive, they have since been shown to carry a considerable risk. None of the psychoactive drugs, in fact, is free from this risk, and all of them carry the additional hazard of side-effects.

Cannabis and other drugs

The illegal (so far), mood-altering drug, cannabis, though in widespread use, presents a less serious threat because it is not addictive to the same degree as tobacco or alcohol. But heroin, cocaine, LSD and a variety of other substances such as glue, remain a worry.

A few of these drugs can be described as addictive, in the sense that they tend to create a craving, making it very hard for anybody who has become habituated to them to stop taking them. With some drugs, such as heroin, the process of "drying out" is emotionally and physically painful and sometimes protracted. Nevertheless on balance it seems as if it is less the drug than the people who take it that is responsible for addiction. For example, there are parts of the world where opium is notoriously a drug of addiction; in other countries, however, it has been consumed freely, and with as few unwelcome consequences as beer and wine. Emphasis on the danger of the drugs themselves, and massive campaigns to try to eliminate them, have failed, or been counterproductive, as Prohibition was in the United States, largely because of a failure to appreciate that it is the addiction-prone personalities rather than the substances they become addicted to, which need to be dealt with.

Orthodox treatment

It has to be said that the medical profession has done little to investigate the problem of addiction at source: to try to find out why certain individuals become addicts. Indeed very few GPs have thought this was their business. It is still not uncommon for addiction to alcohol, for example, to remain unobserved until the alcoholics are past the point of no return. Then, few GPs have any recourse except to refer them to the nearest mental hospital, where they may be dried out, but they are very rarely cured.

The best work in connection with addiction, in fact, has been done by the lay organizations, such as Alcoholics Anonymous. But even they cannot claim that they have any answer to addiction, other than total abstinence.

Appetite reducing drugs for obesity
When obesity was found to be linked with diabetes and high blood pressure, the medical profession began to regard it as a disorder in its own right, and to treat it primarily with appetite-reducing pills. When coupled with self-restraint on the part of the patients, the method could be effective. But the amphetamines, it was soon found, did not just reduce appetite, they could be used to give a ''lift''.

It was not long before doctors were having to deal with the disastrous consequences. The amphetamines proved to be extremely addictive, and often ultimately destructive – the symptoms ranging from minor complaints of brittle fingernails to lethal ulcers, chest infections, liver damage and strokes. The government banned over-the-counter sales, but this led to a massive black market, whose spread was only checked when doctors, realizing that pills of this kind were too hazardous a way of promoting weight reduction, stopped prescribing them, leading to a decline in their availability.

Drastic diets and exercise
Appetite-reducing pills are still in circulation, but the tendency recently has been for the medical journals to frown upon them, except in conjunction with special regimens where they are part of a crash course begun in a hospital and closely supervized thereafter. These courses are designed to temper what is close to being a starvation diet with special protein and vitamin supplements. The method can bring weight down by several stone in a matter of months, but only a tiny minority of obese people care to take advantage of it.

For the most part, the conventional treatment for obesity is a combination of pills (new ones, claimed not to be addictive, are marketed from time to time) and advice to take more exercise. But eating less, for reasons we consider in the therapy section under *Diets* (see pages 28 to 37) is not necessarily helpful, and exercise does not in itself do very much to reduce weight.

Treating drugs with drugs
For a time there were high hopes that heroin addicts could be weaned off heroin gradually on to a less addictive drug, usually methadone. In the mid-1970s, the number of addicts being treated in this way in the United States ran into six figures. However most of them lapsed after the treatment finished, and others became hooked

on methadone; hundreds of deaths from black market methadone have been recorded annually.
Detoxification
Exulting over the collapse of the case for treating addicts medically, *Time* magazine called for a return to tough law enforcement "and 'cold turkey' detoxification of addicts – a tough but effective treatment''. Tough it was, but this total deprivation of the drugs turned out to be just as ineffective as using methadone, and in social terms the side-effects were even more destructive; when heroin's black market price rose, addicts robbed and murdered to obtain the funds to secure their supply.
Special clinics
For a time the British system, allowing registered addicts to obtain a maintenance dose of heroin, worked surprisingly well, keeping the number of addicts down to a manageable handful in most cities. In the 1960s there was a sudden upward jump in the number of addicts, but this was halted when the reason was realized; a few rogue doctors were selling prescriptions for heroin, which then found its way to the black market. When this racket was exposed, heroin prescriptions were banned except through designated clinics, and again, there was a relatively quiet period. Recently, however, the heroin addiction figures have begun to rise again, and it is becoming uncertain whether the clinic system is going to be able to cope with the strain. These clinics, in any case, have the severe limitation that they have been primarily concerned with one particular drug – heroin. As has often been pointed out, addiction to barbiturates, for example, can be just as hard to deal with, and is even more widespread.

Here there is a further problem: far from being of assistance in the campaign against addiction, the medical profession has a heavy responsibility for breeding addicts, or at least for providing them with the material on which to become addicts. The medical journals and the

Department of Health are continually but ineffectively complaining that sedatives, tranquillizers and antidepressants (the whole psychoactive range of drugs) have been, and are being over-prescribed.

Alternative treatment

The basis upon which natural therapists would like to treat addiction is determined by the needs of the individual. For simplicity this can be summed up in the question: "What did the addict *need*, which led to the addiction?"

With sugar and salt the craving is usually implanted by early conditioning. Social conditioning in adolescence is likely to have played some part in connection with addiction to smoking or drinking. With drink, however, other factors – a personality weakness of some kind or reaction to stresses at home or at work – need to be taken into consideration.

Natural therapists insist that the causes of addiction have always to be considered before they decide how to treat an individual case. Obviously the prescription may need to be very different for somebody who has become addicted to smoking – whether tobacco or cannabis – because it is soothing, and somebody else who finds it a stimulant. Similarly it will be different for someone who has become hooked on drugs in the pursuit of a Huxley-style experience, than for a meths-drinker in "Skid Row", or for an alcoholic who, though he or she is normally able to keep social drinking under control, collapses into alcoholism following the loss of a job or the break-up of marriage.

Allowing for the need to suit the treatment to the individual, two general observations can be made: first, that almost any form of therapy can be effective in the short term; second, that no form of therapy can be effective in the long term unless the addict really *wants* it to work.

Nature cure

In principle, the basis for the correction of obesity is nature cure, as natural therapists of all types would agree. In practice, however, some are inclined to feel that nature cure establishments (see *Nature cure*, pages 16 to 18), which have become very profitable largely on the strength of their ability to reduce the weight of their clients, have been too ready to accept those clients on short-term visits, for a fortnight or even for a week. This can do little more for them than make room, as it were, for more gourmandizing when they go back to their homes and their jobs.

The nature cure *principle*, however, is clear. People who are obese, and want to get back to their normal weight, need a preliminary spell of near starvation, perhaps with purges and enemas, before starting on a balanced diet again.

Recently more attention has been paid by naturopaths and other therapists to the role of emotions in connection with weight reduction. This has two aspects: firstly, the common link between addiction to food and an unrequited need for love; and secondly the commoner link between stress and indigestion. Weight gain can be the result of either, or both. In the case of addiction, the appetite is unnatural. With cases affected by stress, the appetite may be natural, but the metabolism is thrown out of gear, so that the digestion does not work properly. One or other of the psychological therapies may be needed, therefore, to assist in the weight-reducing process.

Many naturopathic establishments now have counsellors. They also have begun to offer *Yoga* (see pages 138 to 144), *Massage* (see pages 95 to 100), *Shiatsu* (see pages 133 to 137) and other optional extras not because of any direct influence on their clients' weight, but because they help to "set the clients up", making them feel healthier, emotionally as well as physically, and consequently benefitting their metabolism. Where exercise works as a weight reducer, it is for this reason, rather than the amount of perspiration lost.

Psychological & Oriental therapies

The main types of addiction-breaker in most common use are *Acupuncture*, (see pages 120 to 133), and two of the psychological therapies, *Hypnotherapy* (see pages 166 to 173) and *Behaviour therapy* (see pages 196 to 197).

Acupuncturists and hypnotherapists aim to provide the addict with some kind of prop during the initial stages of treatment (how acupuncture provides this service is not clear, but research carried out in Hong Kong with heroin addicts has given very encouraging results, and trials are in progress in the West to try to find whether the same effects can be obtained in our environment). Behaviour therapy aims to create unpleasant associations in the mind of the patients so that they cease to crave whatever it is they are addicted to.

Acupuncture
In some western countries, there has been a rapid increase in the use of acupuncture against addiction. In a recent interview in the *Guardian*, Sidney Rose-Neil, then Chairman of the British Acupuncture Association, claimed that the success rate is very high: "we reckon to be able to cure 80 to 90 percent of drug addicts, 70 percent of alcoholics, 60 percent of smokers and 40 percent of slimmers" (presumably he was referring to food addicts). Such figures cannot be relied upon unless backed up by follow-ups, and they take no account of differences between acupuncturists – whether some are more successful than others. However, there is now no doubt that acupuncture can assist in the initial stages and acupuncturists claim that there are no withdrawal symptoms.

Psychotherapies
Hypnotherapy (see pages 166 to 173) involves planting the suggestion in the addicts' minds that the desire to take the drugs, or to smoke, will disappear, and if necessary to repeat the process until they

have come to terms with their ability to do without it. *Psychotherapy* (see pages 163 to 166) is sometimes used in the hope of unmasking the reasons for the addiction; sometimes both are used.

Behaviour therapy
This revolves around aversion therapy (see page 196) where the principle is the creation of a mental link between taking the drug and some unpleasant experience.

High motivation is crucial to the success of aversion therapy and the rapport established between therapist and patient may be far more influential in deciding the outcome.

"Motivation" in any case comes in various guises, from a desire to please a loved one to a feeling that money could be better spent; it may be unconscious, simply awaiting arousal. If so, Andrew Weil has argued in *The Natural Mind*, to think of addiction as necessarily something to treat, in the conventional sense, is a mistake. The aim must be to rechannel the impulse which gave rise to the addiction into something satisfying, rather than destructive.

Manipulative therapies

Interestingly, the educationalist John Dewey suggested in his book *Human Nature and Conduct* that a lesson could be learned about the treatment of addiction from F.M. Alexander – whom he greatly admired. "The hard drinker who keeps thinking of not drinking is doing what he can to initiate the acts which lead to drinking", Dewey observed. "To succeed, he must find some positive line of action which will inhibit the drinking series" – this being in line with what Alexander taught about how to remove inappropriate postural habits (see pages 104 to 108).

Health centres

The most successful of the institutions set up to counter addiction have been those in some cities in the United States, which have offered a variety of therapies. In the

1970s, for example, the San Francisco Centerpoint Clinic was offering among other things, *Gestalt, Transactional analysis, Encounter* groups, *Biofeedback* sessions, and various other psychotherapeutic opportunities (see *Psychological Therapies*, pages 162 to 222). Former addicts returned from it to the community with their craving removed, or rendered manageable to gratifying numbers. All too often, unluckily, when they were back where they had come from, they would again fall prey to the same frustrations and the same temptations that they had previously experienced, and would relapse. What is required, therefore, is a combination of physical treatment, which will enable the addict to temporarily shed his or her craving for the drug and *Psychotherapy* (see pages 162 to 165) to help him or her find the need which led to the addiction (and if possible, something to fill that need when the treatment is finished). This is something which society has not been good at making provision for.

Self-help

There is one sound general rule for addicts who want to lose their addiction, and that is not only to think in terms of exercising greater self-control. It *can* work, and in a few cases, it does work, but it is extremely unlikely to continue to work unless it is backed up by something positive to put in the addiction's place. It is not enough, for example, for a smoker simply to take to chewing gum instead of cigarettes. It is more a matter of finding something to do which will distract attention from the urge to smoke or chew. What this distraction is depends on the individual's willingness to explore the natural therapies which are on offer.

ALLERGY

Allergy is a disorder in which the body's homeostatic system goes into action as though to repel hostile invaders, often in a gratifyingly vigorous manner. The trouble is that the invaders or allergens, as they are known, are neither really hostile, nor capable of doing any real damage. In the commonest of allergies, hay fever, the allergen is pollen, yet most of us can breathe in enormous quantities of pollen, and still be none the worse for it.

Causes of allergy
It has gradually come to be realized that we can become allergic to *anything*. Pollen, mysteriously, is the commonest allergen, but house dust (or the mites which attach themselves to it) and cat fur are also often responsible for streaming eyes, running noses and occasionally, rashes and nausea.

Recently, more attention has been paid to another suspect: food. It has long been known that some babies become allergic to cow's milk, or to eggs, reacting by attacks of asthma, or of eczema, or both. A further complication has been the development of the theory of "autoimmune" disease. The more self-explanatory term is "autoallergic", the implication being that some of our symptoms may be caused by our homeostatic system reacting unnecessarily, or even in the wrong way, to one of our body's own constituents.

Inevitably the autoimmune theory of disease causation has been responsible for further confusion, because of the difficulty of deciding whether a symptom is allergic, autoallergic, or simply caused by some pathogen or toxic substance or whether it is psychosomatically induced.

Orthodox treatment

One consequence of this confusion is that until very recently there has been little attempt to treat allergy itself, as distinct from treating its symptoms. Although the need for allergy to be treated as a speciality may be conceded, nothing effective has been done to bring this about – as the *Lancet* has pointed out in a recent editorial. Obviously, the writer argues, if allergy exists, it ought to be treated by specialists; ''but at present, no suitable training exists''.

Even among those few who specialize in allergy, or the rather larger number who, while not specializing, interest themselves in the subject, there is little harmony. As the *Lancet* went on to point out ''there are considerable differences of opinion on the management of common allergic disorders''. Some allergists swear by skin tests; others say that such tests rarely reveal anything that a good doctor (and a sensible patient) cannot find out without them. Many allergists, however, are so wrapped up in their search for food allergies that they can think of nothing else. ''Until clinicians with an interest in allergy can present a more united front'', the *Lancet* primly reminded them, ''there may be difficulty in persuading outsiders that allergy qualifies as a speciality''.

Tranquillizers, painkillers and other drugs

For a time hopes were raised that it would be possible to provide desensitizing injections for allergy victims. To a limited extent, and for a very limited range of allergens, this has worked. Some hay fever sufferers, for instance, can take a course of injections in the spring which, during the summer will make them less susceptible to pollen. The prevention this affords, however, is limited, and it cannot be regulated to fit the erratically changing pollen count.

As a result, the great majority of allergy cases are treated only with the kind of drug which would be given for the same symptoms if they were caused by a pathogen. This is usually a palliative, a painkiller or a tranquillizer. For hay fever, symptom suppressants are commonly prescribed in the form of antihistamine drugs which can be effective in stopping the flow of mucus. But they can also have unwanted side-effects and, because they promote drowsiness, may also be dangerous for anybody who has to work, or drive a car.

Alternative treatment

The growing recognition of how widespread allergies, and more particularly, food allergies, are, has been a gift to the practitioners of alternative therapies; in particular naturopaths who were emphasizing the importance of a wholesome diet long before allergy was recognized for what it is.

Nature cure

Clinical ecologists believe that allergies and autoallergies are frequently the consequence of pollution of the air we breathe and, even more, of the food we eat. They blame additions to food, preservatives, and colouring matter such as monosodium glutamate, on the one hand, and subtractions from food, the removal of fibre from our diet, on the other.

Although naturopaths welcome clinical ecology, they are careful to warn people not to go overboard for it.

The common mistake of the clinical ecologists, naturopath Leon Chaitow argues, is that they ''lose sight of the essence of human disease – the individual''. Allergies are indications that something has gone wrong with the body's defence mechanism. The answer therefore, is not desensitization or drugs, ''nor is it, in the long run, necessary to avoid the substances to which allergy is displayed, unless these foods are of questionable value or are obviously undesirable''. If eating chocolate produces a migraine headache, for example, ''then simply stopping the chocolate is only the beginning of an answer. Ideally the patient should be taught a reformed and balanced pattern of eating and living''.

The great majority of natural therapists would agree with this, while adding that their particular therapy can be a help in restoring the body's defences to normal. Chaitow recommends people with allergies to institute a variety of therapies, citing ''relaxation and stress reduction, osteopathic normalization of spinal and cranial structures, etc''.

People who have become conditioned to the use of antihistamine sprays for hay fever and other similar conditons, but then find that they suffer from side-effects, have reported successful results using *Air ionization therapy* (see pages 38 to 39) instead.

Systems of medicine

In *The Science of Homeopathy*, George Vithoulkas contrasts what happens to two patients with allergic eczema: one treated allopathically; the other homeopathically. The first patient is prescribed cortisone ointments with the result that the eczema was controlled so long as the ointments were applied, but the patient noticed a gradual increase in sulkiness and irritability. Her symptoms are shifted and, worse, they tend to shift to deeper levels. But with the other patient, ''treated by a homeopathic remedy prescribed on the totality of symptoms, the eczema will be found to leave the face and torso out to the extremities, and finally leave altogether'' – clearly a curative direction, ''and the long-term prognosis is excellent''. *Homeopathy*, (see pages 66 to 73) therefore, provides a clear alternative for allergy sufferers.

Psychotherapies

In the treatment of allergy, *Hypnotherapy* (see pages 166 to 172) has proved to be valuable not so much because it can provide an easy cure, but because it can be used to show that the mind often has the power to remove the symptoms. In his book *Natural History of the Mind*, Gordon Rattray-Taylor cited research carried out in Japan which demonstrated that it was possible to induce an allergic reaction merely by pretending to touch a patient under hypnosis with a substance to which he or she was allergic. This research also showed that the patient did *not* have a reaction when touched with a substance to which he was normally allergic if, under hypnosis, he was told it was something else to which he was *not* normally allergic.

Some hypnotherapists make a point of demonstrating to patients that when it is suggested that they will no longer get say, the symptoms of hay fever from pollen, they can be showered with pollen and remain symptom-free – for a time. The hypnotherapist will, however, ordinarily point out that this does not constitute a cure. All it does is reveal that the allergy is not ''organic'', and that it can be banished. It is then up to the patients to try whatever other psychological methods they fancy, along with diet, or other expedients to see whether they can banish the allergy permanently.

Relaxation techniques

Autosuggestion (see pages 173 to 176), *Autogenic training* (see pages 178 to 181) and *Yoga* (see pages 138 to 144) can also relieve allergy, as even some clinical ecologists have emphasized. In his book, *Basics of Food Allergy*, Dr J.C. Breneman, Chairman of the US College of Allergists' Food Allergy Commmittee, has observed that people who cannot eat fish in their everyday lives ''may find they can tolerate fish very well during a happy vacation''. Some women, too, who can ordinarily eat fish and have no problems may come out in a rash if they eat fish during their periods ''or during an episode of marital disharmony''.

Manipulative therapies

Practitioners of *Applied kinesiology and touch for health* (see pages 116 to 118) use extensive muscle tests for the detection of food and other allergies, and report success in the treatment of these disorders using various specialized muscle-balancing techniques.

Self-help

The first step is to try to identify the allergen, which is not difficult where the symptoms come on in such a way as to be distinct from other types of disorder – when snuffles follow a visit to a flat whose owner keeps a cat for example – but it can be frustrating. Having made an identification, by whatever means, the most important point is not to give way to the temptation of simply obeying instructions about what to do and what not to do, while taking symptom-removers. It is worth trying to work out whether there is an underlying emotional reason for the allergic symptoms coming on when they did, and at the same time experimenting with diets designed not just to avoid the food or drink which contains the allergen, but also to reduce the consumption of sugar, animal fat and so on, to find whether that helps.

INFECTIOUS DISEASES

As far as the general public is concerned, the impression is that it is the job of the medical profession to handle most infections and that they are outside the scope of natural therapists. In one respect this is certainly true: only members of the medical profession have the right to prescribe certain drugs which can still, in some disorders, provide the most effective treatment. Moreover in a few cases, immunization has been strikingly successful; notably with polio and a number of different tropical diseases.

Recently, however, it has come to be realized that germs and viruses are not the sole causes of the diseases with which they are identified; and consequently that immunization and drugs cannot provide the complete answer to them. Both immunization, and drugs too, can have unwanted side-effects. Drugs have a further disadvantage: that when over-prescribed, as they have been, they become counter-productive, as they can lead to the spread of resistant strains of germs. Gradually, the emphasis is shifting to give more attention to the body's own resistance mechanism as the best line of defence.

This was originally advocated by the French physiologist Claude Bernard. His theory was that the body's homeostatic mechanism is ordinarily capable, if we look after it, of dealing with hostile pathogens, but that if it is *not* properly looked after – in a community, for example where there is malnutrition, squalid housing, and so on – they all too often win. Moreover the French chemist Louis Pasteur, who had put the germ theory of disease to the forefront of his work, surprisingly admitted on his deathbed, ''Bernard was right. The germ *is* nothing: the terrain is everything'' – the terrain being the body, and the way it *reacts* to the germ.

Since then, pathologists searching for the germ responsible for an outbreak of infectious disease have often also reported that in addition to the germ which they believe to be responsible they have observed swarms of other pathogens – staphylococci, streptococci, and so on – apparently doing no harm. Some of them may even, conceivably be doing good, by affording a measure of protection against more destructive pathogens.

If it is difficult to fit germs into any stable role in the causing of disease, viruses present still more of a problem. It is not even clear what viruses *are* – let alone why they behave in so erratic a fashion. In his book the *Lives of a Cell*, Dr Lewis Thomas, President of the Sloan-Kettering Memorial Center in New York, remarked that viruses, ''instead of being single-minded agents of disease and death, now begin to look more like mobile genes''.

In medical reports, however, they are still commonly referred to as single-minded agents of disease and death. When they are found in connection with a disease, they are still called its ''cause''. More and more, in fact, doctors put the blame on a virus when they do not know what is the matter with a patient.

With infections caused by germs, there is at least some degree of positive identification of the culprit. People do not have TB unless they are harbouring the ''vibrio''. But although specific viruses, too, may be found with specific sets of symptoms, there are many puzzling features about their behaviour. In fact, in 1942, J.E.R. MacDonagh, a former Hunterian Professor of the Royal College of Surgeons, had actually suggested in a letter to the London *Times* that viruses should be regarded not as the cause of disease, but as its consequence – the consequence of a breakdown in the body's resistance.

Another weakness in the conventional assumptions about infection, to which natural therapists are beginning to pay more attention, concerns the mode of transmission. The evidence is piling up that person-to-person transmission of infections – whereby an infected person breathes out or sneezes out germs which are thereupon breathed in by healthy individuals, causing them to become infected – does not satisfactorily explain the course taken by many epidemics (see *Respiratory disorders*, pages 325 to 327).

Unexplained epidemics
The mechanics of infectious disorders is even more baffling in connection with those which are regarded as diseases of the nervous system, as many episodes show.

In the summer of 1976, for example, over two hundred people, most of them staying in a hotel in Philadelphia for an ex-servicemen's convention, contracted a disease resembling a virulent form of flu, and 29 of them died. Later, the outbreak was attributed to a pneumococcal infection; but no explanation has been found for why what is now known as ''Legionnaire's disease'' took the explosive form it did. Why did it spread no further? Moreover, why did it not affect any of the hotel staff?

During the past few years too, there have been several outbreaks of a disorder which has some of the characteristics of polio in its early stages, though fortunately not its long-term effects. The epidemics usually occur in institutions, often in hospitals, where paradoxically it appears to be the patients who are protected; it is the *staff* who are affected. Such outbreaks have been given the name myalgic encephalomyelitis – inflammation of the brain and spinal cord, with muscle involvement – but no pathogen has been found to account for them.

The only disease of this kind for which a vaccine has been found is poliomyelitis. Polio is not quite on a par with the others as it is basically an intestinal infection, which sometimes spreads to the nervous system. The vaccine proved effective against the infection in its intestinal stage. The protection that immunization has provided has made it less necessary to probe the subject further, but the way in which polio is transmitted – sometimes breaking out in epidemics, sometimes picking off individuals – remains a mystery.

It has become obvious, in fact, that neuro-epidemics cannot be accounted for on any straightforward basis, such as spreading from person to person by airborne viruses, or by other forms of contact. Two possible explanations have been suggested: Sir Fred Hoyle's hypothesis that the pathogens fall from the sky, having come from outer space (in which case there is little that can be done about them); and the idea of Dr Lewis Thomas, has put forward in *The Lives of a Cell*, that epidemics may be spread by a process ''something like the panic-producing pheromones that slave-taking ants release to disorganize the colonies of their prey''.

The basis for Dr Thomas's theory is that pheromones (free-floating scent molecules) trigger off epidemics, stirring the germs and viruses which we all harbour (and which ordinarily do us no harm) into rebellion – or, alternatively, into having a dampening effect on our homeostats. But why should the pheromones act in this way? The most plausible explanation is that in some way they transmit what might be described as a psychic infection, of the kind that quite commonly breaks out in schools and is put down to hysteria. Perhaps hysteria is pheromone-activated.

Orthodox treatment
So far, however, all the emphasis, in research into infectious diseases has been placed on pathogenic organisms. This was for a time valuable in detecting dangerous bacteria, and finding drugs which would slay them. But where they are not the cause, so much as the effect (or simply the identifying feature), of the disorder, slaying the bacteria is not enough.

Antibiotic-type drugs remain invaluable as a last resort, where the homeostat has failed and the pathogens are proliferating. In this capacity, drugs have saved countless people who would otherwise have died. However, the indications are that antibiotics are losing their effectiveness so we may not enjoy this protection much longer.

To some extent, the medical profession and natural therapists are in agreement: people who lead a healthy life with a balanced diet, plenty of fresh air and exercise, and a minimum of bad habits such as smoking, are less likely to succumb to an infection – and more likely, if they do, to recover quickly. But the holistic theory requires a role for the mind, too, and it can cite research which suggests that the mind's importance in dealing with infection has been underestimated.

Although this is an area which has yet to be comprehensively explored, the evidence is strong enough to justify looking out for, and if necessary, treating, an emotional component in all infectious diseases, however outlandish this may seem to anybody brought up to think of germs and viruses as *the* cause of epidemics.

Alternative treatment
The confusion which now exists about the way in which infectious

diseases are transmitted; the growing recognition that germs and viruses do not cause disease in the simple cause-and-effect manner which used to be taken for granted; and the decline in the effectiveness of antibiotics, have all been leading to a renewed interest in the possibility that nature cure and other natural therapies can offer a useful alternative.

On one point all natural therapists are agreed. Infectious diseases ought no longer to be regarded as the exclusive preserve of the medical profession. The professional monopoly means that it is essential for anybody suffering from one of the more dangerous types of infectious disease to go to hospital. However, this does not mean that a natural therapist, if you have one on whom you normally rely, is incompetent to advise you, it is merely that, as the law stands now, he or she does not have access to hospital facilities.

Nature cure & Herbal medicine

Naturopaths (see pages 18 to 21) and *Herbalists* (see pages 45 to 57) rely mainly on keeping the body's defences in good order, to make it less likely that their patients will catch an infection – and more likely, if they do, that the attack will be mild. Most natural therapists who use primarily physical treatments (acupuncturists and manipulators, for example) believe that their forms of treatment give protection because they are designed to restore the natural homeostatic balance both psychological and physical rather than to provide a substitute for it.

Systems of medicine

Homeopathic medicine (see pages 66 to 73) is perhaps best placed to provide an alternative, as so many homeopathic practitioners are medically qualified and as such are legally permitted to prescribe an antibiotic, if they feel it is indicated, in an emergency. Normally, though, they work on a different principle.

Their remedies are designed not to seek out and slay bacteria, but to rouse the body's own disease-fighting mechanism. They can point to the fact that in the days before antibiotics, their record in epidemics was better than that of orthodox medicine. In the great cholera epidemics, in particular, the mortality rate in homeopathic hospitals was much lower than in conventional hospitals not just because the treatment was more effective but because of their closer attention to prescribing the appropriate remedies for each individual.

Psychological therapies

A few years ago, the notion that psychological treatment of any kind could be effective in cases of infectious disease would have been dismissed as absurd – as, by some doctors, it still is. Yet Dr Kissen's ingenious research into the various emotional factors connected with TB gave notice that the mind ought not to be regarded as outside the range of possible causes. Work done since, such as the research at England's Common Cold Unit into the way that patients' states of mind can affect the results of their treatment, suggests that psychological factors need to be taken into account not just as an element in making people more susceptible to infections, but as an aid to avoiding them, or recovering from them.

Self-help

The main need, at present, is for a radical change of attitude to infections, a realization that we should not continue to think of them as caused by pathogens which we can do nothing about except smother them with powerful drugs.

There are a few lethal pathogens from which even the most doughty homeostat can provide us with little or no protection, and a few infections which are a menace whenever they are encountered, notably some tropical diseases. Otherwise, however, our homeostats ought to be

capable of keeping order. Where they let us down, we need to ask why and following this, find ways to stop them letting us down again, rather than relying on antibiotics, which should be kept for real emergencies.

CANCER

The term "cancer" is usually applied to growths, or tumours, which become "malignant". Cells proliferate as if out of control, spread through the body's tissues and sometimes produce secondary growths, "metastases", in other areas of the body. The term has also come to be applied to certain disorders of the blood, the *leukemias*; of the bone and muscle system, the *sarcomas*; and of the lymph system, the *lymphomas*. However, by far the most widespread and lethal of the cancers are those of the lining materials of the body (the skin, the gut, and the glands), the *carcinomas*. The most common are lung cancer in men and breast cancer in women, though lung cancer also kills more women every year.

The causes of cancer remain undiscovered. Even when there is a strong presumption of guilt (such as with cigarette smoking, which statistically is closely linked with the risk of lung cancer), some other factor must be presumed to be at work as well, because the majority of people who smoke heavily do not contract the disease. Environmental agents of various kinds are under suspicion; there are indications that some types of personality are cancer prone; and stress has also been indicted.

Orthodox treatment

No way has been found to cure cancer, but three types of treatment have been developed over the years: surgery, radiotherapy and finally chemotherapy.

Throughout history, surgeons have removed tumours – if they can be removed. Towards the end of the nineteenth century it was found that radiation could destroy tumours, and it has been used for that purpose ever since. Periodically, too, drugs have been tried, but it is only within the last few years that they have emerged as serious contenders for primary, as distinct from adjuvant or auxiliary, use.

Surgery and radiotherapy
Examining the statistics in 1974, a medical journalist in Washington, Dan Greenberg, found that over a period of 25 years, the survival rate for the commoner forms of cancer had remained virtually unchanged. Dr Basil Stoll of St Thomas's Hospital, London has recently admitted: "A highly responsible body of scientific opinion has suggested that neither surgical treatment nor radiation therapy is likely to affect the outcome of the disease in the majority of patients". There is even evidence "that extensive surgery or radiotherapy might even accelerate the course of the disease".

Gradually the reasons for this failure are becoming clear, chief among them, that the theory upon which cancer has been treated for the past century has been mistaken. The assumption has been that cancer develops initially in a "rogue" cell or cells. Cancer cells then begin to proliferate, some of them eventually flaking off to be swept away to other parts of the body, there to "metastasize" or "set up" secondary cancer colonies. It seemed natural to believe that if the initial tumour could be detected early enough and removed by surgery or radiation, there need be no secondaries, and with luck there might be no recurrence of the disease. To be on the safe side, some cancer specialists thought, it would also be wise to remove tissue, and perhaps glands and muscles, in the vicinity of the original growth, when it was being operated upon.

The case of breast cancer
Amputation of the entire breast, *mastectomy*, was introduced a century ago and quickly became standard practice. Unfortunately the mortality statistics failed to justify expectations, and from time to time individual cancer specialists expressed doubts about the value of mastectomy. In 1936 a leading British surgeon, Geoffrey Keynes, argued in the *British Medical Journal* that there was nothing to show any advantage for mastectomy over a simple "lumpectomy" which involves removal of the tumour, leaving the breast otherwise intact.

It was argued, however, that the blame for the lack of reduction in mortality figures lay with the delay in detecting breast cancer. Women were advised to palpate their breasts regularly and to seek treatment at once if they found a lump. Later, screening with X-rays, mammography, was introduced so that any growths could be detected even earlier.

For a while, the figures for survival time appeared to show a gratifying improvement – until it was realized that what they reflected was simply the fact that cancer was being diagnosed sooner. The crucial statistics, those which show the general mortality rate from breast cancer (the number of victims and the average age at the time of death), have remained virtually unchanged. A recent *Lancet* editorial stated that it has proved "extremely difficult" to demonstrate that earlier diagnosis leads to improved survival. Moreover, although there has been a great volume of research into the different ways of dealing with breast cancer, "it has so far failed to identify any useful measures that might be adopted for its primary prevention".

It is now coming to be recognized that cancer should be regarded not as an indication that some cells which have become incurably diseased must be eradicated before they spread, but rather as in indication that the body's homeostatic mechanism is out of order. Ordinarily, this mechanism intervenes at some point to stop the actual growth of tumours (as it does with warts) and also what are described as tumours *in situ* (in cases of cervical cancer, for example). It may even reverse the process and cause the growth to regress. However, if it fails to exercise control, although it may be necessary to remove cancerous tissue because it is causing an obstruction, or simply for the patient's peace of mind, surgery and radiation cannot check the spread.

A number of trials in different countries have lent confirmation to this hypothesis. They have compared the results of different types of surgery with or without different types of radiation. The outcome is clear: neither, in whatever form they are given, makes any appreciable difference to the eventual outcome. Some individuals die quickly, others recover completely, irrespective of the medical treatment they have received.

Chemotherapy
The growing recognition that surgery and radiation make no difference to survival has led in recent years to intensified research into chemotherapy for cancer. In one respect it offers more promise: if an effective cytotoxic drug could be found, it could pursue cancer cells everywhere throughout the body, delaying and perhaps staving off the development of cancer altogether. Some trials suggest that chemotherapy can indeed increase survival time. But the side effects are even uglier than those which commonly occur with radiation – and they are bad enough. It has been far from uncommon for patients to beg that the treatment be discontinued, so that they can live, or die, in peace.

Alternative treatment
Cancer cures, as such, can only be prescribed by a member of the medical profession. There are, however, many alternative forms of therapy which individual members of the profession have experimented with, and some which can be used by medically unqualified practitioners without the risk of landing in court.

In the past it has often been argued that by trying any of the alternative methods, rather than accepting orthodox treatment, carcinoma patients jeopardize their chances of recovery. Now that it is so widely recognized that orthodox treatment does not work, this can hardly be maintained any longer. In any case, some of the unorthodox therapies can, if patients wish, be used in conjunction with whatever treatment their specialist has prescribed. Most of them are based on the proposition that there must be forces in us which are ordinarily capable of dealing with cancer cells, but which, for some reason, have let us down (or we have let *them* down). What we need to do is to stir them back into action or, perhaps, remove the obstacle, whatever it may be, that has blocked their flow.

No responsible practitioner of alternative medicine would claim to have a *cure* for cancer (irresponsible practitioners who do could soon find themselves in court). The generally accepted view is that cancer is often terminal in a very real sense; that it is one of the ways in which impending death manifests itself. This does not mean that the victims have a ''death-wish''; the implication is that for some reason – usually advancing age coupled with a loss of zest for living or with some traumatic experience – there is a falling-off of the vital force which keeps people healthy. If they are marked for cancer, rather than for any other disease, by genetic, constitutional and environmental factors, this will determine their fate. But if the vital force can be revived, by psychological, psychic or physical means, or a combination of them, the spread of cancer can be checked, and occasionally even reversed.

Nature cure

The attitude of the nature cure practitioner (see *Nature cure*, pages 16 to 44) to cancer is simple: anybody who sticks to a healthy diet, does not smoke and takes care to keep physically fit will rarely be a victim of the disease. For those who have broken these rules, admittedly, straight nature cure may have little to offer once they have cancer. However, there are a number of therapies derived from nature cure, all of which claim some success, though none provided evidence which will satisfy sceptics.

Of these, the best known are associated with Max Gerson, Josef Issels and William Donald Kelley, all three of which can be described as applied *Naturopathy* (see pages 18 to 22) with quirks attributable to the beliefs or experiences of the founder. Other practitioners follow similar principles but advocate additions to the diet, as in enzyme therapy, in which doses or injections are given of what are regarded as cancer-inhibiting enzymes, or in *Megavitamin therapy* (see *Diets*, page 33).

Although the patients who testified to any such form of cancer treatment may have been deceived, or have deceived themselves, the success of this deception may have been precisely what cured them. The evidence that *any* medicament, or even any diet, can check or cure cancer is still derived mainly from such testimonials. Evidence that cancer is a disorder in the psychosomatic and stress bracket, however, has been building up on the strength of controlled trials. This suggests that there is likely to be a significant, and sometimes powerful, psychological element in a successful form of treatment.

Psychological therapies

In the nineteenth century, it was taken for granted that cancer was a reaction to disappointment and distress. Cases were so frequent in which deep anxiety, deferred hope and disappointment were quickly followed by the growth or increase of cancer, the great surgeon Sir James Paget observed, ''that we can hardly doubt that mental depression is a weighty addition to the other influences that favour the development of a cancerous constitution''.

Research into the relationship between emotional stress or distress, and cancer has since backed this hypothesis. Thirty years ago a survey of women cancer patients in Chicago indicated that the majority of them shared one characteristic – they were unable to release their emotions satisfactorily. Lawrence LeShan, the New York doctor, found the same ''bottling up'' in his cancer patients. Moreover, in an impressive controlled trial carried out in Glasgow in the early 1960s, Dr David Kissen found that ''the poorer the outlet for emotional discharge, the less the exposure to cigarette smoke required to induce lung cancer''.

The evidence that cancer often follows some traumatic experience is also strong. The onset ''in about 80 percent of cases follows the loss of a spouse, death of a child, loss of a job, or an accident'', Dr Alec Forbes has estimated, or it may follow a milder shock, but of a type ''to which they have been sensitized by their past experience to find upsetting''.

There is not much that can be done, as a rule, to avoid such shocks, but much can be done to make them less shocking; to acquire the ability to cope with them. This is not a matter of cultivating stoic endurance – rather the reverse. Psychotherapists in general emphasize the need to release emotions, where appropriate, such as after the loss of a close relative, and how to avoid releasing them where inappropriate through relaxation.

The best-known techniques for use specifically with cancer are: *Visualization therapy*, (see page 184) as developed by Carl and Stephanie Simonton (it might be described as aggressive meditation, patients, having first taught themselves to achieve a relaxed frame of mind, use it to give their homeostatic systems instructions on how to fight the cancer cells); and *Inten-*

sive meditation as taught by Australian psychiatrist Ainslie Meares (see page 185), the emphasis is on restoring the homeostatic system to working order and allowing it to do the fighting.

These methods can also be applied to Hypnotherapy (see pages 166 to 173) or to one of the techniques of Autosuggestion (see pages 173 to 176).

Paranormal therapies

Some of the most spectacular cancer cures have been reported following the visit of a patient either to a healing centre, such as Lourdes, or to a healer (see pages 227 to 230). It has not proved possible to mount an investigation which would indicate how often this method is successful – or even whether it should claim the credit when the healing appears to have worked. The medical term for such cures is still "spontaneous regression". Where it is linked to healing, the cure can then be pronounced a coincidence.

Doctors prepared to accept the possibility that remissions take place often argue that they are simply examples of the power of autosuggestion, arising from the patient's confidence in the healer, rather than in the healer's powers. However, the possibility that there is an as yet undiscovered healing force – analagous to magnetism – has also to be taken into consideration.

SKIN DISORDERS

Nobody, presumably, has ever gone through life, or even childhood, without some skin disorder. Some skin disorders are superficial: rashes which appear and disappear for no discernable reason. Others, such as impetigo, can be traced to specific pathogens. They may also be the consequence of accidents, such as burns. Some represent surface tumours: benign like warts, or malignant like some melanomas. Alternatively, they can arise through expulsion, or attempted expulsion, by the body of toxic matter, acne, boils and cysts.

Skin disorders are the commonest of all maladies and, even when they are not painful, they are among the hardest to bear because they are so often humiliatingly disfiguring. Moreover orthodox medicine's record as far as finding ways to prevent and treat them has not been encouraging.

Orthodox treatment

One reason for the failure of orthodox medicine to give satisfactory results is obvious – or should be: the simple fact that there is this specialty called "dermatology". The spread of specialization has been particularly unfortunate in this area, because what goes wrong with the skin is so rarely related solely to the skin. Its condition is for the most part dictated by what is going on inside the body, in the digestive system in particular, and in the mind. The slightest change of mood is reflected in the action of the sweat glands and the way blood is sent coursing to, or away from, the surface of the body, as well as influencing all the other components of the skin.

Of course it is possible for a consultant dermatologist to become an expert on the interaction of the digestive system with the skin, and of the relationship of psychosocial upsets to skin disorders. A few do. But unfortunately, a dermatologist rarely sees patients until they have already gone through two preliminary stages: self-medication, usually with some over-the-counter remedy, and prescriptions tried out after a visit to a doctor. In other words, dermatologists are most likely to see the established cases, and are unlikely to have the time, even if they had the inclination, to get to know about the circumstances which led up to the skin trouble in its early stages.

Over the past 20 years or so, resistance in the medical profession to admitting the reality of allergy or 'autoallergy" as the cause of symptoms has been slowly broken down. It is now coming to be accepted that many skin disorders are – or can be – allergic; representing a hiccup in the body's self-regulatory system. Dermatologists can from practice become expert in judging whether a skin complaint is caused by a "contact" allergy – when somebody becomes allergic to nylon for example. But they cannot be expected to be expert in detecting, let alone treating, a skin disorder which arises from some food allergy, or from an allergy of an undiscovered source.

The use of steroids and cortisone
Up to a point disorders of the human skin have proved amenable to symptomatic treatment with hormone drugs such as the steroids. Often they can remove rashes or eczema very quickly, and where the cause of the disorder happens to have been some transitory upset, whether in the digestive system or in the mind, the results can be most satisfactory. But steroids applied topically (locally, on the skin surface) can only work topically. If they are employed to treat skin problems arising from a deep-seated dietary deficiency, an allergy, or some psychosomatic source, they may for a time have a cosmetic effect, but the long-term consequences can be unfortunate.

"Topical steroids" began to be widely prescribed in the early 1970s, and to all appearances they were highly effective. Only in the mid-1970s did it become apparent that they were causing rosacea, a roughening and reddening of the skin, in thousands of cases, and in some of them, doing irreparable damage. The record of these skin creams and lotions can in fact be simply stated: the more effective they are at clearing up symptoms, the more dangerous they are likely to be when used indiscriminately.

Alternative treatment

Natural therapists have a very different attitude to skin disorders to that of orthodox practitioners. First, they take it for granted that the symptoms in the great majority of cases are the consequence of some internal upset making its presence felt on the skin. Consequently they do not waste their time treating the skin. Of course, if a palliative is needed – to stop itching for example – there are innumerable herbal creams and lotions which can be tried. They are not, as a rule, briskly effective as symptom-removers in the way steroids are, but they are capable of reducing discomfort more safely. The natural therapist's second important consideration is that the role of the mind in therapy in the form of suggestion or placebo effect, is neither discounted nor regarded as an intruder, it is valued as an ally.

The "internal upset" mechanism
Because more emphasis is put on internal upset as a trigger mechanism, and on the mind as an ally to help put it to rights, less attention is paid by natural therapists to diagnostic details – working out precisely what type of skin disorder each patient has. Identification is recognized as necessary in the rare forms which are passed on by contagion from person to person. For other types, the feeling is that individual susceptibility, perhaps inherited, perhaps constitutional, may be decisive, so that it is more important to consider the individual than the particular type of skin trouble presented.

Understandably, the emphasis differs with the therapist's preconceptions and training.

Nature cure

Naturopaths (see pages 18 to 21), emphasize the need for an accurate diagnosis – but of the condition of the circulatory and digestive systems, rather than the external condition of the skin. They also place more faith than most other therapists, orthodox or unorthodox, in treatments such as Epsom salts baths, which influence the skin by, as they believe, permeating it. They encourage the use of compresses and fomentations which they believe draw out poisons from the body, and make a particular point of warning patients not to try to suppress symptoms. As always, naturopaths are particularly insistent upon the need for a balanced diet.

The dispensers of *Tissue salts* (see pages 42 to 44) and *Bach remedies* (see pages 63 to 65), are all very careful to insist that the remedy must be specific to the patient and not necessarily the symptom.

Herbal medicine

Herbalists (see pages 45 to 58) provide any number of recipes for skin care, both as preventives and as palliatives, though they are now rather more cautious about claiming that they have remedies for skin conditions which work because of some ingredient in the herb itself. The power of suggestion, in this context, has been too well documented to ignore. They are more inclined now to recommend herbs which are designed to purify the blood stream, or improve digestion, than to prescribe palliatives.

The problem here is that there are so many herbs and some disagreement about which are the most affective. For example, in *Health Secrets of Plants and Herbs*, the author, Maurice Mésségué lists 21 purifying agents for use in eczema. Paul Schauenberg and Ferdinand Paris, in their *Guide to Medicinal Plants*, list 18 only two of which feature among Mésségué's list of recommendations.

Systems of medicine

Homeopaths (see pages 66 to 73) have a similar range of remedies, and they are also careful to insist that the selection must fit the patient, rather than the symptoms; as do the dispensers of *Anthroposophical remedies* (see pages 74 to 76).

Manipulative therapies

Many people find it hard to believe that corns, bunions, callouses and the rest can be the consequence of stressful events, but reflexologists (see pages 112 to 115), working as they do on the feet of their patients, realize that this is a common occurrence, which they attribute to the fact that the emotional upheaval affects the hormonal system. Anna Kaye recalls the case of a patient who came to see her with large callouses which had not been there the previous week: "in response to my query as to whether she had had some sort of emotional shock, she said that indeed she had – her marriage had been terminated by her husband, who had moved out to live with a younger woman". That kind of dramatic evidence, Anna Kaye admits, is rare, "but it does serve to remind us that the skin reveals the emotional state – and the consequent acute need for relaxation".

Psychotherapies

In a trial reported in the *Lancet* in 1959, 10 patients had been hypnotized, and while under hypnosis told that the warts on one side of their body would disappear. The warts on that side duly disappeared; the warts on the other side did not. The realization that warts can be removed by *Hypnotherapy* (see pages 166 to 172) – even if not infallibly, because some people are not susceptible to hypnotic suggestion – has encouraged its use, and that of therapies based on *Autosuggestion* (see pages 173 to 176), in the treatment of other types of skin disorders.

Such results can sometimes be startlingly impressive, but the therapist should warn you that merely getting rid of the symptoms, though a gratifying indication of the powers of your mind over your skin, may need to be followed up by an attempt to find out what went wrong with you to bring on the skin trouble in the first place.

Self-help

Self-help in connection with skin disorders is largely a question of a changed attitude of mind: thinking of the whole range of symptoms, from acne to whitlow, as the product of something wrong internally, which is unlikely to be put right by using creams or lotions on the skin. Surveys undertaken in the early 1970s showed that about half the households in Britain have some sort of skin medicament in the medicine cupboard, and that at any given time, about one person in ten of the population is dabbing something on daily, or more often. The great bulk of this self-help treatment is self-medication, using over-the-counter, proprietary medicines.

Only rarely is there anything in these products to justify their cost, though their placebo effect may be powerful. Their chief defect is that they encourage people to continue to think of skin disorders as skin-deep, rather than as an indication of an unbalanced diet, or an unrecognized allergy. The first practical step towards self-help is often to throw away the skin creams and lotions in the house, to concentrate instead on a change of eating habits, along with a decision to take more fresh air and exercise, and to learn how to relax.

BONE AND MUSCLE DISORDERS

In Britain, around eight million people consult their doctors with what are diagnosed as rheumatic, arthritic or related complaints. The statistics are staggering. At any time, for example, more than one million people are, to some extent, incapacitated and between 40 and 50 million working days are lost each year as a result. Yet little progress has been made over the last 30 years in the fields of conventional research, diagnostic procedures, treatment or preventive measures: there has been little or no reduction either of the incidence of bone and muscle disorders or of the suffering they cause.

Rheumatoid arthritis
This degenerative condition used to be attributed to life's wear and tear although periodically evidence was produced which pointed to a

virus as a possible cause, or to crystals which act like pieces of grit in the body's works.

The idea that rheumatism is an autoimmune reaction – the body's self-protective mechanism failing in its duty – is now coming to be accepted.

Back pain
Although it is generally regarded as a minor, and indeed almost laughable, disorder, in its severe forms backache can not merely render sufferers almost incapable of moving, it can produce protracted, nagging pain, and sharp, agonizing spasms. Intravertebral discs (the shock-absorbers between the vertebrae, consisting of a pulpy substance enclosed in an outer cover of cartilage) can rupture, or they can squeeze out between the vertebrae and press on a nerve – the condition is commonly known as a "slipped disc".

Whatever the initial cause of the trouble, it can lead to the ligaments and muscles associated with the spine going taut, as if to afford it some support, and this in itself can be the cause of discomfort and sometimes considerable pain.

Bursitis and gout
Bursas might be described as primitive versions of spinal discs, since they are like small shock-absorbers interposed between moving parts of the body to reduce friction. Bursitis is an indication of a breakdown in the body's lubricating system, sometimes overcompensated for by an accumulation of fluid around the joint or tendon, as in "housemaid's knee".

Excessive indulgence (specifically in port) and general high living is usually blamed for the malady, though not necessarily by the victim, who may insist that not he but his ancestors, were responsible. Gout has, in fact, a strong genetic component, and it does chiefly affect men. The cause usually given is an excess of uric acid in the blood which in itself is often attributable to overindulgence of food, particularly fatty meats, and drink.

Orthodox treatment

Orthopedic physicans and surgeons have long disputed the territory of bone and muscle disorders between them. First one type of treatment has become fashionable, then another. For some years the operations for "slipped" discs, which often involved "fusing" the vertebrae above and below the affected disc to prevent jarring, were claimed to be highly effective and safe. Hundreds of thousands of them were performed all over the world. Gradually, however, it became clear that in many cases, disc trouble could not be held responsible for the pain, and in other cases, where a disc had appeared to be responsible for the pain, repositioning it or removing it made no difference; the pain continued.

In cases of arthritis, replacement of diseased joints by artificial ones has given some impressive results; but this method is suitable only for those most seriously handicapped.

Traction, corsets and plaster casts
Various other alternatives have also been tried in the hope of finding some way to treat backache more successfully. Patients are often subjected to traction, a gentle adaption of the medieval torture chamber's rack, in the hope that separating out the spinal vertebrae will allow the spine to come together again in alignment. Patients who cannot, or will not, stay in bed are often enclosed in plaster casts or surgical corsets which they are expected to wear for varying periods of time. But these devices have made no significant impact. The standard advice to patients with backache is still, as the *British Medical Journal* described it in 1977, "recumbency and analgesics". In other words they recommend that you stay in bed, and when in pain, take some aspirin.

The miracle drugs for arthritis
The other commonly used form of treatment for arthritis has been with drugs. When cortisone was launched, in the late 1940s, orthopaedic physicians assumed it was going to

be the answer to bone and muscle disorders. Patients who had been bedridden for years could get up, and get around; wheelchair cases found they could walk; crutches were thrown aside. The miracle drug, however, was effective only as long as patients continued to take it; but the longer they continued to take it, the more they tended to suffer from ugly and sometimes fatal side-effects. Nausea, rashes and headache were common, and so was endocrine inbalance; women grew beards, while men lost all their hair. Worst of all, cortisone lowered resistance to infection, so that patients contracted influenza, pneumonia or TB and often died. Surveying the evidence after five years, the British Medical Council ruefully recommended that patients would be well-advised to stick to an old and tried remedy for rheumatoid arthritis, namely aspirin.

Aspirin still holds the field today, in spite of the fact that after cortisone's failure, a succession of its derivatives were marketed. Corticosteroids, were ecstatically promoted as having its advantages without the adverse side-effects. But investigations by the American Senate's Kefauver Committee in the early 1960s showed that this was simply untrue – the side-effects, if not quite so lethal, were still severe.

More recently, the anti-inflammatory drugs have been marketed and lavishly promoted as being free from steroid side-effects; but their record has been little better.

In the summer of 1982 one of the most widely prescribed antiinflammatory drugs, Opren, had to be withdrawn when it was found to be causing serious reactions – in Britain alone, there were over 60 fatalities.

Alternative treatment

What has gone wrong with orthodox treatment of the bones and muscles and where do the natural therapies fit in? The trouble can be traced back to mistakes which the medical profession made in the nineteenth century. Traditionally, fractures and dislocations had been left to the local bonesetter who, partly by knack and partly by experience, could deal with them more expeditiously than doctors. Victorian Britain's leading surgeon, Sir James Paget, warned his colleagues that if they did not learn the bonesetters craft, he would steal their patients, and that was what happened; though the bonesetter was soon joined, and eventually largely replaced, by the osteopath and the chiropractor.

The other mistake the profession made a century ago was to begin to believe that back pain, and indeed all forms of bone and muscle disorder, must have an organic cause – as in the efforts to link arthritis, for example, to a virus. The possibility that there might be some psychosomatic component was discounted. Yet there was a mass of evidence from research in the latter half of the nineteenth century that under hypnosis, patients could lose their symptoms. Inevitably it is the manipulators who have benefitted most from the first of these mistakes by the medical profession, and hypnotherapists and healers who have benefitted from the second mistake.

Nature cure

Sufferers from rheumatoid arthritis make up a substantial proportion of the people who try aspects of *Nature cure* in spas and *Hydrotherapy* establishments (see pages 22 to 27). Naturopaths insist that much pain and incapacity can be averted if those sufferers would stop taking painkillers. Desirable though pain relief is, Max Warmbrand pointed out in his *Encyclopedia of Natural Health*, when it is obtained by suppressive measures it is rarely lasting, "and often leads only to greater suffering. *We should seek permanent relief which is obtainable only through the establishment of a normal metabolic pattern*" –

through adopting a balanced diet, and other nature cure precepts.

Herbal medicine

Herbalists (see pages 45 to 57) have a wide range of remedies designed primarily for pain relief but they, too, stress the need for preventive measures such as detoxification, and offer herbal beverages to take instead of, say, coffee and tea, which they believe will delay the onset of degenerative disorders such as rheumatism.

Systems of medicine

Homeopaths (see pages 66 to 73) have long claimed that their remedies are more effective in the treatment of arthritis cases than conventional medicines. In the late 1970s, they had the chance to demonstrate this, and controlled trials set up in Glasgow proved that they were right.

Oriental therapies

Sufferers from back pain, rheumatism and arthritis may benefit from *Acupuncture* (see pages 120 to 133) on the principle that needles inserted in the appropriate acupuncture points restore the balance of the life forces, enabling the system to work smoothly again.

Pain relief is a major aspect of acupuncture treatment, and practitioners report that they have considerable success in the treatment of sciatica and other similarly painful conditions. Often therapists recommend combining acupuncture treatment with manipulation for a mixture of adjustment and pain relief. *Shiatsu* and *Acupressure* practitioners (see pages 133 to 137) can also provide pain relief.

Manipulative therapies

Manipulation is much in demand for the actual treatment of backache and pains associated with it, fibrositis and sciatica. But it is not commonly thought of for prevention. Here, *Massage* (see pages 95 to 100) has been attracting increasing notice, along with the *Alexander principle* (see pages 104 to 108) and *Rolfing* (see pages 101 to 103). By setting the posture to rights, their practitioners claim, the spine and its associated ligaments and muscles are relieved of the strains which gave rise to trouble; all have their devotees.

Exercise/movement therapies

Yoga (see pages 138 to 143) is another method of teaching the body to move and function properly. In his book *Yoga against Spinal Pain*, however, Pandit Shiv Sharma makes the point which yogi in general emphasize – that the exercises should not be regarded simply as exercises designed to relieve aches and pains. "It should be borne in mind that steadiness and strength of mind are closely linked with the fitness of the body". Yoga ought to be taken up for this wider purpose, with freedom from pain as only one of the welcome by-products – though remarkable results have been achieved in helping arthritis patients. The same can be said for *T'ai chi*, *Aikido* and *Dance therapy* (see pages 144 to 153).

Psychological therapies

The idea that there is a psychosomatic component in bone and muscle disorders was put forward by J.L. Halliday, a Scots general practitioner as early as 1937. In many of his patients, he had observed, the onset of lumbago or fibrositis followed a time of emotional tension. If they could recover peace of mind, their symptoms went away.

Recent research in the U.S. has shown that the prospects for relief and recovery are bleaker in those cases of rheumatoid arthritis in which the patients are worried and depressed. If so, a psychological therapy of some kind may be advisable. *Hypnotherapy* (see pages 166 to 173) or one of the *Autosuggestion* procedures (see pages 173 to 176) can also be used to explore what control the mind can exercise over symptoms, and how to exploit this.

Paranormal therapies

Most healers think of the forces they invoke as having a divine, or spirit, source, and of all the different types of disease, rheumatoid arthritis and back pain have provided them with their most spectacular cures (see *Hand healing*, pages 243 to 253). The late Harry Edwards could point to dozens of examples, some filmed and shown on TV programmes, of crippled patients being able to straighten out arthritic backs that had long been bent, or able to walk away from their wheelchairs. The argument that orthopedic surgeons ordinarily use – that such "cures" are almost invariably temporary – is correct, but hardly relevant. The fact that healing can work at all in such cases, even if only for a few hours, ought to have been enough to encourage more research into the links between mind and body.

Other forms of treatment

There are any number of forms of treatment for rheumatism and arthritis which sound eccentric, to put it mildly, but which obviously work for some people, and may be worth trying if other methods fail. One which has had a good deal of publicity lately is an extract from the green-lipped mussel, a denizen of the Pacific. In trials, as many as two out of three arthritic patients have reported improvement in their symptoms: but the trials have been criticized. The value of wearing a copper bracelet, long dismissed as an old wives' tale, has also recently been reconsidered on the basis of a theory that valuable trace elements may indeed penetrate the skin.

Self-help

Little is known about how to prevent the onset of rheumatism and arthritis, but it is generally believed that a balanced diet, fresh air and exercise, and healthy living will delay it. By contrast, there has been far too much in the way of advice on how self-help can be used to prevent back pain, some of it contradictory and a good deal of it of doubtful validity.

"Nowhere in the field of back pain prevention is there greater confusion and speculation than the area of seating design", Paul Branton, a consultant ergonomist, has lamented. Recommendations "usually proceed from wrong or untenable assumptions to incomplete or unwarrantable conclusions, made for unexplained reasons and aiming at unrealistic purposes".

The basic fallacy, Branton contends is that there is an anatomically correct sitting position; whereas each one of us has a different posture and different needs. A chair which is right for you may be wrong for somebody else.

Keep fit exercises
On exercises of this kind there is much controversy. Many of those which schoolchildren are put through as a matter of course are frowned upon by some backache specialists. In his book *You Don't Have to Ache*, for example, Arthur A. Michele, Professor of Orthopedic Surgery at the New York Medical Center, lists exercises you ought *not* to take. These include: press-ups and pull-ups; touching the toes with the legs straight; work-outs on parallel bars; lying face down while raising the arms and legs and arching the back; and lying flat on your back and raising the legs while keeping your knees straight.

Clearly, there are few safe guidelines, however. Self-help is very much a matter of finding what exercises, chairs and beds suit you personally.

CIRCULATORY DISORDERS

Until little more than half-a-century ago heart disease was not regarded with any great concern. The heart, it was believed, was a marvellous piece of machinery. Occasionally something went wrong: the blood clotted, causing apoplexy if the brain were affected, or a heart attack if its blood supply failed. Some people, too, had congenital heart defects. But ordinarily the heart went on beating until it wore out in old age. Even then, it was the general ageing process that was usually held to be responsible, rather than the organ itself.

Heart disease as an epidemic

Between the wars, and particularly after the Second World War, heart disease began to cause growing concern. By the 1960s it had become the most common cause of death among men, and the mortality rate for women, though much lower, was also increasing. Worse: heart attacks were killing off apparently healthy people, very suddenly, in the prime of their lives.

In 1969, the World Health Organisation warned that this would soon mean ''the greatest epidemic mankind has faced, unless we are able to reverse the trend by concentrated research into its cause and prevention''.

That epidemic has materialized. Most people today die of heart attacks, commonly precipitated by cholesterol, a congealed fatty substance which is deposited on the walls of the arteries, reducing the flow of blood to the heart. If the blood should clot, this can cut off the supply altogether. ''Strokes'' – apoplexy resulting from hemorrhage or clotting affecting the brain – are another menace.

Disorders of the circulation, often culminating in a heart attack or heart failure, are also common: angina pectoris, (a severe pain which spreads across the chest to the shoulder); and intermittent claudication (cramp and pain in the calf muscles) are two forms. On an everyday level, there are problems such as: palpitations, heart flutter and irregular heartbeat.

Risk factors

When it began to become clear that the incidence of heart disease was rising rapidly, cardiologists were at a loss for an explanation, and uncertain where to look for one.

Over the years, however, a pattern has begun to emerge. The individuals most at risk from heart attacks are often heavy smokers of cigarettes; they have high blood pressure; and they eat a lot of saturated (mostly animal) fat. Other risk factors have been found: obesity; lack of sufficient exercise; a high salt intake; and a low intake of dietary fibre.

Potentially the most important discovery of all from trials of this kind has been about the role of emotional stress. In the 1960s psychologists in the United States navy found, with the help of questionnaires, that heart attacks among the crews of war ships were statistically related to stressful events, such as a bereavement, a divorce, or being charged with some crime. In the same period two Californian cardiologists, Meyer Friedman and Ray H. Rosenman, realized from their practice that the impact of stressful events was much more dangerous for people of a certain personality type. The Type A male, as they described him (ambitious, go-getting, driving himself hard), is the kind of person who may land himself in a stressful situation, and have a heart attack; whereas the placid Type B males do not.

There is also evidence that emotional stress can precipitate attacks. At a conference held in New York in 1981 to consider the evidence about sudden deaths from heart attacks, a Boston cardiologist, gave the results of a five-year study of patients who had survived cardiac arrest. One in five of them, it had been found, had had acute emotional disturbances (such as humiliation in public, break-up of a relationship, loss of a job, and so on) in the 24 hours before the onset of their symptoms – most of them in the hour before it.

Not merely are the findings about risk factors remarkably consistent in western countries, but there has also been growing evidence that people who stop taking the risks, or at least reduce their risk-taking, live longer as a result. For example, a number of trials in different countries have now shown that a reduction in the consumption of saturated fats lowers mortality.

Orthodox treatment

One might have expected that the medical profession would have taken note of these findings about the importance of psychosocial factors, and up to a point, it has. In Britain, the Royal College of Physicians and other Establishment bodies have issued warnings about the dangers of smoking and eating too much saturated fat. But the medical profession finds it hard to deal effectively with a disease caused not by germs or viruses but, or so it would appear, by our lifestyles. Doctors have tended to go on as before, using drugs and surgery as their main weapons.

Special care units

The majority of patients who die of heart attacks are dead before they can be brought to hospital, but this did not prevent the proliferation, in the 1960s, of elaborately equipped coronary care units. It could always be argued that those patients who survived long enough to reach them must get the best of attention. Some doctors, however, doubted whether ''the best of attention'', which meant being wired up to gadgetry of various kinds, was really what somebody who had had a heart attack needed; they turned out to be right. In the early 1970s, a survey carried out in hospitals in the South of England revealed that patients' chances of survival after a heart attack were slightly better if they were at home than if they were in a hospital unit, a finding that has since been confirmed in other parts of the country. Coronary care units do save some lives, where there are complications which could not be treated in the patients' homes, but the proportion is so tiny that it does not even register on the mortality statistics.

Yet more drugs

The other prong of orthodoxy's campaign against heart disease, the use of anticoagulants, cholesterol-reducers, and anti-hypertensive drugs, has hardly been more successful. The drugs do what they are called upon to do in the short term, but there is nothing to show that they improve life expectancy, and there is all too clear evidence of their unwelcome side-effects. Patients treated with the drug clofibrate to lower blood cholesterol levels had fewer heart attacks but their mortality rate from *all* causes rose, until 20 years later it was 25 percent higher than that of those in the control groups who had not been given the drug.

Nevertheless, drugs have remained the medical profession's chief line of defence against heart disease, along with coronary care.

Surgical operations

In hospitals, an irregular heartbeat tends to be treated as a disorder, with drugs; patients are often then fitted with heart pace-makers. Yet in a trial recently at the Nottingham City Hospital, 260 patients suspected of having heart trouble were divided into two groups, half being given drugs and half treated with placebos, and their hearts were monitored for abnormal rhythms. When the trial was over, it was found that the survival rate was the same, not merely whether or not the patients were on the drug or the placebo, but also whether or not they had abnormal rhythms.

The latest craze is for "by-pass" operations in which veins from a patient's leg are used as substitutes for clogged up coronary arteries. They are relatively simple, and produce quite satisfactory short-term improvement. But are they necessary?

Alternative treatment

The practitioners of alternative medicine are in broad agreement that the "medical model", as applied to heart disease, is unnecessarily expensive, largely irrelevant and often counter-productive. They concede that surgery can be valuable in remedying congenital heart defects or repairing damage caused in accidents, and that there are cases where it may need to be used for running repairs, as in by-pass surgery. But by-pass surgery, and for that matter most heart transplants, would be unnecessary, they claim, if simple changes in lifestyle were adopted.

A crucial difference between the conventional and unconventional attitudes is displayed over the treatment of high blood pressure. There is no dispute that it is a risk factor, but natural therapists assume that, like pain, it should primarily be regarded as a warning. The doyen of the British medical profession in the early years of this century, Sir James Mackenzie, used to remind his colleagues that raised blood pressure is "for the benefit of the organism": it rises to enable us to meet some emergency, which is beneficial, but it should fall as soon as the emergency is dealt with. The trouble today is that many people cannot release the tensions of work or home life which cause the rise, and so it stays up, reflecting the continued tension.

Natural therapists argue that a way should therefore be found to remove the tension, if possible, by finding its source and removing that. Reducing blood pressure artificially, with the help of drugs, is like switching off the burglar alarm without bothering to see if there is a burglar, and the body's resentful reaction can express itself in unpleasant side-effects.

Angina and intermittent claudication are also regarded by natural therapists primarily as an early warning system. The pain is telling us that our hearts are not receiving an adequate blood supply, or that for some reason they are not pumping the blood out satisfactorily. Even palpitations, alarming though they can sometimes be, should not be regarded as menacing. They may be a sign that the heart is actually doing its job, reacting to some stress of which you are unaware; though of course you would be wise to try to find out what is responsible if the palpitations continue.

Nature cure

Many "symptoms" of heart disease, in short, are not "treated" by natural therapists: they are simply taken into account in diagnosis, as useful indicators of what a patient's problems may be and of how to set about solving them. Warning signs indicate that you should switch to a better balanced diet with, in particular, a reduction of saturated fat intake whether in the form of meat or cream, butter and other dairy products.

Psychological therapies

What exasperates natural therapists is that there is no *need* for drugs to reduce high blood pressure. If it is too high, it can be brought down easily and safely by the use of any of the techniques of relaxation which happen to suit the individual concerned. This can involve using *Self hypnosis* (see pages 166 to 173), *Autogenics* (see pages 178 to 181), *Autosuggestion* (see pages 173 to 176), *Meditation* (see pages 182 to 188), and/or *Yoga* (see pages 138 to 143).

Research in numerous centres has demonstrated again and again that with or without the help of *Biofeedback* (see pages 188 to 193) people can easily and quite quickly be trained (or can train themselves) to lower their blood pressure. And it need not simply be an artificial reduction. Many patients have found that their blood pressure stays down, if they keep up the good work, as if the act of self-discovery, the realization that the mind does enjoy such powers, has been an effective therapy on its own.

Self-help

The prevention of heart disease, because it is a disease of lifestyle, *is* largely self-help. Periodic physical check-ups, apart from warning you if your blood pressure is getting dangerously high, are of little value unless the distinction between Type A or Type B personality is incorporated into them.

The British public has been picking up the message quicker than the medical profession. A survey carried out recently by the Health Education Council has shown that over half the population (if the sample was representative) rate stress as being the major cause of heart attacks.

You should, of course, stop smoking, take more exercise, consume less salt and sugar, and a little more fibre, in your meals. If you are a Type A person, you should learn to relax, particularly before occasions which are likely to be stressful. This is advice you are as likely to get from an osteopath as from a teacher of autogenic training; from an acupuncturist as from a hypnotherapist.

DISORDERS OF THE NERVOUS SYSTEM

Diseases of the nervous system, or "neuropathies" are perhaps best classified by the fact that they are ordinarily dealt with, when they reach the specialist level, by neurologists. Such diseases present a wide variety of symptoms. Some may occur sporadically throughout a lifetime, such as epileptic fits. Some, such as multiple sclerosis (MS), myasthenia gravis and Parkinson's disease, follow a gradually degenerative course, often with periods of remission. Some have been attributed to viruses such as *herpes simplex*, of which the most familiar symptoms are cold sores, and *herpes zoster*, or shingles. There is also glandular fever, where periodic rises in the temperature are accompanied or followed by swollen glands in the neck and elsewhere.

Yet another variation on the theme is diabetes mellitus – a disorder of the body's autonomic nervous system where the pancreas

gland ceases to function efficiently. As a result it ceases to produce the hormone insulin, which normally stimulates the cells in the body into absorbing the sugar in the bloodstream, instead the sugar is discharged in the urine.

The chief common characteristic of the neuropathies, so far as orthodox medical science is concerned, is that they are baffling.

Orthodox treatment

In recent decades, the neurological disorders have, as far as possible, been segregated from those which are regarded as in the province of psychiatry. This used to seem a sensible division, in that the neuropathies can, and often do, arise without any clear indication of a mental, or emotional, as well as a physical breakdown. So long as patients objected to being told that their symptoms could be related to their personality structure, or to their inability to cope with their psychosocial problems, they were happy to be assured that their illness was organic.

As a result research into the neuropathies has concentrated upon the investigation of their organic aspects, in the hope of finding culprits such as viruses or some chemical mix-up. Yet although a great deal has been discovered about the physical *effects* on the nervous system, the *causes* have proved elusive. The identification of the virus merely enables the name herpes to be attached to the disorder, but thereafter, as Geoff Watts, the British medical journalist and broadcaster, has put it, "understanding and agreement melt, respectively, into confusion and discord" – a verdict which could be applied in the case of most of the neuropathic disorders.

Surgery and drugs

There has been widespread use of surgery for these disorders, but with little success. Neurologists have consequently relied heavily on drugs, and they, too, have been disappointing.

When larodopa (L Dopa) was

introduced for Parkinson's disease in the 1960s, it was hailed as the major breakthrough in that otherwise bleak decade for pharmacology. Ecstatic reports of patients making full recoveries were put about, and for a time it appeared to do for the disorder what insulin had done for diabetics. Since then its limitations have gradually become apparent. Between a third and a half of patients derive no benefit from L Dopa or from other such drugs. Of those that do, many are afflicted with side-effects, both physical – nausea and vomiting – and mental – emotional ups and downs. These have necessitated prescribing more drugs, to prevent the nausea or the depression, and these in turn can have their own side-effects.

Insulin replacement

Sixty years ago the Canadian physiologist Frederick Banting and his colleagues introduced insulin treatment for diabetes. As it is a comparatively easy matter to keep the body supplied with insulin through injections, enabling diabetics to lead otherwise normal lives, this was regarded as one of the great achievements of medical science. Two Nobel Prizes were awarded and replacement insulin has been the mainstay of the treatment of diabetes ever since. But there have always been snags.

The record of the proprietary drugs marketed for diabetes has been unhappy. Their manufacturers were singled out for critical comment by the US Senate commission under Estes Kefauver, whose report in 1961 revealed, among other things, how widespread and sometimes sinister adverse reactions to the treatment had been.

In the course of trials two drugs, tolbutamide and phenformin, produced such serious adverse effects that their use had to be abandoned. (Phenformin was actually taken off the market altogether by the command of the Secretary of State for Health, Joseph Califano. This was the first time the power to ban a drug on the grounds that it was "an imminent hazard to public health'' had ever been used.) Moreover, remarkably, the trials showed that for adults, treatment with insulin was in fact no more effective than simple dieting.

Disease management replaces treatment

Recently, patients have been getting restless. With Parkinson's disease, the relief which drugs bring from the symptoms may be sufficient to outweigh the irritation at the side-effects, but for other neuropathies, no drugs have been found. In cases of MS, in particular, neurologists have had to abandon the idea that they are *treating* patients. Instead they have fallen back on the term ''management'' of the disease, which means that they can do little more than recommend that the patient goes to a physiotherapist.

Physiotherapy is also on standard offer for myasthenia gravis, though there is no clear evidence that it is effective except as a palliative. For herpetic cold sores there are soothing lotions. For shingles, there are painkilling drugs. As for glandular fever, there is no effective remedy at all, which has meant, all too often, dosage with antibiotics. These have no effect on the course of the disease, but are commonly prescribed on prophylactic grounds – to prevent infection (though most pharmacologists now dismiss this justification as spurious).

Recently there has been a growing realization that this failure to provide any effective treatment, let alone offer any hope of prevention, may be accounted for by an error that medical science has made, in regarding the symptoms of neuropathies as proof that they are diseases. The possibility remains to be explored that the convulsive symptoms associated with a fit, for example, represent not illness but our homeostatic mechanism's desperate bid to *avoid* illness – that they are in fact, a reaction to stress. Convulsions in themselves, after all, can be the very reverse of a

disorder. For example, fits of laughter are a joy, as, for that matter, are orgasms.

For the present, this argument can be taken no further than to suggest that a disruption of the nervous system, whatever form it takes, may initially indicate a reaction to stress. Only later does it indicate a failure on the part of the homeostatic mechanism to cope with the crisis. If this hypothesis proves to be correct, the need will be to explore ways of removing sources of strain, and getting the homeostat back into working order.

Alternative treatment

Growing dissatisfied with conventional ''management'' of their disorders, some MS victims have been exploring what natural therapies have to offer, and in Britain a new association has come into being – ARMS (Action for Research into Multiple Sclerosis). Unlike most fund-raising organizations of the kind this one has actually dared to support research which has been unable to get any financial backing through conventional sources.

Between them, the therapies offer a wide range of possibilities, from which patients can select whatever appeals to them. However, there is an indication from a research project carried out in Canada that they should take account of the likelihood that one of the risk factors involved in their illness is emotional stress, engendered by reaction to some prolonged emotional disturbance.

The stress factor

Seeking to check whether there is such a link, researchers at McGill University, Montreal found in 1958 that in the 40 patients they examined, all but five had suffered prolonged emotional stress before the onset of their symptoms, and relapse was commonly associated with some renewed strain. Although the researchers uncovered no evidence of an MS-prone personality, the relationship with protracted stress was sufficiently marked to suggest that this aspect

of the disease needs a great deal more research.

For the present, MS victims need to find ways of enabling themselves to reduce tension in situations where it cannot be avoided.

Choosing several therapies

The practitioners of most natural therapies have tales of patients who, arriving in despair, have been relieved of some of their symptoms of MS or of myasthenia gravis, and remained free of them for years. Total remissions remain rare, but there is general agreement that where patients are strongly motivated to recover their health, they have a better chance of doing so, particularly if they combine measures to improve their physical condition, such as diet and exercise, with *Psychotherapy* (see pages 163 to 165) or *Autosuggestion* (see pages 173 to 175).

With shingles and glandular fever, the problem is different: patients understandably want treatment which removes the symptoms as quickly as possible. In the case of glandular fever it is not easy to make recommendations, as so often it is not firmly diagnosed, but only guessed at. In many cases it turns out to be little more than the syndrome of ''just being sick'' with swollen glands as an added contribution to the range of symptoms.

Herbal medicine & Homeopathy

For shingles, there are some well-tried homeopathic remedies, and several recommended herbs. Maurice Mességué's list of purifying and cleansing agents includes garlic, basil, lemon, rosemary, sage and thyme, and he offers as a nightcap, ''an infusion of a pinch of thyme, a pinch of rosemary, a pinch of lavender, a pinch of lime flowers and a pinch of chervil to a cup of water''.

For diabetic adults, there are also herbal and homeopathic remedies with the more positive function of stimulating the pancreas to renewed activity.

Nature cure

Diabetes in adults is an obvious candidate for nature cure. The onset of diabetes in adults is usually gradual, and appears to be the consequence of a gradual wearing down of the pancreas's ability to cope with the quantity of carbohydrates consumed. If this is realized soon enough, and the consumption of carbohydrates reduced, this will usually suffice to remove the symptoms.

Diabetes in children often presents a more serious problem. The symptoms are usually more definite: a perpetual thirst, leading to frequent urination, along with general ill-health. There may be no alternative to a spell in hospital, during which an estimate is made of the level of insulin replacement which will be needed, and the child is taught how to provide it with regular injections.

These should not, however, be regarded as a life-sentence. For a start, it is known that children's blood sugar levels can vary considerably. This is a nuisance, as it means that a constant watch has to be kept on them; too high a level of insulin replacement can be just as dangerous as too low a level in the first place. Yet it is also a hopeful sign, because if the causes of any changes can be tracked down, ways may be found to stabilize or, better still, permanently lower the blood sugar level.

The existence of the links between the ups and down of blood sugar levels and emotional ups and downs (blood sugar is as susceptible to tension as blood pressure – it rises with emotional conflict, and falls when the conflict is over) suggests that parents need to consider whether there may be some cause for tension – perhaps not immediately apparent, as some children often have worries and fears that they keep to themselves. For adult diabetics, too, the possibility that there may be a psychosomatic component always needs to be considered.

Self-help

In her book *Multiple Sclerosis*, Judy Graham, a young journalist and TV researcher who contracted MS in her mid-twenties, has described what she and some of her fellow MS sufferers have chosen to do – often in conjunction with ARMS (Action for Research into Multiple Sclerosis). Her brief experience of "what is considered to be the top-notch neurological hospital in Britain" turned out to be "nothing short of dire" and as the neurologists she encountered were "remote, arrogant and totally lacking in helpful advice of any sort", she decided in future to give them a miss. Instead of settling for their recommended "management", therefore, she began to try natural therapies: a diet low in animal fats, regular exercise in a gym, yoga, acupuncture, deep massage, and a herbal remedy, nightly capsules of evening primrose oil. She could not claim they had cured her, she realized – and even if they had, she would not know how to allocate responsibility for a cure between them. But seven years after MS had been diagnosed, she was feeling distinctly better than she had when she started on her self-help course.

RESPIRATORY DISORDERS

When the symptoms are mild, respiratory disorders fall into the category of *Just being sick* (see pages 303 to 304). Some of the characteristics of the common cold, in particular, occur in many everyday illnesses. The tendency of medical science, however, has been to stress the differences between the various disorders for the purposes of diagnosis.

Colds and flu

In laboratory tests, colds can be distinguished from flu by the different types of virus involved. In practice, however, the distinction is normally made by rule of thumb. The rule differs from household to household, but generally a cold is regarded as a nuisance rather than as a real illness, whereas anybody whose symptoms are bad enough to have to go to bed has flu.

The designation of the condition as "a cold" usually means that they have taken the form of making the victim feel "bunged up" for a time, with a streaming nose to follow. Flu has a wider range of symptoms which usually include a sore throat, temperature, headache and dizziness, and is eventually dissipated in much the same way as a cold.

Bronchitis

Although several disorders have been awarded the title of the English disease, (including the medieval plague, "the sweating sickness" and venereal disease), none has a better claim to the title than bronchitis. Twice as many people die of it annually in the United Kingdom as in any other western country – 10 times more than in Norway, Sweden or Japan. This high mortality rate, admittedly, is to some extent misleading, because elderly people who suffer from bronchitis are likely, in the absence of any other obvious cause of death, to go down on the records as having died from it.

Bronchitis can be either acute, with attacks of breathlessness, wheezing and coughing which come and go like flu, or chronic, when the free flow of air is blocked for days or weeks by what, to the sufferer, feels like accumulated mucus in the lower respiratory tract, which coughing does little or nothing to dislodge. For patients with either the acute or the chronic type of bronchitis, orthodox medicine has little to offer.

Emphysema

Emphysema is distinguishable from bronchitis for purposes of diagnosis by the fact that the airways have lost their "give and take" and, as a consequence, the victim's lungs tend to remain in a state of near-inflation, instead of working like an automatic bellows.

Where there are no obstructions,

such as accumulated sputum, emphysema is also distinguishable from bronchitis by its victims, who find themselves taking short and fast breaths to obtain the necessary amount of oxygen, though they may not otherwise have any so-called bronchitic symptoms.

Asthma

The asthmatic condition greatly interested Dr Flanders Dunbar, a protagonist of psychosomatics, and in her book *Mind and Body*, she gave a succinct description of it. Asthma, she recalled "derives from a Greek word which means 'panting'. The victim has difficulty in breathing, wheezes, chokes, nearly suffocates". The physical cause of the condition is inflammation and swelling of the linings of the air passages, and sometimes spasm in the bronchial muscles, which further obstruct the passage of air. "In any case," says Dr Dunbar, "the important fact for the victim is that he finds it hard to breathe, the difficulty ranging from a gentle wheeze which is hardly noticeable to rather acute paroxysms".

Orthodox treatment

It has long been recognized that there is no cure for the common cold and no way to prevent it. When a "rhinovirus" was first discovered, the hope was that a vaccine could be found to provide immunization. However, soon, scores of rhinoviruses were discovered, leaving no prospect of finding any all-purpose vaccine.

Flu vaccines

With flu, the hope has been sustained for longer, partly because there are fewer flu viruses, but also because epidemics tend to be related to a particular virus strain. Theoretically, people can be given an immunizing injection of the strain which is going to be the danger if the epidemic spreads. Trials, however, have shown that such protection as may be given is not sufficiently effective to make mass immunization worthwhile, and doubt even remains about the value of immunization of those

people who are most at risk.

Antibiotics and bronchitis

When it was discovered that acute attacks of bronchitis were often accompanied by a proliferation of bacteria, it was labelled infectious. When antibiotics came on the market they were lavishly prescribed – not only to treat the symptoms, but sometimes also as a prophylactic, in the belief that they would prevent the bacteria from congregating in the respiratory tract. For a time, as has so often happened, gratifying results were reported. But gradually it has come to be realized that antibiotics are useful only when there happens to be some more serious infection. They are useless for bronchitis except for their placebo effect.

Use of inhalants for asthma

Asthma is much less common, and its mortality rate far lower than bronchitis, yet it has aroused far more interest and research – perhaps, it has unkindly been suggested, because it so often attacks the children of the upper classes. It is often encountered in children who have eczema, leading to the belief that it is the consequence of an allergic or autoallergic reaction. But this, in turn, may also have an emotional origin.

The only effective way which has been devised to treat attacks of asthma has been the use of inhalants, which enable some adrenaline-type drug to be sniffed in to clear the airways. For a time it was hoped that a better solution had been found in the form of the "pressurized aerosol bronchodilator", which could spray the drug up the nostrils. Millions of containers were sold before it was realized that the death rate from asthma, instead of going down, was rising suspiciously fast. Even after the *Lancet* warned that the bronchodilators might be responsible, another two years were to go by before the Committee on Safety of Medicines circularized doctors about the risks. Bronchodilators then went out of fashion – and the death rate from asthma fell again.

Alternative treatment

The theory most widely held by natural therapists is that viruses are not the *cause* of colds or flu, they are simply the *agency* which determines the nature of the symptoms. At a signal, viruses multiply and go into action to create sore throats and other symptoms.

What gives the signal? For the present, we have no answer. Still, the essential point, natural therapists argue, is that we ought to stop putting the blame on viruses which are in us and around us all the time; normally they give no trouble. The blame for their sudden activity ought to be put on the failure of our own homeostatic mechanism to keep them under control. Some natural therapists go further and argue that colds and flu, as part of the syndrome of *Just being sick*, represent the equivalent of what happens when an electrical fuse wire "blows" because too heavy a load had been put on the circuit. They are a warning signal, and should be welcomed as such.

There is fairly general agreement, in fact, that no attempt should be made to suppress the symptoms. If anything, they should be encouraged, because they represent the body's own way of regaining control by flushing out toxic waste matter. Above all, it is agreed, antibiotics should be shunned. Unluckily, in the first enthusiasm for them 30 years ago they were freely prescribed by the medical profession for sore throats and for bronchitis, even for colds. Yet they have no effect on the viruses involved. Antibiotics work, when they work at all, through placebo effect, through autosuggestion on the part of the patients themselves.

Nature cure

The old tag "feed a cold and starve a fever" is not now approved. More commonly the natural therapist's advice is: take plenty of liquid – water or fruit juice – but eat sparingly; do not go to work, if you can avoid it, and take the opportunity to rest. Some naturopaths advocate assisting the course of nature by sweating out the waste products with the help of a hot bath (with Epsom salts), followed by a stay in bed with plenty of blankets. Air ionizers (see pages 38 to 39) may also be of help in cases of breathing difficulties, and to promote sleep.

Natural therapists assume that bronchitis is multi-causal. Heredity, constitution and environment all have a share in the responsibility, but what *does* greatly increase the risk is cigarette smoking. Significantly, people who live or work in places where atmospheric pollution is high, and who *also* smoke, are at much greater risk than would be expected from simply adding the two risk factors together. It is as if smoking and breathing-in polluted air work on each other, to make bronchitis more likely.

This does not necessarily imply a causal connection, any more than it does with lung cancer or heart attacks. There remain the possibilities of the kind Professor Hans Eysenck has suggested – that proneness to bronchitis and addiction to cigarettes both, to some extent, reflect certain personality traits. Natural therapists generally emphasize the need to keep a watch for a psychosomatic element.

Relaxation techniques

The natural therapies do not commonly make any distinction between bronchitis and emphysema in suggesting preventive or palliative measures, but it is claimed that any of the techniques of relaxation (*Meditation*, see pages 182 to 187; *Autogenics*, see pages 178 to 181; *Yoga*, see pages 138 to 143; and *Autosuggestion*, see pages 173 to 176), are of value in acquiring breath control for emphysema.

Herbal medicine & Homeopathy

Herbalists and homeopaths have remedies designed, they insist, not to remove they symptoms but to make them more bearable and assist the body's own resistance mechanism. But a general prescription for colds and flu is "let them take their course", making yourself as comfortable as possible.

Recently evidence has been appearing that indicates stress can be an element in the production of colds. Ingenious tests have shown that the severity of a cold can be related to the level of anxiety of the patient. Natural therapists are consequently emphasizing the need for a tranquil mind, among their recommendation for ways to prevent colds and flu, or to lessen their impact if they cannot be prevented.

Psychological therapies

Most natural therapists would agree that there is often a powerful repressed emotional component in asthma. Some of them, however, feel that the continuation of attacks of breathlessness can often be more in the nature of a straightforward allergic reaction. Their proposition is that emotional stress may have triggered the attacks in the first place, but that the attacks may become attached to some physical substance, such as a scent or even food, which can then trigger the later allergy.

Manipulative & Movement therapies

Bad posture is often associated with attacks of asthma, some of the therapies such as the *Alexander Principle* (see pages 104 to 108), *Dance therapy* (see pages 150 to 153) and *Shiatsu* (see pages 133 to 137) can sometimes be used to help patients.

DIGESTIVE DISORDERS

Gastrointestinal disorders are usually labelled according to the part of the digestive tract in which they are sited. The commonest are inflammations: gastritis, of the stomach; enteritis, of the small intestine; colitis, of the large intestine. As usual the suffix "-itis" leaves no indication of the cause of the trouble. Sometimes specific bacteria will be found and indicated, sometimes not.

Ulcers and appendicitis

Of the disorders which require medical attention, the commonest are ulcers. Though labelled by their site – gastric ulcers, duodenal ulcers, ulcerative colitis and so on – ulcers are sometimes loosely described as "peptic", that is pertaining to the digestion. Here, it is as if the digestive juices, which ordinarily break down the food which is passing down through the stomach and the intestines, have turned their attention to the mucus membrane, and are trying to break that down, as well as the food.

Also common, though less so than it used to be, is appendicitis. This is inflammation of the appendix, an organ which, for some obscure reason, remains as a relic of an earlier evolutionary epoch, though it no longer does us a service, and it can on the other hand do us a lethal disservice.

Hemorrhoids

Also known popularly as piles, hemorrhoids, are another common "disease of civilization". These are a varicose condition of the veins at the lower end of the rectum, sometimes external, sometimes internal. They have no single cause, but are often associated with obesity, constipation (and its treatment by purging), and disorders of the digestion.

Gallstones

Cholecystitis, inflammation of the gallbladder, can be accompanied by cholecystolithiasis, or gallstones in the bladder.

Gallstones have long baffled specialists, because neither their number nor their size bears any known relationship to the pain, which can be considerable. The gallbladder may be full of stones, without the patient suffering; and the stones may come and go, for no discernible reason. They can be cleared out easily and with minimal risk by surgery, and may have to be if they cause an obstruction, but this will not prevent a new crop emerging. "Neither medical nor surgical treatment", the Lancet has recently admitted, "offers a permanent remedy for the underlying metabolic abnormality of which gallstones may be only one consequence".

What, then, is the cause of the underlying metabolic abnormality? Surveying the evidence from all over the world, K.W. Heaton, a senior lecturer at the University of Bristol, has come to the conclusion that the answer is civilization, "especially the modern western variety. No civilization, no gallstones; and the more urbanised and technologically advanced a country becomes the more gallstones it gets". But this, he explains, does not mean it is a disease of affluence. If anything, the poor are more at risk. The likely culprit, he feels, is refined carbohydrates, "by which I mean chiefly white flour and all the products of the sugar beet and cane (refined in this sense means separated from fibre; brown sugar is as refined as white)".

Jaundice

The most familiar symptoms of jaundice are a yellowing of the skin and the whites of the eyes, indicating an excess of bile in the blood. These can be a consequence of a variety of disorders, ranging from the blocking of the normal bile outlets to atrophy of the liver. But because the type of jaundice most commonly encountered was found to be accompanied by a particular virus, it was described as infectious – in medical terminology "infectious hepatitis". Inevitably, though, a second virus was later identified, and the disease was then divided into two categories, either hepatitis A or hepatitis B. Recently virologists have come across yet another variety, which has led them to suspect that there may be still more viruses lurking in the background.

Stress and other risk factors

The weakness of conventional medical treatment in the prevention and treatment of disorders of the digestion can also be traced to a serious omission from the list of risk factors related to the onset of symptoms. The orthodox assumption has been that ulceration and inflammation are "organic", physicochemical in origin, and that consequently they need to be treated by drugs and diet, with surgery as the back-up. But everybody has experienced the way in which "nerves" can affect the process of digestion. The problem with modern life, A.T.W. Simeons has explained in his book *Man's Presumptuous Brain*, is that people have become creatures of habit. They ordinarily have meals at fixed times, and eat what is put in front of them, whether or not they are hungry. But if they are not feeling hungry, the reason may be that they are worried or angry about something. Either can disrupt the digestive process, which is obeying an old instinct, and trying to close down.

Proponents of psychosomatic medicine have argued for many years that the pain of appendicitis is likely to be nervous in origin. Monitoring over a hundred cases of appendix operations, Dr Creed, a psychiatrist at the London Hospital found that nearly half of them had been unnecessary. Before they were operated upon, however, before it was known whether there was anything the matter with their appendixes, he had interviewed all the patients to find out whether they had suffered stressful experiences shortly before the onset of the supposed appendicitis. Comparing the answers, he found that in the group whose appendixes were *not* diseased, twice as many patients had just had some "severe life crisis".

Examinations, trouble with the police, a court appearance, serious rows at work or at home, an enforced change of job – these were "the principal life crises" which Dr Creed found among those who developed "apparent" appendicitis.

Does this mean that anybody who has a pain in the region of the appendix should run to a psychiatrist? Of course it does not. If the appendicitis *is* real, it could be extremely dangerous to delay surgery, and even if it is only "apparent", the operation is so simple that it can be regarded as a sensible form of insurance. Anybody whose appendicitis turns out to be only "apparent" could well consider trying some form of psychological therapy – particularly as in some cases the pains continue after the healthy appendix has been removed.

Orthodox treatment

The disorders which require medical attention are ordinarily first treated with drugs and diets, and where these fail, they are treated with surgery.

Drugs

Where drugs have been most effective is in dealing with infections. It is now coming to be recognized, however, that although they may relieve some of the symptoms of inflammation and ulceration, they are not cures. Even the drugs used to counteract bacterial infections have shown some limitations. It has come to be realized that the bacteria responsible for cases of food poisoning, for example, are not necessarily invaders taken into the stomach in contaminated food. Often they are present in the body all the time, but for some reason the body's self-regulating system goes awry, allowing them to go on the rampage. In such cases, it is the system that needs to have an overhaul.

Even that old standby, bicarbonate of soda (and other similar antacids) no longer holds the position it once did, though it is still widely used. A report in 1975 in the *American Journal of Digestive Diseases* described how ulcer-threatened patients in any army medical centre had been divided into two groups, one treated with antacids and the other with a placebo. No difference was found in the recovery rate of the two groups.

Surgery

This may become advisable, and indeed essential in emergencies – when the stomach wall is perforated or the appendix "bursts" – but it does nothing to remove the cause of ulceration. An article on "Hemorrhoidectomy" in a recent issue of *World Medicine* has told more about the deficiencies of conventional treatment than you would be likely to learn from a textbook on the subject. It used to be one of the commonest operations, and, as the writer, Harold Ellis, Professor of Surgery at Westminster Medical School, put it, it is: "boring and bloody for the surgeon, tedious to the residents, a nuisance to the nurses" and, above all, "greatly feared by the patients", as it is extremely painful.

After performing it for years as a matter of course, Ellis was suddenly confronted with the realization that a simple injection, with a substance that was virtually a placebo, could be surprisingly effective. Since then not only has he almost given up the operation, but he has also been casting a cool eye on the alternatives that have been introduced – all of which, to him, have serious disadvantages. The vast majority of cases of hemorrhoids, he has found, can be treated "by simple injection therapy in the outpatient clinic".

Diets

Their application to ulcers, according to Mark Bricklin, in his *Encyclopedia of Natural Healing*, "could profitably be studied as a case history in medical blundering" – a verdict which few gastroenterologists would now dispute.

For many years the stock diet for the treatment of ulcers was "slops" – bread and milk, and the like. All this did was to make digestion less painful, it did nothing to heal ulcers, and often the pain returned as soon as the patient went back on solid food. "Roughage" on the other hand, was frowned on. Not until the late 1970s did the advocates of fibre begin to get a hearing for their case that fibre is an essential ingredient in the diet, without which digestion cannot function properly and ulcers are unlikely to heal.

Even the injunction to avoid spicy food, for so long almost automatic in ulcer cases, has now been demolished. Spicy foods have "not been shown to affect the gastric mucosa in any way, and people who eat highly-seasoned food do not suffer an increase in gastric ulcers", the US army medical centre investigators found. "We feel it is sufficient to advise patients with gastric ulcers to avoid only those foods that tend to give them "heartburn" or pain.

Alternative treatment

Among the practitioners of natural medicine there is universal agreement on one point: that orthodox medical treatment has been sadly misguided. As Harry Benjamin put it nearly half a century ago in his *Everybody's Guide to Nature Cure*, in a discussion on the treatment of stomach ulcers "the fundamental cause of the trouble – the wrong feeding habits of the individual – are left entirely unaffected". Surgery can make a weakened stomach even weaker: and "merely to cut out the ulcer and leave it at that can hadly be called *curative* treatment, can it?" Benjamin added. Dosing with antacids, though it may give temporary relief, prevents the proper digestion of food: "What we have to do is to *get rid* of the underlying acidity altogether, not neutralize its effects by introducing alkaline chemicals into the stomach".

Natural therapists insist that where there is a risk that surgery may be needed, as in appendicitis, a doctor must always be consulted. They concede that for some infections, modern drugs can be effective – unless resistant strains of bacteria have emerged. In most cases, they believe that natural therapies are more effective than drugs.

Nature cure

Naturopaths understandably feel that they have earned the right to be regarded as the experts in the diagnosis and treatment of all forms of gastrointestinal disorder, except those which are attributable to poisoning, or which have gone too far to be controlled except by surgery. They do not concern themselves so much as doctors do with identifying, say, the particular organ which is giving trouble. They believe that their advice, if followed, will set the digestive system to rights, the organ will recover, and the symptoms, wherever they are, will vanish.

Naturopaths tend to put the blame for hemorrhoids partly on constipation, and partly on the way it is treated with purges. They disapprove of operations or of injections because, as Harry Benjamin put it, "in either case the underlying cause of the condition is not in the least affected by such treatment, so that further trouble of the same kind may be expected to occur again at any time, whilst habitual constipation becomes more stubborn". The only effective treatment, Benjamin argued, is to get rid of the constipation by the standard nature cure method; a cleansing of the intestines by abstinence followed by conversion to a balanced, healthy diet. As a palliative he offered "a cold sitz-bath every morning", a remedy which some of us might find almost as unwelcome as the symptoms, though it is designed to make more bearable.

The remedy for gallstones recommended by Dr Heaton of Bristol University, a low calorie diet with especial emphasis upon a restricted intake of refined carbohydrate, is what nature cure practitioners have been recommending for over half a century. They commonly advocate a protracted nearfast to start with, longer than the one they normally prescribe, with only a few drops of fruit juice in hot water, along with frequent enemas and hot compresses to ease the pain while it lasts. The stones, they claim, gradually dissolve – a belief which used to be disputed by orthodoxy, but which has been supported by some X-ray findings.

It has to be added that some naturopaths have their own individual methods of dealing with gallstones small enough to be discharged in the excreta. One such, for example, involves a fortnight's preparation on a balanced diet, followed by three days on fruit juice, before beginning the specific treatment which consists of half a pint of olive oil, followed by half a pint of lemon juice once a day, with only water to drink the rest of the time. The outcome, where it works, is the evacuation of the stones. It is almost as if the oil, by lubricating them, facilitates their departure.

Rest in bed, a fat-free light diet and avoidance of alcohol happen to be what virtually all natural therapists have long recommended for the treatment of jaundice. It is recognized that the epidemic variety cannot always be avoided, but the belief is that a combination of external cleanliness and a balanced diet will cut down the number of people who catch it, and make the symptoms of those who do less acute.

Herbal medicine

Herbalists have an almost embarrassingly wide range of remedies for stomach trouble. In their *Guide to Medicinal Plants*, Paul Schauenberg and Ferdinand Paris list about 50, 20 of them for stomach ulcers including some that are readily available: garlic, chickweed, marigold, sage and the common nettle. Most of these are temporary expedients, to be taken to soothe the occasional upset, but some can be used as preventives.

Of the recommended herbal remedies, one has the distinction of actually being named after the disorder it is used to treat: the lesser celandine, or pilewort. "Behold here another verification of the warning of the ancients", Culpeper wrote in his herbal, "that the virtue of an herb may be known by its 'signature', as plainly appears in this; for if you dig up the root of it, you shall perceive the perfect image of the disease which they commonly

call the piles". According to Hilda Leyel, the root is made into an ointment with hog's lard. Alternatively, an infusion can be made by adding a teaspoonful of herb to a teacupful of boiling water, and infusing it for 15 minutes; the mixture is taken three times a day.

Systems of medicine

Homeopaths (see pages 66 to 73) also have a sizeable range of remedies for gastrointestinal disorders, but, as always, they stress the need to treat the patient, not the symptoms, and this requires a preliminary consultation to select the appropriate treatment for you, rather than for your symptoms. Once a particular homeopathic remedy has been decided upon, however, you may return to it in cases where it has been effective.

Manipulative therapies

Osteopaths and *chiropractors* (see pages 80 to 94) believe that gastrointestinal disorders are often related to a spinal defect, because either the blood supply or the nervous system may be affected, or both. Their services are not often called upon in this connection, however, except when patients who have gone to them with backache are surprised and delighted to find that manipulation sets their digestion to rights, too. All postural and manipulative therapists, whatever their beliefs, take for granted that their methods can benefit impaired digestion processes by toning up the system.

Oriental therapies

All forms of gastrointestinal disorders can be treated by *Acupuncturists* (see pages 120 to 133). There is a "stomach meridian" and a "large intestine meridian", each with its acupuncture points into which needles will be inserted according to the therapist's interpretation of the source of the disorder, as revealed from pulse diagnosis and other indicators.

Psychological therapies

All the various groups offering psychological therapies agree that whatever physical mood may be used to relieve or remove stomach disorders, an essential prerequisite of prevention is to realise that the process of digestion is dependent upon a tranquil mind – something which in our workaday world we all too rarely take into consideration. "Grace" before meals, in the form of a few minutes meditation, some of them argue, is essential.

That hemorrhoids can be a stress disorder may sound surprising, but a reason for thinking of them in these terms was given in the form of a case history in one of the early surveys of psychosomatic medicine, Alfred J. Cantor's Handbook, published in New York in 1951. A 67-year-old Polish nobleman who "had an excellent insight into his condition" presented himself for treatment. Hemorrhoids, he explained, ran in his family; but "the bleeding occurred only during emotional crises, and he indicated that he had no symptoms whatsoever at any other time". The reason, he had realized, was that during an emotional crisis he became constipated, and it was only then that the hemorrhoids emerged, and bled. In other words, if *Psychotherapy* (see pages 162 to 165) or *Autosuggestion* (see pages 173 to 175) can be employed successfully to deal with the emotional stresses which have given rise to a disordered digestion, hemorrhoids may cease to be a problem.

Research has even shown that it is possible for individuals to use *Biofeedback* (see pages 188 to 193) to learn to control bowel movement. In his *Mind as Healer, Mind as Slayer*, Kenneth Pelletier has described a method in which a stethoscope is used, attached to the stomach, the sound being amplified so that the patient can learn how to distinguish between fluctuations: "once an individual is made aware of the activity in his intestinal tract, he can then learn how to maximise it or minimise it in order to allow that part of his body to function more freely". By noting an increase in this audible signal, a patient can learn to overcome chronic constipation, alternatively he or she can decrease this activity in order to self-regulate diarrhea.

Self-help

The most valuable form of preventive medicine which can be practised in the home and at work is to pay more attention to appetite. Your appetite is largely responsible for making the digestion work smoothly, from salivation to evacuation.

Admittedly there are difficulties. Appetite can be psychologically disordered: there are people who cannot stop eating, just as there are people who through neurosis cannot bear to eat. Appetite can be artificially stimulated, as with cocktails. Appetite can also be conditioned to take certain courses which are unhealthy, like a craving for sweets. If appetite is to be allowed to dictate when to eat and how much to eat, it must be natural, and the food (and drink) must be of a kind that is both digestible and nutritionally balanced.

Given sound eating habits, there will be no need to fear ulceration or inflammation – or, for that matter, constipation. Conventional medicine and natural therapies are in agreement that contipation in all but a tiny fraction of cases does no harm to anybody, whereas purges do. It is possible to go for a week, or even a month, without evacuating the bowels, and the only reason for worry will be worry itself – because most of us have been conditioned from childhood to assume that the bowels must move daily, which simply is not true.

Diarrhea (and nausea for that matter), can often be a sign that the system is working efficiently by getting rid of toxic matter. Of course, it can also be a nuisance, as it commonly is on visits abroad. Here, the explanation appears to be

that the body's protective system encounters strange bacteria and decides to take no risks, though often they are harmless. In any case, it is wise to avoid the drugs marketed to control travel diarrhea, if that is possible – their track record in terms of adverse reactions is not good.

Another golden rule is to throw out all medicines of a kind which are used to treat chronic, or recurring, disorders such as constipation or dyspepsia. An exception may have to be made for bicarbonate of soda, for people whose lifestyle renders them susceptible to occasional over-indulgence in food and drink, with the inexorable consequences of heartburn or hangover. But the dose should be considered as a temporary expedient to deal with a self-inflicted injury. To take purges or indigestion tablets regularly, or even irregularly but frequently, should be recognized as self-destructive. Doing the digestion's work for it, in this way, eventually leads to the digestion being unable to do its work.

UROGENITAL DISORDERS

In Britain, only medically qualified practitioners are permitted by law to treat venereal diseases – syphilis and gonorrhea. But there is a range of symptoms which are described as urogenital (or genito-urinary) in textbooks which do not fall into this category – though there has been controversy during the past years over whether some of them ought to be regarded as venereal, and they are commonly referred to as sexually transmitted diseases (STD).

Urethritis and NSU
In men, the most common symptom is urethritis, usually beginning with a slight "nip" feeling during urination at the tip of the penis, sometimes accompanied by cloudy urine which may cause discomfort. In the majority of cases where tests are made, no organism is found which

can be held responsible, and the urethritis is termed non-specific (NSU). Sometimes specific bacteria are found, but it remains doubtful whether they are the cause.

Thrush and "trich"
Women can harbour these bacteria following intercourse with a man who has urethritis, but they rarely cause symptoms. Women can also have a non-specific infection which is labelled vaginitis, but more commonly they harbour identifiable microorganisms which are held to be the cause of their symptoms: the fungus *candida albicans* associated with vaginal thrush, which produces a white discharge, itching and discomfort during urination; and trichomonas ("trich") gives rise to similar symptoms, though the discharge is heavier, with a bilious colour, and malodorous.

Just as women rarely present symptoms even if they are infected with the microorganisms associated with urethritis, so men may harbour the microorganisms from the vaginal discharge of their sexual partners without suffering from them. It used to be assumed that they could reinfect their partners as a result (a frequent occurrence with gonorrhea), but recent research has cast doubt on this assumption, as it appears to make no difference whether a male partner is, or is not, given treatment for trichomonas at the same time as the female.

The most plausible explanation is that "trich" and thrush are not (or not necessarily) sexually-transmitted: they are internal infections which come and go, like herpes. Some venereologists have even been arguing that the fungus and the parasite are not the cause of the infections but a symptom of it. Certainly they are both frequently found in the vaginas of women who are experiencing none of the familiar symptoms; itch and discharge.

Cystitis
Technically a bladder infection, the term cystitis is commonly applied to symptoms of which the most notorious are a nagging need to urinate

and a burning sensation while urinating. The common assumption has been that it is caused by pathogens passing up through the vagina; but even this has been disputed, and the hard fact remains that very little is known about the causes.

Prostate

As orthodox doctors freely admit, very little is known about the prostate – a group of glands which surrounds the male urinary tract at the point it leaves the bladder. If the prostate becomes enlarged, as it tends to do with advancing age, urination can become more difficult. This in itself is usually no more than a minor inconvenience; but some men find that it is accompanied by an increased desire to urinate, as if the body was in some way trying to compensate for its disability, in spite of the fact that there is no real need, as the amounts of urine on each occasion are small.

Unless the condition becomes serious, with the prostate so enlarged that it is difficult to urinate at all, doctors commonly tell patients that prostate trouble is self-limiting; it may last only for a few days.

Orthodox treatment

Scores of drugs have been marketed to treat urogenital infections, and from time to time there are boasts that they are effective. Some drugs are effective for some people, but they can have unwelcome side-effects, and no satisfactory preventive has yet been found.

Alternative treatment

There has been some reluctance on the part of natural therapists to offer treatment for urogenital disorders; in Britain this may be because of uncertainty about whether they would be within the law. But there is general agreement among them that the cause lies deeper than an invasion by pathogens. If the homeostatic system has failed to clear up an infection, the assumption is, you should look for possible psychosocial reasons.

Significantly, a few decades ago family doctors used to refer to "honeymoonitis", a non-specific infection, producing itching and discharge which often occurred in the weeks immediately following the marriage. As in those days the bride was often a virgin, and the groom of "good" character, it became hard to believe that honeymoonitis was a venereal disease in the usual sense of the term. And in those times doctors were still willing to accept the possibility that a traumatic emotional experience, as the first sexual encounter could often be – particularly for the wife, who frequently was totally ignorant of what could be involved – might be responsible.

Nature cure

Inevitably, *Naturopaths* (see pages 18 to 21) tend to look for dietary deficiency (or imbalance), but most therapists now accept that there may also be a stress component.

Naturopaths attribute prostate trouble to faulty living habits, and prescribe a regime that may include a special diet, abdominal exercises, hot and cold sitz baths.

Herbal medicine & Homeopathy

Herbalists (see pages 45 to 57) offer a variety of remedies, among others, parsley, ladies' mantle, horse chestnut, golden rod, couch grass, rosemary and nettles. *Homeopaths* (see pages 66 to 73), too, have a variety of remedies, their selection being made with reference to the patient rather than of the patient's prostate.

MENSTRUAL DISORDERS

In women of child-bearing age, the menstrual flow takes place fairly regularly every four weeks, lasts four or five days, and causes little more than inconvenience. But a variety of disorders are associated with menstruation, and although they are widespread, no convincing explanation has been found for them.

The conventional process by which these disorders are split up for purposes of identification has led to their division by doctors into amenorrhea (absence of periods); dysmenorrhea (irregular, difficult or painful periods); menorrhagia (excessive menstrual flow); and metrorrhagia (bleeding outside the menstrual period). It is doubtful, however, whether this division into categories provides much of a therapeutic benefit, except in the few cases where some specific defect, such as womb displacement, is responsible. Nor can they readily be separated out from what has recently come to be known as the premenstrual syndrome.

The premenstrual syndrome

Pain, swellings, headaches, backache, skin rashes, irritability, lethargy, depression, loss of appetite, sexual disinterest, tension, accident proneness – this galaxy of symptoms is now known collectively as the premenstrual syndrome. It became front-page news in Britain in 1981, when a woman who could have expected a heavy sentence for a crime received a light one following a plea by her lawyer that she was suffering from premenstrual tension at the time.

Orthodox treatment

The common assumption of the medical profession when concerned with menstrual disorders has been that there is often a close relationship between changes in hormone levels and the appearance and disappearance of the symptoms of PMT, the main cause of the symptoms must be hormonal inbalance. It has seemed to follow, therefore, that the aim should be to employ hormone remedies to put the balance back to rights. Hormone treatment can work, but often it doesn't, and there are also the usual problems of side-effects. Knowing this, many GPs prefer to prescribe diuretics and tranquillizers to their patients but these, too, are disapproved of by a great many specialists.

Alternative treatment

The only item of orthodox treatment which most natural therapists accept for menstrual disorders is vitamin B6. For some PMT sufferers, it works well – presumably because vitamin deficiency is at the root of their symptoms.

Herbal medicine

Innumerable herbal remedies have been advocated for menstrual disorders. In his book *Health Secrets of Plants and Herbs*, Maurice Mésségué even separates out the 19 which he recommends for amenorrhea, from the 14 for dysmenorrhea and the 16 for metrorrhagia; nettle and sage are the only plants which are common to all lists.

Systems of medicine

Homeopaths (see pages 66 to 73) use a different classification. Ruddock's *Homeopathic Vade Mecum* divides menstrual disorders into membraneous (varying), painful, irregular or infrequent, scanty, excessive, recurring too early or lasting too long, suppressed and vicarious. The emotional condition of the patient is given particular consideration; patients who are diffident or nervous receive different remedies from those who are outgoing.

Nature cure

Naturopaths argue that the commonest cause of PMT is "toxic accumulations which a desperate body is trying to get rid of by vicarious means", as naturopath Leon Chaitow has put it. "The cure lies in detoxification as well as in providing help to the organs which have borne the brunt of the battle to prevent the body from drowning in its own waste products". What is needed, then, is a better balanced diet, with periodic cleansings.

Psychological therapies

This aspect of menstrual disorders has recently been receiving more attention, because it has proved possible to treat them satisfactorily with placebos, with suggestion under hypnosis (see *Hypnotherapy*, pages 166 to 173) and with *Autosuggestion* (see pages 173 to 176). The theory is that although the hormonal inbalance is the precipitant of the symptoms, this imbalance is itself the result of emotional stress. The "tension" in premenstrual tension, in other words, is cause as well as an effect.

The likelihood that it is the tension which activates (or suppresses) the hormones, rather than vice-versa, has since been well-documented. In *New Mind, New Body*, Barbara Brown, one of the American pioneers of *Biofeedback* (see pages 188 to 193) describing research carried out into the relationship between heightened activity of the autonomic nervous system and menstruation, remarks that it has shown "the relative ease with which important body hormones are altered by emotion". In one such study, a large number of subjects were "chastised verbally" while their skin resistance response was being monitored. "Both before and after the experiment, two hormones, adrenaline and noradrenaline, the stress-anxiety related substances of the nervous system and ANS (autonomic nervous system) were measured, and were found to increase" – this increase being related directly to the change in the subjects' skin resistance.

Self-help

"Self-help is women sharing experiences, knowledge and feelings – women supporting each other and learning together", Angela Phillips and Jill Rakusen claim in their book *Our Bodies Ourselves*, which originated in the Boston's Women's Health Book Collective. "Self-help begins by working from a practical base, starting with learning from physical self-examination, finding out what we *do* know, what we do *not* know, what we *want* to know and exploring from there".

Phillips and Rakusen emphasized the need for women to learn how to make and exercise choice – which involves accepting Ivan Illich's premise, as set out in *Medical Nemesis*, that the need is now for a demystification of medicine. Their main emphasis, however, is on women getting together to insist upon a better performance by the medical profession and its auxiliaries rather than on the desirability of looking for alternatives. *Our Bodies Ourselves* could do with a supplement pointing to those areas where natural medicine has more to offer than orthodoxy. Still, it provides a useful starting point from which to explore the possibilities for self-help in the prevention and treatment of women's disorders.

CHILDBEARING AND MENOPAUSE

Nobody regards puberty as a disease, nor, in theory, can childbearing or menopause be described as disorders. But giving birth has become increasingly medicalized, with women being made to understand that they are antisocial if they prefer to have their babies at home; and the tendency has been to make women regard menopause as, potentially at least, a threat to health.

Childbearing

Until little more than a century ago, bearing a child could indeed have been regarded as a disorder, all too often a fatal one, as puerpural fever carried off great numbers of mothers. When in 1847, the Hungarian obstetrician Ignaz Semmelweiss warned that the fever was "caused by conveyance to the pregnant women of putrid particles derived from living organisms, through the agency of the examining fingers" – and introduced antisepsis – he was derided by his colleagues; but it turns out that he was right after all.

The trend over the past century has been to make childbirth as safe as possible not simply by insisting upon antisepsis, but by exploiting all the benefits of modern technology. Unluckily, the outcome has been to create a production-line mentality, in which the mothers (and, eventually, their babies) are treated as if they were automatons. "From the moment that an expectant mother passes through the doors of a hospital", Michael House of the West London Hospital has observed, "she ceases to be a healthy woman and becomes a patient".

Menopause
The onset of the time when a woman ceases to be able to bear children is signified by the termination of their menstrual periods, sometimes gradually over a period of years, sometimes abruptly. For some women, this is accompanied by the symptoms which have come to be known as menopausal, the most distinctive being 'hot flushes'. The others are usually variants of the syndrome of just being sick – headaches, palpitations, dizziness, diffuse pains, and malaise.

Orthodox treatment
Although practice varies considerably from hospital to hospital, many obstetricians have introduced practices based on "high-tech" childbirth. This technological approach can entail induction of labour with the help of drugs, fetal heart monitoring (which requires the mother-to-be to be wired up, so that she cannot move around); forceps delivery; caesarians; epidural anesthesia; and "episiotomy" – a cut made in the entrance to the vagina in order to facilitate the emergence of the baby.

Induced childbirth
Some idea of the extent to which these practices may be used has been provided by recent investigations. For example, according to a recent article in London's *Sunday Times*, the rate of induced births at St Mary's Hospital, Manchester, has been 25 percent of the total: "all women have fetal heart monitors attached unless there is a specific request not to; rupturing of the membranes is routine; caesarians

last year accounted for 18 percent of births; the epidural rate is 40 percent".

Recently, however, there has been a reaction. It began with the realization that in some maternity units, induction was being carried out for the convenience of the staff – to avoid births at weekends or in the small hours of the morning, and although obstetricians argued that this was also for the convenience of the mother (and the father, too) they did not sound convincing.

The statistical evidence, too, began to suggest that the vaunted greater safety to hospitals over homes for childbirth was marginal, and had its risks – the widespread practice of early separation of mother and baby into different wards, for example, could have adverse long-term effects. In 1976, researchers in Cleveland published a report showing that close sensory contact between mother and baby in the period immediately after the birth was highly desirable for "bonding" (the important psychological link between mother and newborn baby) of the two.

Positions for delivery
Another bone of contention is the issue of whether a mother in hospital should have the right to decide, as she has at home, in what position she would like to deliver the baby. Obstetricians who employed fetal monitoring were necessarily compelled to insist that the mother lay in bed in what is colloquially known as the "stranded-beetle position". But many leading obstetricians, notably Professor Caldeyro-Barcia of the World Health Organization disapprove of the practice. "Making a mother lie on her back", he argues, "reduces the maternal blood-flow to the placenta, which is the route whereby oxygen is supplied to the fetus".

Recently women's organizations have begun to protest at what they complain is the high-handed manner in which doctors and hospital hierarchies dictate to mothers-to-be in this way. There is an increasingly widespread feeling that

mothers should be given the right to make their own decisions over childbirth in maternity hospitals and units everywhere.

Drugs in the treatment of menopause
Most doctors realize that the menopause is not a disease, and that the symptoms associated with it are commonly related to an emotional reaction to the "change of life". But some prescribe hormone-replacement pills; some dish out tranquillizers or anti-depressants, and some refer patients to surgeons who perform hysterectomies.

The case for hysterectomies
There is little evidence that hysterectomies bring any benefit, on balance, but in the United States they have become one of orthodox medicine's leading rackets. Surgeons justify them with the same argument that they use to justify operations to remove an appendix even when they are sure that it is not the cause of a patient's symptoms: that a woman after menopause has no further use for her womb, and might as well have the grapes and sympathy of friends which accompany a hospital stay.

Alternative treatment
During the 1970s, a resistance movement was developing in favour of what came to be known as natural childbirth. In the influential book, *Birth without violence*, which was first published in 1977, the French obstetrician Frederick Leboyer urged a reassessment of child-birthing techniques: mothers and babies, he insisted, must both be treated as people with feelings. Two years later, British author and specialist on childbirth, Sheila Kitzinger called for the "demedicalization" of birth, including the en—couragement of women who want to have their babies at home to get their wish. "Many hospitals", she wrote in her book *Birth at home*, "are not good enough to provide an environment suited for a peak experience of one's life, not for the birth of a family. But more than this,

they are sometimes frankly dangerous places in which to have a baby''.

Natural childbirth

The term ''natural childbirth'' does not refer to any particular method, but to the general principle that mothers should be given the chance to decide for themselves how and where they would like their babies to be born. Legally, they have this right, but in practice, many have been overawed by obstetricians into accepting that they must do what doctors and nurses tell them to do. Certainly, there is a great deal of pressure on expectant mothers not to have their first child at home.

The maternity unit of an ordinary local hospital at Pithiviers, not far from Paris, is today the pioneering centre of natural childbirth in Europe. The unit is run by Dr Michel Odent, who believes that each women knows how it is best for her to give birth and that she should be allowed to do it without any unnecessary interference from the medical staff in the hospital.

Of over 1,000 mothers who had been through his unit early in 1982, only two had opted to have their babies lying down. Most of them had their babies in the ''supported squatting position'', with Dr Odent or one of his midwives supporting them under the armpits (or with a midwife holding the woman on one side, the father-to-be on the other). Some women chose to relax in a warm pool until the delivery (certain women even chose to have their babies delivered in the water).

Anesthetics are not used at all at Pithiviers, and mothers are encouraged to scream, if they feel like it, the idea being that they learn to deal naturally with their own pain and often find this a welcome release. If there is an emergency, all the facilities of a modern hospital can be activated in minutes.

Odent achieves better results than most with a minimum of interference; his unit has fewer stillbirths, fewer deaths and fewer caesarians than in hospitals in Britain and the United States. And because the hormone balances of the mothers have not been affected by drugs, post-natal depression at the Odent's unit is almost unknown.

Relaxation techniques

Of the therapies that are being used in conjunction with pregnancy, relaxation techniques are the most extensively employed. There are specific *Yoga* techniques (see pages 178 to 181) designed to prepare the pelvic region for labour and to prevent or ease low back pain and hypertension. *Massage* can also be used to reduce tension and promote relaxation (see pages 95 to 99). In their book *New Life*, Janet and Arthur Balaskas have provided a succession of simple breathing exercises to help dilate the cervix, before the birth (for which the mother can chose one of the squatting positions or whatever she feels will be right for her). There are also post-natal yoga exercises to get the body back in trim.

In cases of menopause, most practitioners of natural medicine assume that the direct need is to give aid and comfort through what may be a difficult few months, whether by promoting relaxation through massage or by counselling, and if necessary psychotherapy.

Psychotherapies

Hypnosis (see *Hypnotherapy*, see pages 166 to 173), is now coming into common use to reduce, and in some cases remove altogether, labour pains. Moreover, recent research has shown that it may be possible to use hypnotherapy to shorten the duration of labour.

Herbal medicine & Homeopathy

All natural therapists urge the cessation of smoking, drinking and any form of drug-taking (including drugs designed to suppress morning sickness) during pregnancy, along with a reduction in the consumption of tea and coffee. Homeopathic and herbal preparations and tissue salts are available for pre- and post-natal conditions.

There are traditional herbal remedies for menopausal symptoms, usually the same as they would be if the symptoms arose from other causes. Homeopathic remedies, on the other hand, are prescribed in relation to the individual, rather than the symptoms.

Oriental therapies

Analgesia using acupuncture is being increasingly often employed to enable women to have a pain-free birth while fully conscious.

Self-help

The chief need – as many doctors would agree – is for recognition that menopause need not in itself make any difference to your life, other than removing the inconvenience of menstruation, as this realization often in itself effectively banishes menopausal symptoms.

IMPOTENCE AND INFERTILITY

The inability on the part of a man to have sexual intercourse with his partner, or of the partner to conceive (if she wishes to) can both be accounted for by constitutional defect, but this is rare. By far the commonest causes of impotence and infertility are emotional problems, and these are frequently at a subconscious level.

Impotence

In the common sense of inability to obtain an erection, impotence is basically the consequence of a loss of sexual appetite, whether temporary or permanent. Such a loss can be traced to a great variety of possible causes, ranging from simple boredom with the sexual partner to deep-seated, repressed emotional conflicts. It can arise out of organic defect, or as a by-product of disease, but this is rare. Unhappily, among the increasingly common causes of impotence are the side-effects of powerful drugs.

Infertility

Inability to bear children has been the source of much worry, as scores of accounts from the Old Testament on up to our own times have shown. The impression now growing is that the worry itself is often the reason for the infertility, or at least a contributary factor.

Orthodox treatment

Few general practitioners are suited by temperament or training to deal with impotence, and the tendency until very recently has been to prescribe drugs – either those marketed specifically to stimulate the sex glands or those which reduce anxiety or tension. But these are now widely recognized as unsatisfactory.

Fertility drugs and hormone injections

In some cases, where women attend clinics to find if anything is the matter with them, a structural fault may be found and where possible put right. In others, hormone injections may be prescribed or one of the "fertility drugs" which have received considerable publicity in the last few years. But the injections can have unwanted side-effects, and the fertility drugs are apt to lead to triplets (or more).

Fertilization outside the womb

The technique of removing an ovum, artificially fertilizing it and putting it back in the womb has been developed for cases where there is a block between ovary and uterus, but it is too early yet to assess its long-term value.

Alternative treatment

The basic assumption of practitioners of holistic medicine is that an impotence is almost always a psychological or psychic disorder, the cause must be looked for in the individual's personality and problems. But it has also often been found that any form of treatment designed to restore good health in general, whether through diet, manipulation or acupuncture, can exert a beneficial side-effect by restoring appetite and potency.

Loss of sexual appetite

Except where impotence can be traced to some genetic or constitutional defect, natural therapists assume that it is the consequence of a loss of sexual appetite. Like the loss of appetite for food, this may arise for various reasons, social, emotional or psychic, and the appropriate remedy cannot be found unless and until these are uncovered. But some temporary expedients are available for use as aids in the short term, most of them of the old wives' tale kind.

Subconscious factors affecting conception

Where conventional methods fail to treat infertility, the first need is to consider the possibility of subconscious factors operating to prevent conception. Many women still find this difficult to accept; yet it is well known that there is a parallel, showing the astonishing power of the mind over the body. This is "pseudocyesis", false pregnancy.

If intense desire to conceive – the most plausible explanation – can produce a false pregnancy, it is not difficult to surmise that a fear of conception, or a desire not to conceive, perhaps unconscious, can prevent conception, or cause miscarriage. "It should not be surprising that the bodily machinery of conception and pregnancy is especially sensitive to emotional conflicts", Flanders Dunbar observed in her book, *Mind and Body*. "In the families in which most of us were brought up, the genital organs were the subject of more taboos, warnings, fears and discipline than all the rest of the body put together". Many women, Dr Dunbar commented, are subconsciously ashamed of the whole sexual process, and its outcome, and they were the ones who were most likely, she found, to suffer from morning sickness or miscarriage. Again, the only way out is a better understanding of the subconscious urges and inhibitions responsible.

Herbal medicine

Literally hundreds of different kinds of food and drink have been recommended, in different places and in different eras, for their aphrodisiac potential – ranging from fungi to oysters. A few, such as "Spanish Fly" or cantharides (a drug made from dried beetles, ground up) have won a considerable reputation, but are extremely dangerous to employ. The vast majority seem to owe their success to autosuggestion, or placebo effect. Maurice Mességué, the French herbalist, recommends, among other herbal remedies, garlic, basil, hogweed, celandine, mint, rosemary, sage and even cabbage, but other herbalists produce very different lists. The only sensible policy is to take whatever herb works for you – provided, of course, it works also for your partner (see *Herbal medicine*, pages 45 to 65).

Impotence can also be temporarily dealt with by taking a drug which removes inhibitions, as alcohol does – in moderate quantities: in excess, "Lechery, Sir, it provokes and unprovokes", as Macbeth's porter put it in Shakespeare's play. "It provokes the desire, but it takes away the performance". Cannabis can have a similar, but often even more powerful aphrodisiac effect.

Psychological therapies

All these therapies take for granted that impotence and other sexual hang-ups are treatable either by providing individuals with insight into the unconscious processes responsible, or, as in the case of, say, *Encounter groups* (see pages 201 to 203), liberating repressed emotions through the kind of release which can be obtained through a controlled, therapeutic version of mass hysteria.

Self-help

The most important role self-help can play usually lies in recognizing that impotence is neither a physical deficiency nor a reflection of incompetence as a lover, but an indication that something has gone awry with a relationship. If this can be discussed candidly with the partner, this in itself may promote the recovery.

MENTAL ILLNESS

That conventional forms of treatment for mental illness have proved disappointing, to put it mildly, is now accepted, even by psychiatrists, throughout the West. Psychiatry's reputation is now unenviable, and rightly so.

"The average standard of psychiatric practice in Britain is abysmally low", the Royal College of Psychiatry admitted in a memorandum to the Department of Health in 1974. Since then a succession of ugly scandals have been reported from mental hospitals and, as Virginia Bradshaw has shown in her *Conscientious Objectors at Work*, others have been hushed up, thanks to collusion between the hospital authorities and the trade unions, protecting their members who work in them.

In the United States, though psychiatry has improved since the notorious "snake pit" era of the 1950s, the situation is no more encouraging. The public's image of it was reflected in the book and the film *One Flew Over the Cuckoo's Nest*, and within the profession, the efforts of psychiatrists to prove that they are "scientific" have become a standing joke. This is particularly true in connection with diagnosis of mental illness.

No longer are there thousands of long-stay (usually a lifetime stay) patients locked up in wards in jail-like asylums built in the last century. But the expectation that the new drugs would enable patients to lead normal lives has turned out to be an illusion. Far fewer patients stay in hospital for the duration of their lives, but patients continue to arrive, be treated, leave for a while

and then, having found life impossible in the outside world, they will return.

Compartmentalizing mental disorders

A century ago, when psychiatrists began to bring their discipline into line with the rest of medicine, efforts were made to divide up mental disorders into diagnostic compartments: schizophrenics were differentiated from manic depressives, psychotics from neurotics. ("A neurotic builds castles in the air, a psychotic lives in them", medical students were jocularly told.) To the embarrassment of leading psychiatrists, however, when a few years ago these categories were tested – for example, by showing a film of a patient to a number of psychiatrists, and getting them to give their diagnoses – the results showed total confusion.

Even more embarrassing, and a source of much amusement to the rest of the medical profession, has been the result of a trial in the United States, in which a number of sane people arranged to present themselves at mental hospitals, saying only that they "heard voices". All were admitted, diagnosed as schizophrenic (except one, who was told he was a manic depressive) and kept in for periods ranging from a week to two months, in spite of the fact that they behaved normally. Invariably their fellow patients rumbled them, but not the psychiatrists or the nurses.

The question of sanity

Psychiatry differs from conventional medicine in that there is a strong element of doubt about the whole concept of mental illness *as* illness. In his book *The Myth of Mental Illness* the Professor of Psychiatry at the State University of New York, Thomas S. Szasz, has described how he became exasperated with "the vague, capricious and generally unsatisfactory character of the widely used concept of mental illness and its corollaries, diagnosis, prognosis and treatment", and came to the conclusion that one fundamental mistake

has been to think of mental and emotional disturbances in terms of illnesses, in the same mould as physical illness. This has inexorably kept psychiatrists as second class citizens in the profession, he argues, because mental and emotional disturbance simply do not fit the medical model.

The British psychiatrist R.D. Laing has gone further, arguing that insanity may represent not a breakdown, but a breakthrough – at least, potentially. It can reflect the unconscious mind's rebellion when consciousness can no longer deal with the problem which confronts it. If the problem can be understood and acted upon, he believes, the apparently chaotic pronoucements of the schizophrenic may be found to serve a valuable therapeutic purpose. Neither Thomas Szasz nor R.D. Laing, however, has had much appreciable influence on orthodox psychiatry.

Orthodox treatment

Psychoactive drugs – sedatives, tranquillizers and antidepressants – are now defended, primarily as providing a breakwater, giving patients some protection from the stormy emotional seas which have driven them to seek treatment. But they do not in themselves equip patients for their return to the turbulence from which they have sought shelter. Even in their breakwater role, drugs can now be seen to have grave disadvantages. The tranquillizers, marketed for years with the boast that they are not addictive, have been shown to be capable of "hooking" addiction-prone people, with destructive consequences. Some of the stronger psychoactive drugs which have been dispensed almost as a matter of course in mental hospitals have been found to cause "persistent tardive dyskinesia", with its endless ugly facial contortions, which (as the word "persistent" only gently intimates) can be a life-sentence.

Electroconvulsive therapy

Since the beginning of the century, various forms of treatment have been tried: insulin coma therapy, for example, and brain surgery in the form of lobotomy or leucotomy. Initially, successes were claimed, but in time, they have fallen into discredit. Only one has managed to retain any respect among psychiatrists – ECT (electroconvulsive therapy). But recent reports on the way it has been used in hospitals has shaken even some of its firmest advocates.

Electroconvulsive therapy is based on the principle that giving patients an artificial fit shakes up their brains, breaking up congealed thought and behaviour patterns. This is not as odd as it may sound, as in many tribal communities, the inducing of fits to cure the sick has been standard practice. However, it depends very much on careful selection of patients as well as, of course, careful handling of the actual electric shocks.

Psychiatry's record in this respect has been shocking. The most notorious case on record is of a hospital in Britain where the new ECT machine was employed for a couple of years before it was discovered that it had never in fact delivered any current. The patients there, however, could consider themselves lucky, compared to some who have been compulsorily given ECT as a punishment. Leonard Roy Frank's *History of Shock Treatment*, published in 1978, has given chapter-and-verse source references for some of the ways in which ECT has been misused and abused, and it constitutes an appalling indictment not just of psychiatry, but of the medical profession as a whole, for permitting such horrors.

Psychiatry and psychotherapy
For many GPs, psychiatry is not a therapy, but a last resort. They refer patients to a psychiatrist in desperation, for lack of an alternative. Having themselves received hardly any training in psychiatry and none in psychotherapy, they realize that there is actually little they themselves can do.

The divisions within psychiatry about psychotherapy are marked and quite public. Psychotherapists in the Freudian tradition have conducted a vigorous slanging match with the behaviourists for years. And until quite recently were feuding sourly among themselves.

Psychotherapy of any kind is not easy to come by on the National Health Service, and when it is obtainable, patients have no choice of therapist. He or she may turn out to be a dedicated Freudian, or a behaviourist, impatient of other forms of psychological medicine.

Alternative treatment
Because conventional psychiatry is in such an obviously chaotic condition, there is less resistance at the general practitioner level to the idea of patients seeking alternative therapies. "Alternative", however, is not necessarily different.

Psychological therapies
Many therapists who are not connected with the medical profession practise one or other of the forms of psychotherapy used by practitioners who *are* in the profession, using techniques derived from Freud, or Jung, or sometimes from the behaviourist school.

Psychotherapists of this type, however, are in a minority, as the trend over the past decade has been away from conventional psychotherapies of any kind to those which are described as *Humanistic* (see pages 198 to 219) and *Transpersonal* (see pages 220 to 222). Here, however, there are marked differences between Britain and the United States. In the United States the humanistic and transpersonal schools have been dominated by clinical psychologists, many of them doctors. In Britain, those clinical psychologists who work in a medical capacity are ordinarily assistants to the medical profession. If they wish to hold salaried posts, they cannot take patients except on referral from a doctor. Although this is beginning to break down, most practitioners of the humanistic, transpersonal and other psychological therapies in Britain have no formal qualification, and often only a sketchy training.

Understandably, this has led to uneasiness about the risk that people with, say, an incipient neurosis or psychosis, will try some therapy which has the effect of pushing them over the top. Or, as in the case of therapies which have become cults, of sucking them into the organization, in the way the Scientologists and the "Moonies" have been acused of doing, by brainwashing.

In 1971, Sir John Foster, who had been asked to conduct an inquiry into risks of this kind, reported that it was "totally easy for the unscrupulous therapist, who knows enough to create dependence in the first place, to exploit it for years on end to his own advantage in the form of a steady income, to say nothing of the opportunities for sexual gratification". He recommended that the practice of psychotherapy should be restricted to duly qualified persons. And later, a working party endorsed this view.

One of the participating bodies, however, the British Association for Behavioural Psychotherapy, disagreed on various grounds, with arguments which effectively disposed of the illusion that "qualification" would be meaningful. "There is no general agreement as yet on what constitutes a valid psychotherapeutic training, nor is there good evidence that patients benefit from treatment by most qualified psychotherapists, with a few exceptions", its dissenting report pointed out. Registration "is likely to do more harm than good by unnecessary restriction of access to those treatments which are useful, and by retarding innovation in a field which is changing rapidly".

Things might improve, the dissenters hope, and then, registration on the basis of some agreed training might become feasible. All the indications since then, however, have been that traditional psychotherapy is being eroded by humanistic and transpersonal psychology. How far this trend will continue, and whether there will be fusion or more fission as a result remains to be seen.

Nature cure

Although the obvious alternative to orthodox psychiatric treatment, in cases of mental illness, would appear to be a trial of one of the psychological therapies, this is not the only possible approach. It is coming to be accepted that some mental disorders are "somatopsychic", in that they are primarily the consequence of a particularly unbalanced diet.

Examining the diet of a 12-year-old schoolboy who was suffering from over-excitability, aggressiveness, lack of concentration and associated symptoms, Professor Jeffrey Bland, Director of the Bellevue-Redmond Medical Laboratory in Washington, found that it was "full of empty calories: sugared cereal, chocolate, milk, pies, soft drinks, cookies". The parents were advised to change his diet to cut out candy, doughnuts and ice cream, and substitute food rich in vitamins and minerals. Within three weeks the aggro had diminished, and his schoolwork had improved.

"Obviously not all human aggression is explained by diet", Professor Bland has commented in a recent issue of *Psychology Today*. It does appear, however, that some abnormal behaviour may depend on eating habits that upset delicate biochemical balances in the brain".

Other natural therapies

Homeopaths (see pages 63 to 73), *Acupuncturists* (see pages 120 to 133), and *Manipulative therapists* (see pages 77 to 118) all, from time to time, report satisfactory results with patients who have been suffering from the milder forms of neurosis, tension, anxiety, and depression.

TERMINAL ILLNESS

Until about half a century ago, it was taken for granted that people dying from terminal diseases should be looked after, even if there was nothing that could be done for them except relieve their pain and loneliness. There were hospices for the dying in every large town. Gradually, however, the notion began to spread, among the public as well as through the medical profession, that it was humiliating for people to be admitted to such institutions. This attitude became more widespread as the advance of medical science held out the hope that cures might be found for illnesses previously considered terminal.

Orthodox treatment

Gratified by the success of antibiotics and other drugs in preserving lives which previously would have been lost, doctors, have felt increasingly disturbed by cases they can *not* help. The development of specialization has also tended to make the specialists, in particular, more interested in those they can, or might, help, at the expense of those whom they can not help.

The hospice movement
There are, however, "winds of change sweeping through the country for terminal patients" claims Harvey Humann in his book *New Realities*. They are emerging through the hospice movement. Humann, a patient-care volunteer in Hospice Care of Mid-America, which is among the oldest organizations in the country, gives the main credit to three women who inspired the movement – Dr Elizabeth Kubler-Ross in the United States, Mother Teresa of Calcutta, and Dr Cecily Saunders, founder of St Chistopher's Hospice, in London.

Some hospices in Britain are funded by the state, but most have been established with the aid of charities and run with voluntary help. As Dr Derek Doyle, Medical Director of St Columba's Hospice in Edinburgh, has observed, although the lay public is enthusiastic, hospices are "still viewed with caution, and occasionally distrust, by many members of the medical profession". Even where their usefulness is recognized, "much of their research and teaching, often of a high standard, is commonly ignored". St Christopher's Hospice has a mildly religious aura about it, but of an unobstrusive Anglican-cum-ecumenical kind. It is run on the same lines as a hospital, but with the emphasis on informality. Patients can do what they want, within reason, – go for a walk, drink, even smoke in bed. The chief aim is to create a friendly, relaxed atmosphere, for patients and visitors.

Alternative treatment

Alternative medicine does not have any specific recipes for the way to deal with dying patients, but therapists in general accept the Elizabeth Kubler-Ross/Mother Teresa/Cecily Saunders model, which is indeed consumer-based.

Working in the psychiatric department of the University of Chicago, Dr Kubler-Ross came to the realization, as she described in her book *On Death and Dying*, that what terminal patients most needed was emotional help.

Kubler-Ross hopes to furnish more than consolation. She helps her patients to not just die in peace, but to make the most of whatever time they have to live – including dealing with "unfinished business". As far as possible they are kept free of pain, and fully in possession of their faculties. It can also mean helping them to release bottled-up tensions. She advocates the installation of a sound-proofed "screaming room" where they – or friends, or relatives – can externalize their anger at what they feel has been the unfairness of the death sentence. "To help somebody to die with dignity and serenity does not mean to help them die in a state of acceptance", she argues. "It means to love them unconditionally and to help them die in character".

Resources

The following list of organisations is by no means comprehensive, it is a list of the main centres where you can find out about any of the therapies you are interested in. We have kept everything in the same order as the book to make it easier for you to follow. Many of the organisations are registered charities so it is advisable to enclose a stamped, addressed envelope.

NATURE CURE

BRITISH COLLEGE OF NATUROPATHY AND OSTEOPATHY BRITISH NATUROPATHIC AND OSTEOPATHIC ASSOCIATION
Frazer House
6 Netherhall Gardens
London NW3
01·435 8728

The college runs a four-year course in naturopathy and osteopathy. The association has clinics of its own and keeps a register of its practitioners.

VEGETARIAN SOCIETY
53 Marloes Road
London W8 6LA
01·937 7739

The society offers cookery courses, lectures, conferences, and publishes its own journal. It also publishes an International Vegetarian Handbook *annually – this includes an up-to-date list of health farms.*

VEGAN SOCIETY
47 Highlands Road
Leatherhead
Surrey
0372 372089

The society offers advice, holds meetings and publishes its own journal.

McCARRISON SOCIETY
23 Stanley Court
Worcester Road
Sutton
Surrey
01·643 2812

The society was formed to study the relationship between health and nutrition. Membership is open to "those qualified in medicine, dentistry, vetinary sciences and related professions".

BATES ASSOCIATION OF EYESIGHT TRAINING
49 Queen Anne Street
London W1

Training sessions are available as well as publications.

HERBAL MEDICINE

NATIONAL INSTITUTE OF HERBAL MEDICINE TUTORIAL SCHOOL OF HERBAL MEDICINE
148 Forest Road
Tunbridge Wells
Kent
0892 30400

The institute has a complete list of practitioners and the school runs a full-time four-year course as well as correspondance courses for professional training and lay people.

WEALDEN NATURAL HEALTH CLINIC
1 Clanricade Gardens
Tunbridge Wells
Kent
0892 45443

This is an aromatherapy clinic within a larger natural health clinic. It can provide a list of other British aromatherapists.

DR EDWARD BACH CENTRE
Mount Vernon
Sotwell
Oxon OX10 0PZ
0491 39489

The centre supplies remedies, books and advice on treatment.

SYSTEMS OF MEDICINE

BRITISH HOMEOPATHIC ASSOCIATION
27a Devonshire Street
London W1N 1RJ
01·935 2163

The association has a list supplied by the Faculty of Homeopathy of all the homeopathic doctors and hospitals throughout the UK. They also run courses in First Aid and homeopathy for the lay person.

ANTHROPOSOPHICAL ASSOCIATION
Rudolf Steiner House
35 Park Road
London NW1
01·723 4400

The association keeps a list of all the registered practitioners in the UK.

MANIPULATIVE THERAPIES

REGISTER OF OSTEOPATHS
1–4 Suffolk Street
London SW1
01·839 2060

The register has a list of qualified osteopaths in all parts of the UK.

ANGLO-EUROPEAN COLLEGE OF CHIROPRACTIC
13–15 Parkwood Road
Bournemouth
Hants
0202 431028

The college offers a four-year full-time course in chiropractic.

BRITISH CHIROPRACTORS' ASSOCIATION
5 First Avenue
Chelmsford
Essex
CM1 1RX
0245 358487

The association has a register of practitioners, a clinic and a number of publications on chiropratic.

CITY AND GUILDS INSTITUTE
46 Britannia Street
London WC1
01·278 2468

The institute keeps a list of approved colleges providing courses in beauty therapy – which includes massage.

ROLF INSTITUTE
PO Box 1868
Boulder
Colorado 80302
USA

The Rolf Institute in America offers three year courses in Rolfing to graduates. It has a directory of all its graduates worldwide.

SOCIETY OF TEACHERS OF THE ALEXANDER TECHNIQUE
3b Albert Court
Kensington Gore
London SW7
01·584 3834

The society will provide a directory of all recognized teachers in the UK.

FELDENKRAIS GUILD
4 The Broadway
Wimbledon
London SW19
01·947 4410

The guild has a list of all the recognized therapists in the UK and Europe.

INTERNATIONAL INSTITUTE OF REFLEXOLOGY
PO Box 34
Harlow
Essex CM17 0LT

The institute can supply a list of all qualified therapists in the UK and Europe.

TOUCH FOR HEALTH FOUNDATION
39 Browns Road
Surbiton
Surrey
01·399 3215

This is an Applied Kinesiology clinic and it also provides training courses and has a list of all Touch for Health instructors in the UK.

ORIENTAL THERAPIES

BRITISH COLLEGE OF ACUPUNCTURE
44 New Market Square
Basingstoke
Hants
0356 65333

The college offers a two-year postgraduate course for doctors, dentists, physiotherapists and practitioners of natural medicine.

BRITISH ACUPUNCTURE ASSOCIATION AND REGISTER
34 Alderney Street
London SW1 4EV
01·834 1012

The association has a register of members, mostly graduates of the British College of Acupuncture.

TRADITIONAL ACUPUNCTURE SOCIETY
TRADITIONAL ACUPUNCTURE SCHOOL
Queensway
Royal Leamington Spa
Warwicks CU32 5EZ
0926 22121

The society has a register of all graduates from the school.

SHIATSU SOCIETY
3 Elia Street
London N1
01·278 6783

The society publishes a newsletter and has a list of practitioners and teachers in the UK.

EXERCISE/MOVEMENT THERAPIES

BRITISH WHEEL OF YOGA
General Secretary
80 Lechampton Road
Cheltenham
Glos

This organization has a list of all the qualified teachers of yoga throughout the country as well as information about the British Wheel of Yoga teaching diploma courses.

Your local education authority will also have details of courses run by qualified teachers.

BRITISH T'AI CHI CHUAN ASSOCIATION
7 Upper Wimpole Street
London W1M 7TD
01·935 8444

The association offers beginner, advanced and teacher training courses and also a six-year healing course.

BRITISH AIKIDO FEDERATION
29 Abberbury Road
Iffley
Oxford
0865 777022

This is the headquarters for Aikido in Britain and can put you in touch with teachers all over the country.

MARTIAL ARTS COMMISSION
First Floor
Broadway House
Deptford Broadway
London SE8 4PS
01·691 3433

The commission has a list of T'ai chi and Aikido teachers in the UK.

LABAN ART OF MOVEMENT GUILD
Boynnes
Hadley Common
Herts EN5 5QG
01·449 5268

The guild is the headquarters of the Laban dance movement.

NATURAL DANCE ASSOCIATION
14 Peto Place
London NW1 4DT
01·278 6783

The association runs courses and workshops in natural dance.

SENSORY THERAPIES

BRITISH ASSOCIATION OF ART THERAPISTS
13c Northwood Road
London N6 5LT
01·348 6143

ASSOCIATION OF PROFESSIONAL MUSIC THERAPISTS
22 Ermine Street
Caxton
Cambs CB3 8PQ

The association keeps a register of music therapists in the UK.

PSYCHOTHERAPIES

ASSOCIATION OF CHILD PSYCHOTHERAPISTS
Burgh House
New End Square
London NW3
01·450 5014

This is the only professional organization for child psychotherapists.

BRITISH ASSOCIATION OF PSYCHOTHERAPISTS
121 Hendon Lane
London N3 3PR
01·346 1747

This association provides training in psychotherapy and has a register of trained and approved therapists.

BRITISH PSYCHO-ANALYTICAL SOCIETY
63 New Cavendish Street
London W1
01·580 4952

This society, too, runs training courses for therapists.

INSTITUTE OF GROUP ANALYSIS
1 Bickenhall Mansions
Bickenhall Street
London W1
01·487 5374

The institute runs training courses and workshops.

SOCIETY OF ANALYTICAL PSYCHOLOGY
30 Devonshire Place
London W1
01·486 2321

The society runs training courses for therapists and a clinic.

ASSOCIATION OF HYPNOTISTS AND PSYCHOTHERAPISTS
BLYTHE TUTORIAL COLLEGE
25 Market Square
Nelson
Lancs
0282 699378

The college offers training for both the medically-qualified and the lay person. The association keeps a register of practitioners.

BRITISH SOCIETY OF DENTAL AND MEDICAL HYPNOSIS
c/o Ms M. Samuels
42 Linke Road
Ashstead
Surrey KT21 2HY
27 73522

The society keeps a list of members in various parts of the country who are willing to accept patients for treatment with hypnosis – patients must be referred through their own doctors.

SILVA MIND CONTROL (UK) LTD
BCM Learning
London WC1N 3XX

The centre can provide information about courses.

CENTRE FOR AUTOGENIC TRAINING
15 Fitzroy Square
London W1
01·388 1007

The centre offers group and individual tuition.

HUMANISTIC PSYCHOLOGY

ASSOCIATION FOR HUMANISTIC PSYCHOLOGY IN BRITAIN
62 Southwark Bridge Road
London SE1 0AU
01·928 8284

The association has a list of therapists throughout the UK and can provide information about particular therapies such as Gestalt, Co-counselling and Transactional Analysis.

THE GESTALT ASSOCIATION

11 Weech Road
London NW6
01·435 0581

The association has been set up for practitioners and trainees in Gestalt. Its activities include organizing workshops, study groups and public seminars all over the United Kingdom.

HOLWELL CENTRE FOR PSYCHODRAMA

East Down
Barnstaple
Devon EX31 4NZ

Training courses and treatment are available at the centre.

INSTITUTE OF TRANSACTIONAL ANALYSIS

12 Kings Hall Road
Beckenham
Kent
01·778 2916

The institute holds courses and workshops.

HUMAN POTENTIAL RESEARCH PROJECT

c/o Diana Lomax
Adult Education Department
University of Surrey
Guildford
Surrey
04835 71281

The project organizes short courses and workshops in Guildford and London which include some work with co-counselling.

POLARITY THERAPY ASSOCIATION OF THE UK

2 Leys Road
Cambridge
0223 316364

This association has a list of practitioners working in the UK.

METAMORPHIC ASSOCIATION

67 Ritherdon Road
London SW17 8QE
01·672 5951

The association offers evening and weekend courses and has a list of therapists practising in the UK.

TRANSPERSONAL PSYCHOLOGY

PSYCHOSYNTHESIS AND EDUCATION TRUST

50 Guildford Road
London SW8 2BU
01·720 7800

The trust has training courses for professionals, lay people, young people and children. They keep a list of therapists all over the UK.

PARANORMAL THERAPIES

HARRY EDWARDS SPIRITUAL HEALING SANCTUARY

Burrows Lea
Shere
Guildford
Surrey
048641 2054

The centre organizes both contact and absent healing.

CHURCHES COUNCIL FOR HEALTH AND HEALING

Marylebone Road
London NW1 5LT
01·935 7315

This is an interdenominational organization representing British

churches and allied professions "for mutual consultation and cooperative action".

FOUNTAIN TRUST

3a High Street
Esher
Surrey KT10 9RP
78 67331

The trust offers information on the charismatic movement worldwide. It holds meetings and conferences.

CHRISTIAN SCIENCE

108 Palace Gardens Terrace
London W8 4RT
01·221 5650

This centre gives information on Christian Science and its healing work and keeps a list of the churches throughout the country.

NATIONAL FEDERATION OF SPIRITUALIST HEALERS

Church Street
Sunbury-on-Thames
Middx TW16 6RG

This organization has a list of member healers in all parts of the country.

THE RADIONIC ASSOCIATION

16a North Bar
Banbury
Oxfordshire OX16 0TF
0295 3183

The association has a list of registered practitioners and can give you details of the courses run by the affiliated school of Radionics.

PARANORMAL DIAGNOSIS

IRIDOLOGY RESEARCH CENTRE

188 Old Street
London EC1
01·254 4076

FACULTY OF ASTROLOGICAL STUDIES
2 Four Acres
127 Holden Road
Finchley
London N12
01·445 0975

The faculty runs correspondence and evening courses. It also keeps a list of astrological consultants.

ASTROLOGICAL ASSOCIATION
Bay Villa
Plymouth Road
Torquay
South Devon TQ9 59Q

The association has list of registered astrologers and holds regular meetings and lectures.

ASTROLOGICAL COUNSELLING FORUM
21 Greystone Gardens
Kenton Harrow
Middx HAF 0EF

This forum works to promote astrology in a counselling framework.

CHILDBIRTH

NATIONAL CHILDBIRTH TRUST
9 Queensborough Terrace
London W2
01·221 3833

The trust provides ante-natal classes, breastfeeding counselling and support. There are 250 branches throughout the UK.

ACTIVE BIRTH CENTRE
32 Cholmeley Crescent
Highgate
London N6 5JR
01·348 1284

Encourages freedom to assume natural positions during labour. Can provide information about other natural childbirth organizations.

HOSPICES

ST. JOSEPH'S HOSPICE
Mare Street
Hackney
London E8

This is a working hospice, dealing particularly with cancer patients. It has a list of hospices elsewhere in the UK.

GENERAL ADDRESSES

If you are unable to find the therapist you need in the resources list you can contact one of the following organizations.

HUMAN POTENTIAL RESOURCES
LFG Ltd
HP 12
Subscription Department
PO Box 10
Lincoln LN5 8XE
1522 31631

This is a quarterly magazine which provides a directory information service and guide covering the Human Potential Movement. Many therapists also place advertisements here.

INSTITUTE OF COMPLEMENTARY MEDICINE
21 Portland Place
London W1N 3AF

This is a public information and documentation service.

Bibliography

GENERAL REFERENCE

Annet, S. *The Many Ways of Being: A Guide to Spiritual Groups and Growth centres in Britain* (London 1976)
Hastings, Arthur C. (ed) *Health for the Whole Person* (Boulder CA 1980)
Hill, Ann (ed) *A Visual Encyclopaedia of Unconventional Medicine* (London 1979)
Kaslof, Leslie K. (ed) *Wholistic Dimensions in Healing: A Resource Guide* (New York 1978)
Kogan, Gerald (ed) *Your Body Works: A Guide to Health, Energy and Balance* (Berkeley CA 1980)
Popenoe, Cris *Wellness* (Washington 1977)

NATURE CURE

Airola, Paavo *How to Get Well* (Pheonix Arizona 1974)
Bates, W.H. *Better Eyesight Without Glasses* (London 1940)
Bircher, Ruth *Eating Your Way to Health* (London 1961)
Bricklin, Mark *The Practical Encyclopaedia of Natural Health* (New York 1962)
Eagle, Robert *Eating and Allergy* (London 1979)
Ernst, Sheila and Lucy Goodison *In Our Own Hands: A Book of Self-Help Therapy* (London 1981)
Huxley, Aldous *The Art of Seeing* (London 1943)
Inglis, Brian *Natural Medicine* (London 1980)
Ledermann, E.K. *Good Health Through Natural Therapy* (London 1976)
Lindlahr, Henry *Natural Therapeutics* (Saffron Walden 1981)
Stanway, Dr Andrew *A Guide to Biochemic Tissue Salts* (Redhill 1982)
Sokya, Fred *The Ion Effect* (New York 1977)
Warmbrand, Max *Encyclopaedia of Natural Health* (New York 1962)

HERBAL MEDICINE

Chancellor, P.M. *Handbook of the Bach Flower Remedies* (London 1971)
Griggs, Barbara *Green Pharmacy: A History of Herbal Medicine* (London 1981)
Griggs, Barbara *The Home Herbal* (London 1982)
Thomson, W.A.R. *Herbs that Heal* (London 1976)
Tierra, Michael *The Way of Herbs* (Santa Cruz 1980)
Valnet, Dr Jean *The Practice of Aromatherapy* (London 1980)

SYSTEMS OF MEDICINE

Coulter, Harris L. *Homoeopathic Science and Modern Medicine: The Physics of Healing and Microdoses* (CA 1981)
Pelikan, Wilhelm *Healing Plants* (London 1976)
Steiner, Rudolf and Ita Wegman *Fundamentals of Therapy – an Extension of the Art of Healing Through Spiritual Knowledge* (London 1967)
Vithoulkas, George *The Science of Homeopathy* (New York 1980)
Voegeli, Adolf *Homoeopathic Prescribing* (Wellingborough 1976)

MANIPULATIVE THERAPIES

Alexander, F. Mathias *The Use of Self* (New York 1941)
Barlow, Wilfred *The Alexander Principle* (London 1943)
Chiropractic in New Zealand – Report of a Commission of Enquiry (Wellington 1979)
Downing, George *The Massage Book* (New York 1972)
Feldenkrais, Moshe *Awareness Through Movement* (New York 1972)
Gleb, Michael *Body Learning: An Introduction to the Alexander Technique* (London 1981)
Kaye, Anna and Don C. Matcham *Reflexology: Techniques of Foot Massage for Health and Fitness* (Wellingborough 1978)
Kerr, Irvin *The Physiological Basis of Osteopathic Medicine* (New York 1970)
Klein, Lawrence and Sharon Meyer *Chiropractic: an International Bibliography* (Iowa 1976)
Maisel, Edward (ed) *The Alexander Technique* (London 1974)
Maxwell-Hudson, Clare *Your Health and Beauty Book* (London 1979)
National Institute of Neurologic and Communicative Disorders and Strokes: *The Research Status of Spinal Manipulative Therapy* (Washington DC 1975)
Palmer, D.D. *The Science, Art and Philosophy of Chiropractic* (Portland, Oregan 1910)
Rolf, Ida F. *Rolfing: The Integration of Human Structures* (Santa Monica 1977)
Still, Andrew Taylor *Autobiography* (Kirksville 1908)
Stoddard, Alan *Manual of Osteopathic Technique* (London 1959)
Thie, John F. and Mary Marks *Touch For Health* (Santa Monica 1973)

ORIENTAL THERAPIES

Acupuncture: A Comprehensive Text (Shanghai 1980)
Bewith, George T. *The Layman's Acupuncture Handbook* (Wellingborough 1981)
Veith, Ilza *The Yellow Emperor's Classic of Internal Medicine* (London 1972)
Waturu, Ohashi *Do-it-yourself Shiatsu* (London 1977)

EXERCISE/MOVEMENT THERAPIES

Balaskas, Arthur *Bodylife* (London 1977)
Balaskas, Arthur and Janet *New Life* (London 1979)
Huang, Al Chung-liang *Embrace, Tiger, Return to Mountain: The Essence of T'ai Chi* (Utah 1973)
Iyengar, B.K.S. *Light of Yoga* (London 1976)
Tohei, Koichi *Aikido in Daily Life* (San Francisco 1966)

SENSORY THERAPIES

Priestley, Mary *Music Therapy in Action* (London 1975)
Tibbs, Hardwin *The Future of Light* (London 1981)

PSYCHOTHERAPIES

Benson, Herbert *The Relaxation Response* (London 1976)
Black, S. *Mind and Body* (London 1968)
Brown, Barbara B. *Stress and the Art of Biofeedback* (New York 1977)
Carrington, Patricia *Freedom in Meditation* (New York 1978)
Coué, Emile *How to Practice Suggestion and Autosuggestion* (New York 1923)
Eliade, Mircea *Patanjali and Yoga* (New York 1975)
Edmonston, William E, (ed) *Conceptual Hypnosis and Hypnotic Phenomena* (New York 1977)
Green, Elmer and Alyce *Beyond Biofeedback* (New York 1977)
Pelletier, Kenneth R. *Mind as Healer, Mind as Slayer* (New York 1977)
Popenoe, Cris *Inner Development The Yes! Bookshop Guide* (London 1979)
Schultz, J.H. and W. Luthe *Autogenic Therapy Vols 1–6* (New York 1969)
Schwartz, Gary and Jackson Beatty (eds) *Biofeedback Theory and Research* (New York 1977)
Shattock, E.H. *Mind Your Body* (London 1979)

Silva, José and Philip Miele *The Silva Mind Control Method* (London 1978)
Storr, Anthony *The Art of Psychotherapy* (London 1979)
Ullman, Montague *Working with Dreams* (London 1983)
Waxman, David *Hypnosis: A Guide for Patients and Practitioners* (London 1981)
White, John (ed) *What is Meditation?* (New York 1974)

BEHAVIOURISM

Wolpe, J. and A.A. Lazarus *Behaviour Therapy Techniques* (London 1966)

HUMANISTIC PSYCHOLOGY

Berne, Eric *Games People Play* (London 1963)
Birth and Rebirth: Self and Society magazine vol 6; no. 7 (July 1978)
Clare, Anthony and Sally Thompson *Let's Talk About Me* (London 1981)
Gordon Richard *Your Healing Hands: The Polarity Experience* (Santa Cruz 1978)
Jackins, Harvey *Fundamentals of Co-Counselling Manual* (Rational Island 1970)
Janov, Arthur *The Primal Scream* (London 1973)
Lowen, Alexander *Bioenergetics* (New York 1975)
Maslow, Abraham *The Farther Reaches of Human Nature* (London 1976)
Moreno, Jacob L. *Psychodrama Vols 1 and 2* (New York 1959)
Perls, Fritz *Gestalt Therapy Verbatim* (New York 1969)
Rogers, Carl R. *Encounter Groups* (London 1971)
Rogers, Carl R. *On Becoming a Person* (London 1962)
Rowan, John *Ordinary Ecstasy: Humanistic Psychology in Action* (London 1976)
Saint-Pierre, Gaston and Debbie Boater *The Metamorphic Technique: Principles and Practice* (Wiltshire 1982)
St. John, John *Travels in Inner Space* (London 1977)
Schultz, William C. *Joy: Expanding Human Awareness* (London 1971)

TRANSPERSONAL PSYCHOLOGY

Assagioli, R. *Psychosynthesis: A Collection of Basic Writings* (London 1975)
Ornstein, Robert (ed) *The Nature of Human Consciousness* (San Francisco 1973)
Tart, Charles T. (ed) *Transpersonal Psychologies* (London 1975)

PARANORMAL THERAPIES

Barbarell, Maurice *I Hear a Voice: A Biography of Ted Fricker* (London 1962)
Edwards, Harry *Spirit Healing* (London 1980)
Krippner, Stanley and Alberto Villoldo (eds) *The Realms of Healing* (California 1976)
Leshan, Lawrence *The Medium, the Mystic and the Physicist* (New York 1974)
MacNutt, Francis *The Power to Heal* (Indiana 1977)
Maddocks, Morris *The Christian Healing Ministry* (London 1981)
Meek, George W. (ed) *Healers and the Healing* (California 1976)
Mermet, Abbé *Principles and Practice of Radiesthesia* (London 1975)
Netherton, Morris and Nancy Shiffrin *Past Lives Therapy* (New York 1978)
Peel, Robert *Christian Science* (New York 1958)
Playfair, Guy *The Flying Cow* (London 1975)
Russell, Edward, W. *Report on Radionics* (London 1973)
Wambach, Helen *Life Before Life* (New York 1979)
York Report on the Ministry of Deliverance and Healing (York 1974)

PARANORMAL DIAGNOSIS

Davidson, William *Set of Lectures on Medical Astrology* (New York 1973)
Gettings, Fred *Palmistry* (London 1966)
Jensen, Bernard *The Science and Practice of Iridology* (CA 1952)
Karagulla, Shafica *Breakthrough to Creativity* (CA 1967)
Krippner, S and D. Rubin (eds) *Galaxies of Life: The Human Aura in Acupuncture and Kirlian Photography* (New York 1973)
Luce, Gay Gaer *Bodytime: Physiological and Social Stress* (New York 1971)
Mayo J. *Astrology* (London 1964)
Shap, Mark and Alan Kahn *The Biorhythm Decision Maker* (New York 1978)

DISORDERS

Benet, Lin *Patients and their Doctors* (London 1975)
Bradshaw, John S. *Doctors on Trial* (London 1979)
Burnet, Sir Macfarlane *Auto-immunity and Auto-immune Disease* (Lancaster 1972)
Cairns, John *Cancer, Science and Society* (San Francisco 1978)
Cohen, John and John H. Clark *Medicine, Mind and Man* (Reading 1979)
Cousins, Norman *Anatomy of an Illness* (New York 1979)
Cox, Tom *Stress* (London 1978)
Dixon, Bernard *Beyond the Magic Bullet* (London 1979)
Dubos, René *Mirage of Health* (New York 1959)
Eynsenck, H.J. *Uses and Abuses of Psychology* (London 1953)
Frank, Leonard Ray *The History of Shock Treatment* (San Francisco 1978)
Freidman, Meyer and Ray H. Rosenman *Type A Behaviour and Your Heart* (New York 1974)
Garner, Lesley *The NHS: Your Money or Your Life* (London 1979)
Grof, Stanislav *Realms of the Human Unconscious* (New York 1975)
Guirdham, Arthur *A Theory of Disease* (London 1957)
Horrobin, David F. *Medical Hubris: A Reply to Ivan Illich* (New York 1977)
Illich, Ivan *Medical Nemesis* (London 1976)
Inglis, Brian *The Diseases of Civilisation* (London 1981)
Inglis, Brian *The Book of the Back* (London 1978)
Kothari, M.L. and L.E. Mehta *Cancer* (Boston and London 1979)
Kübler-Ross, Elizabeth *On Death and Dying* (New York 1969)
Laing, R.D. *The Divided Self* (London 1959)
LeShan, Lawrence *You can Fight for Your Life* (New York 1977)
Lynch, J.L. *The Broken Heart* (New York 1977)
Mackarness, Richard *Not all in the Mind* (London 1978)
Meares, Ainslie *Relief Without Drugs* (London 1976)
Phillips, Angela and Hill Rakusen (eds) *Our Bodies Ourselves* (London 1978)
Roberts, C.J. *Epidemiology for Clinicians* (London 1978)
Sacks, Oliver *Awakenings* (London 1973)
Schrag, Peter *Mind Control* (London 1980)
Selye, Hans *The Stress of Life* (New York 1956)
Simeons, A.T.W. *Man's Presumptuous Brain* (London 1960)
Szasz, Thomas *The Myth of Mental Illness* (New York 1961)
Thomas, Lewis *The Lives of a Cell* (New York 1974)
Thomson, A.R. *The Searching Mind in Medicine* (London 1960)
Todd, John W. *Health and Humanity* (Oxford 1970)
Totman, Richard *Social Causes of Illness* (London 1979)

Index

A

Abrams, Albert, 258–59
Abrams box, 259
Absent healing, 227, 242
Achs, Ruth, 277
Acupressure, 133
Acupuncture, 120–33
  and addiction, 308
  definition of, 17
  and gastro-intestinal
    disorders, 330
  and orthodox medicine, 11–12
  and pain, 305
Addiction, 306–09
  and acupuncture, 124, 173
  and art therapy, 159
  and autogenic training, 181
  and hypnotherapy, 173
  see also Aversion therapy
Agpaoa, Tony, 271
Ahimsa, 32
Aikido, 147–49
Alcoholism, 306
  and aversion therapy, 196
Alexander,
  F. Mathias, 104–07, 110
  principle, 104–08
Allergy, 309–311
  and asthma, 327
  causes of, 309, 310, 326
  and skin, 316
  treatments, for 309–10
Alternative medicine,
  revival of, 10–11
American Dance Therapy
  Association, 150
American Holistic Medical
  Association, 15
Amphetamines, see Appetite
  reducing drugs
Anesthesia,
  and acupuncture, 121–23
Angina pectoris, 322
Animal Magnetism, 167, 168
Animals,
  and acupuncture, 131
  and healing research, 250
  and health instinct, 17
Anthroposophical Medicine,
  74–6
Antibiotics, 312–13, 326
Aphrodisiacs, 336
Appendicitis, 327, 328
Appetite, 36–7, 331
  and metabolism 36
  reducing drugs 307
Arigo, Dr, 269
Aromatherapy, 58–63
  and herbal medicine, 45, 60
Art therapy, 156–59
Arthritis, 318–19
  and acupuncture, 120
  drugs for, 7, 319
  and hypnosis, 72
  statistics of in USA, 7
Asana Yoga, 142

Aspirin,
  and arthritis, 7, 72, 319
  side-effects of, 319
Assogioli, Roberto, 220–22
Asthma, 326
Astral Body, 75
Astrology, 286–91
  and herbal medicine, 46
Atavistic regression, 185, 166
Autogenic training, 178–81
Autohypnosis, 179
Autoimmune disease, 309
Autonomic nervous system,
  and colours, 155
  control of, 11, 177, 190–91, 192
Autosuggestion, 173–76
Aversion therapy, 196
Awareness through movement,
  109, 110

B

Bach, Dr Edward, 63–4
Bach flower remedies, 63–5
Back pain, 318, 319
  and chiropractic, 89, 90
  and kinesiology, 116
  and osteopathy, 84, 86
  and posture, 320
Balint, Michael, 217
Banting, Frederick, 323
Barker, Sir Herbert, 78, 297
Barlow, Dr Wilfred, 105–107
Barton, Rita Page, 158, 159
Bates, Dr William H, 40–2, 16
Bates eyesight training, 40–2
Beecham, Thomas, 47
Behaviour therapy, 196–97
  and addiction, 308
Benedict XIV, Pope, 230
Benjamin, Harry, 18–9, 329
Benson, Professor Herbert, 183, 190, 197
Beresford-Cooke, Carola, 136
Berger, Hans, 189
Bernard, Claude, 311
Berne, Eric, 206
Bernheim, Professor Hippolyte, 168
Biocurrents, 258–59
Biodynamic psychology, 211
Bioenergetics, 209–11
Bioenergy, 210, 245, 253
Biofeedback, 188–93
Biorhythms, 282–85
Bio-Strath elixir, 52
Birthwort plant, 48
Blance, Juan, 270
Bland, Professor Jeffrey, 339
Blood pressure
  and biofeedback, 190
  control of, 192–93, 322
Bloxham Arnall, 265
Bloxham tapes, 265–66
Boadella, David, 209
Boater, Debbie, 214
Bohr, Neils, 302

Bonesetters, 78
Boot, Jesse, 47
Boyd, W.E., 263
Boyesen, Gerda, 211
Boyle, Robert, 244
Braid, James, 148, 167
Brain waves
  frequencies of, 191
  and mind control, 177
Brazilian "surgeons", 269–70
Breath, rhythmic cleansing, 142
Breathing,
  and bioenergy, 210
  and primal therapy, 219
  and relaxation, 115, 142
Brezhnev, Leonid, 244
Brinton, Daniel, 77
British Vegetarian Society, 32
Brocklesby, Richard, 160
Bronchitis, 326–7
  and antibiotics, 326
  and nature therapy, 327
Bronchodilators, 326
Buchman, Frank, 201
Bursitis, 316
Butler, Brian, 116

C

Cade, Maxwell, 190
Califano, Joseph, 323
Cancer, 313–16
  and Bio-Strath, 52
  of the breast, 314
  and fear of dying, 185
  and meditation, 183–84
  risk factors in, 9
  statistics of in U.S.A. 7
  terminal, 297
  and visualization therapy, 184
  and vitamin C, 34
Cancer cells, influencing, 253
Cayce, Edgar, 272
Chace, Marian, 150, 153
Charcot, Jean-Martin, 223–24, 168, 174
Charismatic healing, 236
Chemotherapy and cancer, 314
Chi, 129, 131, 133, 146
Childbearing, 333–35
Childbirth,
  high technology, 334
  natural, 335
Children,
  and acupuncture, 130
  and alternative medicine, 300
  and diabetes, 325
  handicapped and dance
    therapy, 152
  retarded and Bio-Strath, 52
  and veganism, 32
Chirognomy, 276
Chiromancy, 276
Chiropractic, 88–95
  versus osteopathy, 88
Cholesterol, 321, 322

Christian healing, 226–27, 231, 233
  and Christian science, 237
  and hand healing, 243
  and Spiritualism, 239
Christian Science, 237–39
Church
  and exorcism, 231
  and healing, 226, 227
  investigations by, 234–35
  and the medical
    establishment 233–34
Churchill, Winston, 303
Circadian rhythms, 282, 283
Claudication, 321
Co-counselling, 208
Colds, 326
Colour,
  and diagnosis, 273
  effects of, 154–56
  Manning's codes, 247
  and personality, 155
Conscious will, 221
Consciousness, levels of, 191
Constipation, 329
Convulsions, 209
Copper bracelet, 27, 320
Copper salicylate solutions, 27
Cortisone, 48, 316
Coué Emile, 173–76
Couéism, 173–176
Creed, Dr, 328
Cripps, Sir Stafford, 107
CSM see Meditation, clinically
  standard
Culpeper, Nicholas, 46, 55–6, 330
Cummins, Professor Harold, 276
Cyriax, James, 79
Cystitis, 331

D

Dance therapy, 150–53
Davitashvili, Dzunha, 245, 253
Depression
  and aromatherapy, 62
Dermatoglyphics, 276
Dermatology, 316
Detoxification
  for addiction, 307
  in naturopathy, 19–20
Dewey, John, 107, 309
Diabetes, 323, 325
  and children 325
Diagnosis,
  and art therapy, 156
  and astrology, 291
  and horoscopes, 289
  and hypnosis, 185
  and iridology, 279–81
  and kinesiology, 118
  and palmistry, 276
  psychic, 272
  and radiesthesia, 261
  and radionics, 261
  visual clues to, 84

Index

O

Obesity, 306, 307, 308
  see also **Weight reducing
  diets**
Opren, 319
Organicism, 168
Orgone, 209
Orr, Leonard, 219
Orthodox medicine,
  and acupuncture, 11, 121–23
  and bonesetters, 78
  and chiropractic, 92, 94
  and herbalism, 52
  and holism, 15
  and homeopathy, 69, 73
  and natural therapies, 9, 12,
    78, 294–95
  and paranormal therapies,
    226, 233–34, 296
Oshawa, George, 31
Osteopathy, 80–6
  and chiropractic, 88
  cranial, 86–7

P

Paget, Sir James, 78, 319
Pain, 304–06
  value of, 85, 98
Pain relief,
  and acupressure, 136
  and acupuncture, 121
  and autosuggestion, 176
  and couéism, 176
  and electrical stimulation,
    129–31
  and hypnosis, 167–68
  and manipulation, 319
  and the mind, 12, 305
  and reflexology, 115
  and self-help, 304–05
Palmer, David Daniel, 88
Palmistry, 276–78
Parkinson, John, 46
Pasteur, Louis, 311
Past lives therapy, 264–67
Patanjali, 138
Patel, Chandra, 193
Pauling, Dr Linus, 33–34
Pavlov, Ivan, 196
Peczely, Ignatz, von, 279
Pedler, Dr Kit, 253
Pentecostal type healing, 226,
  233, 236, 239, 241
Perls, Friedrich, 204
Personality
  and disease, 9
  types, 323
Pestalozzi, Fred, 52
Petrissage, 98
Pheromones and epidemics, 312
Phillipines, psychic surgery in,
  270
Piles, *see* **Hemorrhoids**

Planetary

Planetary position and birth, 288
Plants,
  active ingredients of, 49
  energy field of, 57
  extracts, 46
  remedies, revival of, 48
  research into, 55
  see also **Herbs**
Playfair, Guy Lyon, 269
Polarity therapy, 211–13
Popenoe, Cris, 147
Posture
  and the Alexander principle,
    104, 105, 107
  and applied kinesiology, 117
  and emotions, 101
  and feldenkrais, 109
  and manipulative therapies,
    319–320
  and osteopathy, 80
  in polarity therapy, 213
  and rolfing, 101
  and touch for health, 117
  in yoga, 142
Potencies,
  in homeopathy, 67–68, 71
  in tissue salts, 44
Prana, 74
Prayer
  experiment with, 250
Premenstrual syndrome, 332
Prenatal therapy, 214–16
Priessnitz, Vincent, 24
Primal scream, 217–18
Primal therapy, 217–19
Prostate, 332
Protestant healing, 233–35
Pseudocyesis, 336
Psychic diagnosis, 272
Psychic surgery, 268–71
Psychodrama, 205–06
Psychosocial medicine, 301
Psychosomatic illness, 301
Psychosynthesis, 220–22
Psychotherapy, 163–66
  and allergy, 310
Pulses
  in acupuncture, 125
  in shiatsu, 135

Q

Quimby, Phineas, 237
Quin, Dr, 68
Quinine,
  and Hahnemann, 66

R

Radiesthesia, 257–64
Radionics, 257–64
Radiotherapy, 314
Rebirthing, 217–19
Red Light, effects of, 155
Reflexology, 112–15
Reich, Wilhelm, 209–10
Relaxation,
  and autogenics, 181
  and biofeedback, 192
  and reflexology, 115
  and yoga, 142
Reston, James, 121, 122, 128
  Sally, 128
Rheumatism,
  and acupuncture, 121, 319
  and aromatherapy, 63
  and homeopathy, 72
  and nature cure, 318, 319
Rheumatoid arthritis, 318
Rivers, William Halse, 77
Rogerian therapy, 199–201
Rogers, Carl, 199–201
Rolf, Dr Ida, 101–04
Rolfing, 101–04
Ryde, Dr, 173

S

St. John, Johnny, 203
St. John, Robert, 214
Saint-Pierre, Gaston, 214
Salt-water treatments, 25
Sauna baths, 25–6
Saunders, Cecily, 339
Schiff, Jacqui and Lee, 207
Schultz, Johannes, 179, 161
Schüssler, Dr, 44
**Scientific support for alternative
  therapy**, 297
Self-actualization, 200
Self-hypnosis, 166, 173
Selye, Hans, 303
Shaman, 225–26, 257
Shamanism, 257–58
Shaw, Bernard, 32, 194, 321
Shiatsu, 133–37
Shingles, 324
Shiv Sharma, Pandit, 320
Siegel, Bernard, 184, 185
Sigerist, Henry, 139
Silva, José, 177–78
Silva mind control, 176–78
Simian crease, 277
Simonton, Carl and Stephanie,
  184
Skin,
  and diet, 317
  mood and resistance to
    electricity of, 189, 191
Sleeplessness, 302, 303
Smith, Sister Justa, 251
Snellgrove, Brian, 275

Somatopsychic

Somatopsychic disorders, 339
Somnambulism, 166
Sorcerers, 226
Soubirons, Bernadette, 228
Soviet Union,
  and hand healing, 244
Spas, 23–4
Spezzano, Charles, 216
Spine,
  lesions of, 81
  see also **Back pain and
    Vertebral manipulation**
Spirit possession, 236
Spiritualist healing, 239–43
Spontaneous regression, 316
Steiner, Rudolf, 74–6
Steiner schools, 75
Stevens, Donald, 62
Stevenson, Professor Ian, 267
Still, Andrew Taylor, 80–81
Stone, Randolph, 212–213
Stradonitz, Kekulé von, 302
Straten, Michael van, 52
Stress,
  and aromatherapy, 63
  and atavistic regression, 185
  and autogenics, 179
  and autosuggestion, 176
  and biofeedback, 193
  and biorhythms, 285
  and cancer, 315
  and digestion, 330
  and heart disease, 9
  and hypnosis, 173
  and insomnia, 304
  and meditation, 144, 187, 188
  and metamorphic technique,
    216
  and nervous system, 324
  and obesity, 308
  and psychosomatic symptoms,
    301
  and psychosynthesis, 322
  and shiatsu, 136
  and skin, 317
  and unborn child, 216
  and yoga, 144
  see also **Fight or flight
    response** and **Holistic
    principle**
Strokers, 244
Structural integration, 101
Stuart, Malcolm, 49
Surgery,
  and cancer, 314
  for heart disorders, 322
  for mental disorders, 338
  for neuropathies, 323
  for pain, 304
  for ulcers, 329
Sutherland, William, 87
Swartley, William, 218
Swoboda, Professor Herman,
  282
Sydenham, Thomas, 67

Acknowledgments

Author's acknowledgments
Our thanks must first go to Warren Kenton for introducing us to Dorling Kindersley and then to all those friends who variously checked the manuscript for us, demonstrated their therapies and modelled for us. But we would particularly like to thank Yvonne McFarlane, Jemima Dunne, Derek Coombes and Gillian Della Casa and the rest of the staff at Dorling Kindersley who patiently bore with us whilst the original idea became structured, and then worked away all those necessary hours to produce the book in its final form.
Brian Inglis and Ruth West.

The therapists: Judith Ashton (*Bioenergetics*); Dr Wilfred Barlow (*Alexander Principle*); Carola Beresford Cooke (*Shiatsu*); Sybil Beresford-Pierce (*Music therapy*); Brian Butler (*Touch for health*); E.L. Buxton (*Palmistry*); Antonia Carr (*Hypnotherapy*); Vera Carruthers (*Art therapy*); Christopher Connolly (*Feldenkrais technique*); Susan Farwell (*Osteopathy*); Flo and Dick Farmer (*T'ai chi*); Karl Francis (*Hand healing*); Teresa Hale (*Yoga*); Ian Hutchinson (*Chiropractic*); Dr Dolores Kreiger (*Therapeutic touch*); Joanne Lepage-Browne (*Yoga*); Sandra Levy (*Astrology*); Clare Maxwell-Hudson (*Massage*); Walli Meir (*Dance therapy in special education*); John Morley (*Iridology*); Roger Newman-Turner (*Acupuncture*); Harry Oldfield (*Kirlian photography*); Adele Peronne-Dodds (*Herbal medicine*); A.J. Porter (*Reflexology*); Michael Ronan (*Bates method of eyesight training*); Carole Rudd (*Polarity therapy*); Gaston St. Pierre (*Metamorphic technique*); Carole Shaw (*Dance therapy*); Stephen Silver; Donald Stevens (*Aromatherapy*); Cathy Webster (*Rolfing*); Hein Zeylstra (*Herbal medicine*).

We would like to thank the following organizations and authors for permission to quote from their publications in the text.

P.17 Good Health through Natural Therapy, *Dr E.K. Ledermann*, Kogan Page Ltd. 1976; p.20 Good Health through Natural Therapy, *Dr E.K. Ledermann*, Kogan Page Ltd. 1976; p.28 The Mechanic and the Gardener, *Laurence Le Shan*, Holt Rinehart and Winston; p.33 and p.34 Here's Health Magazine; p.38 New Scientist, *Lois Wingerson* 14 May 1981; p.40 The Art of Seeing, *Aldous Huxley*, reprinted by permission of Mrs Laura Huxley and Chatto and Windus Ltd; p.56 Green Pharmacy: A History of Herbal Medicine, *Barbara Griggs*, Jill Norman and Hobhouse 1981; p.60 The Practice of Aromatherapy, *Dr Jean Valnet*, The C.W. Daniel Co Ltd; p.63 The Medieval Discoveries of Edward Bach, Physician, *Nora Weeks*, The C.W. Daniel Co Ltd; p.64 Handbook of the Bach Flower Remedies, *Philip Chancellor*, The C.W. Daniel Co Ltd; p.70 Homoeopathic Prescribing, *Adolf Voegeli*, Thorsons Publishers Ltd; p.75 Work Arising from the Life of Rudolf Steiner: chapter 6, *Dr Michael Evans*, Rudolf Steiner Press London 1975; p.77. Extract from History of the Melanesian Society, *W.H. Rivers*, reprinted by permission of Humanities Press Inc, Atlantic Highlands, N.J. 07716; p.81 Osteopathy: An Explanation *Harold Klug and Robert Lever* published by The Society of Osteopaths, September 1981; p.84 The Holistic Approach of Osteopathy, *Harold Klug*, The Journal of the Society of Osteopaths published by The Society of Osteopaths, Autumn 1981; p.93 Sounding Board: The Future of Chiropractic by *Walter Wardell*, reprinted by permission of the New England Journal of Medicine 20 March 1980; p.94 British Medical Journal Editorial/Chiropractic in New Zealand, Report of the Commission of Enquiry, Wellington Government Printer 1979; p.95 Your Health and Beauty Book, *Clare Maxwell-Hudson*, MacDonald General Books; p.107 extract from The Alexander Technique by *Edward*

Acknowledgments

Maisel reprinted by permission of University Books Inc, 120 Enterprise Ave, Secaucus, N.J. 0794, USA; p.107 Ends and Means *Aldous Huxley*, reprinted by permission of Mrs Laura Huxley and Chatto and Windus; p.116 Touch for Health, *John F. Thie and Mary Marks*, De Vorss and Co; p.131 Report by *Ronald Melzack and others* originally published by Elsevier Biomedical Press in Pain 2 (1976); p.138 Effortless Being, *Alastair Sheaver*, published by Wildwood House London 1982; p.139 A History of Medicine Volume 2, *Henry Sigerist*, published by Oxford University Press, New York 1961; p.142 Reprinted by permission of Schocken Books Inc. from Patanjali and Yoga by *Mircea Eliade*, French Edition Copyright © 1962 by Editions du Seuil, Translation copyright © 1969 by Funk and Wagnalls; p.144 School of T'ai Chi Chu'an, *Beverley Milne*, handout; p.145 The Many Ways of Being, *Stephen Annett*, Thorsons Publishers Ltd; p.151 Claire Schmais, Wholistic Dimensions in Healing, *Leslie J. Kaslof* (ed), © Leslie J. Kaslof reprinted by permission of Doubleday and Company Ltd; p.155 Colour for Architecture *Tom Parker and Byron Mikellides* (eds), chapter ''Colour currency of Nature'', Nick Humphrey, Published by Studio Vista 1976; p.157 Times Health Supplement 25th December 1981; p.162 The Farther Reaches of Human Nature, *Abraham Maslow*, Viking/Penguin; p.163 Sunday Times Magazine, London, 13th December 1981; p.175 Suggestion and Auto-Suggestion, *Charles Baudouin*, George Allen and Unwin Ltd; p.177 Here's Health Magazine; p.181 Applications of Autogenics, London Centre for Autogenic Training; p.184 Getting Well Again, *Carl Simonton, Stephanie Matthews-Simonton and James L. Creighton*, copyright © 1978 by O. Carl Simonton and Stephanie Matthews-Simonton, Bantam Books Inc; p. 185 New Age Magazine August 1982 © 1982 New Age Communications; Working with Dreams, *Dr Montague Ullman*, Delacorte; p.198 Joy, *William C. Schutz*, Souvenir Press Ltd; p.200 The Courage to be, *Paul Tillich*, James Nisbet and Co Ltd; p.202 In our own Hands, *Sheila Ernst and Lucy Goodison*, The Women's Press; p.203 Travels in Inner Space, *Johnny St. John*, Victor Gollancz Ltd; p.208 Ordinary Ecstasy, *John Rowan*, Routledge and Kegan Paul Ltd; p.209 *David Boadella*, The Language of Bioenergy in Your Bodyworks, edited by *Gerald Kogan*, published by And/Or Press and Transformations Press, Berkeley, California USA; p.209 Sex Literature and Censorship, *D.H. Lawrence*, Twayne Publications/College and University Press; p.211 *Pierre Pannetier*, Polarity Therapy in Your Body Works, edited by *Gerald Kogan*, Published by And/Or Press and Transformations Press, Berkeley, California, USA; P.214 The Metamorphic Technique: Principles and Practice, *Gaston Saint Pierre and Debbie Boater*, Element Books; p.216 Psychology Today, May 1981, Volume 15 number 5, Ziff Davis Publishing Co; p.219 An article by *Anne Dominique Buidschedler* in Self and Society, Volume 6, number 7 (July 1978) a special issue; Birth and Rebirth; p.221 Interview of Assagioli by *Sam Keen*, in Psychology Today, Ziff Davis Publishing Co; p.221 Psychosynthesis and Education Trust; p.250 Invisible writing, *Arthur Koestler*, Hutchinson, reprinted by permission of A.D. Peters and Co. Ltd; p.257 Radionic Association; p.264 Past Lives Therapy, *Morris Netherton and Nancy Shiffrin*, William Morrow and Co; p.282 *Bernard Gittleson* in Wholistic Dimensions in Healing, *Leslie J. Kaslof* (ed), copyright © Leslie J. Kaslof, reprinted by permission of Doubleday and Company Ltd; p.291 *Dr Mario Jones* in Wholistic Dimensions in Healing, *Leslie J. Kaslof* (ed), copyright © Leslie J. Kaslof reprinted by permission of Doubleday and Company Ltd; p.303 *Hans Selye*, The Stress of Life, McGraw Hill Book Co.

Picture credits

P2 *Mary Evans Picture Library*; p.7 *Popperfoto*; p.8 *Popperfoto*; p.11 *Mary Evans Picture Library*; p.12 *Camera Press*; p.15 bottom *Rex features*; p.17 *Mary Evans Picture Library*; p.19 *Daily Telegraph Colour Library*; p.21 *Daily Telegraph Colour Library*; p.23 *Mary Evans Picture Library*; p.25 top *Warwick District Council, Leamington*, bottom *Mary Evans Picture Library*; p.26 *Warwick District Council, Leamington*; p.30 *Bonnie Freer*; p.44 *Homeopathic Trust for Research and Education*; p.46 *Mary Evans Picture Library*; p.48 *Anglia Television*; p.49 *The Iris Hardwick Library of Photographs*; p.54 *Anglia Television*; p.59 *Aromatic Oil Company*; p.60 *Aromatic Oil Company*; p.64 *Edward Bach Centre*; p.67 top *Mary Evans Picture Library*, bottom *Homoeopathic Trust for Research and Education*; p.70 *Anglia Television*; p.71 *Anglia Television*; p.75 *Architectural Association*; p.77 *Alan Hutchison Library*; p.80 *British School of Osteopathy*; p.81 *Oxford Orthopaedic Engineering Centre*; p.88 *Dr Schofield*; p.89 *Brian R. Hammond*; p.93 *Palmer College of Chiropractic*; p.101 and p.102 *Rolf Institute*; p.107 top *Constructive Teaching Centre*, bottom *Mary Evans Picture Library*; p.108 *Dr Wilfred Barlow*; p.110 and p.111 *Bonnie Freer*; p.112 *A.J. Porter, International Institute of Reflexology*; p.120 *Mary Evans Picture Library*; p.122 *Popperfoto*; p.139 top *Michael Holford*, bottom *Camera Press*; p.147 *Mrs Ros Loft*; p.153 *Laban Archives, Lisa Ullmann*; p.158 *Vera Diamond, Jerry Mason*; p.160 left and right, *Arlene Restaino*; p.164 *Mary Evans Picture Library/Sigmund Freud Copyright*; p.167 *Radio Times Hulton Picture Library*; p.168 *Mary Evans Picture Library*; p.172 *Ann Ronan Picture Library*; p.183 *Bonnie Freer*; p.186 *Camera Press/Dmitri Kasterine*; p.190 *Vision International/Anthea Sieveking*; p.192 *Maxwell Cade and Geoff Blundell, Institute of Psycho-Biological Research*; p.196 *Wellcome Institute for the History of Medicine*; p.197 *Wellcome Institute for the History of Medicine*; p.199 *Constable Publishing Co Ltd*; p.202 *Steve Beck*; p.205 *Marcia Karp, Holwell Centre*; p.218 *The Churchill Centre*; p.225 *Robert Harding Associates Agency*; p.226 *Robert Harding Associates Agency/Robert Cundy*; p.227 *Popperfoto*; p.228 *Vision International/P.Tetrel*; p.231 *Mary Evans Picture Library*; p.232 *Camera Press*; p.235 *Christian Fellowship of Healing (Scotland)*; p.327 *Christian Science Board of Directors*; p.240 *Associated Newspapers*; p.241 *National Federation of Spiritual Healers*; p.244 *Camera Press*; p.245 *Matthew Manning*; p.252 *Thames Television*; p.256 *Bonnie Freer*; p.257 *Mary Evans Picture Library*; p.270 *Psychic News*; p.272 *Psychic News*; p.273 *Harry Oldfield*; p.274 *Professor Leonard Konikiewicz*; p.275 *Harry Oldfield*; p.276 *Mary Evans Picture Library*; p.285 *Biomate Ltd*; p.287 *Mary Evans Picture Library/Harry Price Coll., University of London*; p.289 *Ann Ronan Picture Library*.

Dorling Kindersley would like to thank: AcuMedic Centre; Philippa Briggs; Matthew Carroll; Daphne Crabtree; John Dyer; Lesley Gilbert; Keith Goddard; Vee Hale; Robin Hayfield; John Hudson; Lucy Lidell; Fiona McIntyre; Debbie MacKinnon; Melanie Miller; Stephanie Mills; Mysteries Ltd; Mrs Newman Turner; Sue Rose; Anna Selby; Martin Solder; Michelle Stamp; Elizabeth Walton; Sheila Willitt.

Main illustrations:
Russell Barnett
Other illustrations:
David Ashby and Andrew Farmer

Special photography:
Jan Baldwin; Rodger Banning; Geoff Dann; Heini Schneebeli; Anthea Sieveking.

Jacket photography:
Paul Williams

Typesetting:
Servis Filmsetting Limited, Manchester
Elements, London

Reproduction:
Repro Llovett, Barcelona

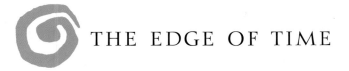

THE EDGE OF TIME

THE
EDGE
OF TIME

PHOTOGRAPHS OF MEXICO BY

MARIANA YAMPOLSKY

UNIVERSITY OF TEXAS PRESS ❧ AUSTIN

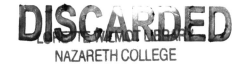

WITTLIFF GALLERY SERIES

This series originates from the Wittliff Gallery of Southwestern & Mexican Photography, an archive and creative center established at Southwest Texas State University to celebrate the photographic arts. BILL WITTLIFF, SERIES EDITOR

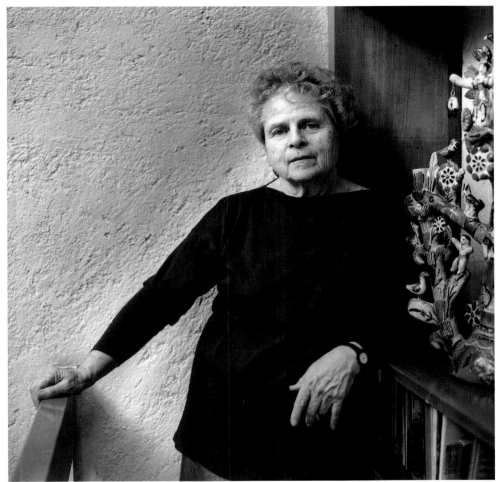

ROGELIO CUELLAR

Mariana Yampolsky

The introductory essay by Sandra Berler was originally published in *Mexico: The Artist Is a Woman*, Occasional Paper #19 (1995) of The Thomas J. Watson Jr. Institute of International Studies, Brown University.

LIBRARY OF CONGRESS CATALOGING-IN-PUBLICATION DATA

Yampolsky, Mariana, 1925–
The edge of time : photographs of Mexico by Mariana Yampolsky / Mariana Yampolsky. —1st University of Texas Press ed.
p.   cm. — (Wittliff Gallery series)
Includes bibliographical references.
ISBN 0-292-79604-8 (cloth)
1. Photography, Artistic.   2. Photography—Mexico.
3. Mexico—Pictorial works.   4. Yampolsky, Mariana, 1925– .
I. Title.   II. Series.
TR654.Y353   1997
779´.9972—dc21   97-6581

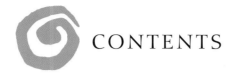

CONTENTS

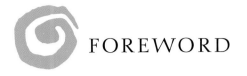 FOREWORD

BY ELENA PONIATOWSKA

She walks ahead of me, hands on her hips like the handles of a little jug, in the way of country women—elbows bent so that the camera and film bag won't slip off her shoulders. She carries her own equipment. Edward Weston mentions several times in his *Daybooks* that when he and Tina Modotti went out into the field to photograph they were accompanied by young boys who carried their tripods and photographic plates for them. But their Graflex was so heavy—the Hasselblad, on the other hand, is not. Mariana takes the film out of the camera, conscientiously wets the end of the roll with the tip of her tongue to seal it, and puts it in her leather bag. There. Sixteen captured images join the other rolls. They look cheerful at the bottom of the bag—a promising harvest. Mariana shoulders her gear and sets out again like a strong *campesina* headed for home with her sheaf of wheat at the end of a hard day's work.

Mariana Yampolsky's work is essential to her life. When she opened the window on her very first morning in Mexico City and saw a bougainvillea blooming against the white wall outside, she decided, "This is my country." And when she walked through the bustle and energy of the downtown streets—Cuauhtemoctzin, Donceles, San Juan de Letrán— among the lottery ticket vendors, the street peddlers, the deliverymen shouting, "Careful there! Give me room!" she chose her people without a second thought.

Albert Camus says in one of his *Carnets:* "The moment I am no more than a writer I shall stop writing." The same can be said of Mariana, because if she were no more than a photographer, she would give up photography. No worries there, for just as printed images surface in a darkroom, many Marianas have come to light over the years: the teacher, the engraver, the curator of exhibitions, the book designer, the editor, the photographer.

When she photographs in the field, Mariana approaches the people in a village as if she's carrying a white flag in her hands. She pauses under the pale cotton canvases of the marketplace; she knows how to listen and how to ask questions, absorbed by a reality that is always new and always surprising. Men, women, and children respond because they see the seriousness in her eyes, the respect in her attentions, the commitment of this quiet woman who speaks slowly, deliberately, never faltering. She considers, waits, and weighs each situation. She never rushes. (I'm just the opposite—I spill the beans at the least provocation.) Mariana doesn't just think twice, she thinks seven times before she speaks. Gradually, as she describes a scene—a simple hut, an empty pot on the fire—she captures us. The stories she tells with her camera and her words leave us no escape. There we are, and we can't pretend we don't see.

Her relation to those she photographs is direct and vital: to the old carpenter explaining his craft, to the bride in short skirt and white ankle socks, to the four old women waiting for the priest. They come right through the camera and say to our face, "Look! Here I am and there you are. And what are you going to do about it? What are you going to do about my wrinkled hands, my ragged shawl, my eyes like embers? How will you be as you were before?"

You should see Mariana take her pictures: how she gets excited, makes a decision, takes a shot, looks for the right light, goes and comes, always smiling, afraid that the moment will get away from her. A key in a wooden door illuminated by a particular ray of light, a lace doily on the back of a rocking chair, a *campesina* who protests, "Wait a minute. Let me comb my messy hair" (we're always messy when someone wants to take our picture)—it's all part of the creative process. After she finishes the roll, Mariana searches her bag for another. This gives her time to reflect. And once again, enthusiasm animates her face, the face of a woman who becomes involved, who knows how to see, who sees and understands critical essences, who captures and—above all—who loves her country with a profound, sorrowful love. Over there is a pregnant woman with a child in her arms. How can she have the strength to bear another? But strength she has; and Mariana and she, face to face, both bear the dearest of fruits. We look at them drawn to each other: the photographer and the mother, a river of light between them. Then Mariana continues on, borne by the strength of a woman who knows where she must go.

As she drives along in her small Volkswagen, Mariana is cradled in the lap of the landscape, comforted and diverted by it. She looks ahead steadily. Nothing escapes her gaze—not the flower of the maguey, nor its stalks used for building houses, nor the marvelous aqueduct of Padre Tembleque waiting in the distance. "Look at the mountains, look at that wide powerful gap between them, look at the roof of maguey spikes, look at the pulque worker." Mariana knows the maguey plant inside out. She can name all its uses and can quote its virtues. She appreciates it just as she appreciates the grace of the peasant mother with a child on her hip or the bold attitude of a young Mazahua woman. To Mariana, everything is art—as it was for Leopoldo Méndez and Pablo O'Higgins, her strongest influences. She sees those who work the land as part of a great ongoing poem in which harvesting alfalfa, gathering corn, embroidering a handkerchief are not simply part of life but are also acts of creativity. It is this way of seeing that is Mariana's greatest contribution to the culture of our country. She, too, incorporates into her work the days and the hours, the fiestas and the everyday objects, the labor and the sorrow that Diego Rivera painted in his murals—as well as the rage and indignation that Orozco captured in his. Mariana is less violent but equally incisive: the face of the young pulque worker reflects the age-old weariness of exploited children, and the desolation of the old-young girl of *Niña con maguey* has a similar air. Other recurring themes include the survival of syncretic pre-Hispanic forms, the weight of religion, and the omnipresence of art in Mexican daily life. Mariana's whites, immaculate whites, emerge from the shadows—the little girl in her first communion dress, the woman retreating in a flowing head cloth, the girl with her hair tied up in a rag who turns and suddenly becomes Joan of Arc or a novice ready to surrender her soul to God.

Soul? There was a time when we thought a photograph stole a bit of the soul. Now, having a personal photo hanging on the wall is like declaring oneself, like saying, "Look at me, this is who I am; look at me, here I stand; look at me, I exist in the world." Mariana confirms this: "People's attitudes have changed. Now they ask me for photos all the time. Even in Ocumicho, Michoacán, girls followed me down the street, giggling and calling out, 'Seño, steal us a picture.' People ask me, 'What kind of pictures do you take?' And I don't know how to answer, because I can't stand the word 'artistic'—it's not important to me if something is art or not. When I see a photograph that moves me, I don't wonder if it's art, but rather how vital these people are, captured by the wizardry of someone like Cartier-Bresson or Eugene Smith. It doesn't occur to me to ask whether or not something is documentary or any of the other labels people tend to put on photography."

Forty years ago, architect Hannes Meyer asked Mariana to photograph her fellow engravers for a memorial edition published on the twelfth anniversary of the Taller de Gráfica Popular (Popular Graphic Arts Workshop) in Mexico City. "I had taken few photographs up to that time and it flattered me when he asked me to take these portraits." She used her Rolleflex with trepidation and took great care with each roll of film. Besides working at the Taller, Mariana took a class given by photographer Lola Alvarez Bravo in the Academy of Fine Arts, San Carlos. "We worked in a damp, windowless room—a storeroom, really—where we took turns practicing with a huge, old glass-plate camera. I was terribly frustrated because, since we were several students, my turn came up only once a week, and I was anxious to learn how to develop and print. On the weekends I went out to take pictures using just one roll of film. I now think that extraordinary practice was very good training, because I was forced to judiciously consider every shot. When I look at the images of the great photographers of the past, I realize that to have the most modern equipment is incidental; the important thing is what is taken. Cartier-Bresson works with the same Leica that he used as a young man. I really began to like photography because behind the lens I discovered secret and surprising places; and I found myself drawing less and photographing more. I've never been interested in expressing my own ego; on the contrary, I was interested in reflecting a moment in the lives of people that others perhaps don't see or don't value.

"People, always people. In Europe I saw splendid parks and museums that speak for the past; but on my last trip there I took one roll of film during an entire month's stay. When I got home, I went out to the country and took four rolls in less than two hours—moved by seeing people so close to the earth and living in a sort of loving disorder. Mexico is surprising, forceful; the people, often kind, sometimes brutal, always graceful. To me, Mexico is light. I must admit that when I got back, things I usually considered in bad taste moved me as never before. Even the plastic flowers seemed to have character.

"How do I know if a photograph will be good? I don't have to see it printed. I know it at the moment that I click the shutter. Form and content have to express my feelings when the image is recorded. Above all, I want to share what I see with others. If they like my vision, that's wonderful; and if they don't, it bothers me, but it doesn't stop me. I always try to go beneath the surface, although many photographers find that to be painful."

Possessed of a keen social conscience, Mariana sometimes postpones her own work to attend to the interests of others, to be more than a photographer, to share, to give, to meet societal obligations. She was an engraver at the Popular Graphic Arts Workshop when the Workshop put up protest posters in the streets; she was a teacher, an editor in charge of designing free textbooks for the Ministry of Education. It wasn't enough for her just to do engravings and portraits of Mexico's children; she also had to help teach them to read. Later, when she edited the *Enciclopedia Infantil Colibrí*, she demonstrated her profound concern for the needs of children living in the countryside, quite different from those of urban children. It was not only a question of producing good material but also one of becoming involved with the children themselves. To give one's life—heart, energy, action, suffering—Mariana gave it all; because to her, every child's portrait is a personal experience: a conversation, a trip to the home village, a study of expressions and attitude—those things which produce an image that will live in memory.

"In the publishing house Fondo Editorial de la Plástica Mexicana," Mariana says, "Leopoldo Méndez, Manuel Alvarez Bravo, and Rafael Carrillo decided to do a book about Mexican popular arts; and so a project that was very important to me was born, producing two volumes entitled *The Ephemeral and the Eternal in Mexican Popular Art* (Lo efímero y lo eterno del arte popular mexicano). I not only helped Leopoldo choose objects but I also searched in private collections for suitable things to photograph, and I was able to go out into the field to take pictures. During three years of intense work I traveled to remote villages to document dances, ceremonies, costumes: people living their lives and expressing their inexhaustible creativity through their everyday objects and in the celebration of their fiestas. I took what touched and thrilled me. It's always been that way—I take what I feel.

"Often my best photographs are the ones that I didn't take. I want to capture a certain moment, but at the same time I feel like an intruder. So first I try to create a kind of accord and explain what I'm doing. Only when people invite me into their homes and are willing to be photographed do I continue. They have the right to reserve for themselves their deepest emotions, and as a consequence, I find it impossible to photograph them. I get angry with myself afterward for not having taken a particular photograph, but my feelings of reserve are greater than my disappointment. If I determine beforehand that I'm going to offend someone, I simply stop. I've gone out on trips with photographers who don't have this problem, who get right in a person's face and snap a picture. Personally, I've never been able to do this. To me, the person's feelings are more important than taking the picture."

Always with infinite respect, Mariana has chronicled the people of Mexico and their creative expression. She is not interested in reporting violent confrontations or looking to go "where the action is." Her war is another and it is profoundly felt. Sometimes she regrets not having immersed herself in an urban life and dedicated more time to the contradictions of the city: the crowding, the smog, the aggression, the lack of love. The great cities are a reality of our times that we should ponder; but one of the few rights left to us is that of choice, and Mariana has chosen the measured cadence of the Mexican countryside: the sounds of the bells and the grinding stone, the smell of the cilantro and onion, the warmth of the hearth, the sight of children bathing in the river. Because she is her own woman, she will not exploit, she will not ride roughshod, she will not deceive. She travels the hard and dusty roads of a Mexico she chose on the day she opened the bougainvillea window and said, "This is my country."

—TRANSLATION BY CONNIE TODD

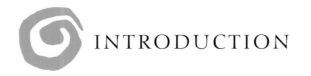 INTRODUCTION

Mariana Yampolsky:
An Artistic Commitment

BY SANDRA BERLER

The figure is centered with her back to the camera. Her head is covered in a rough white triangular cloth. Barefoot, she steps away from the viewer across the cobblestones of her village. A rural stillness emanates from the picture; intense light and shadow wash the image. In this picture, *Huipil de tapar* (a simple cotton garment used as a head covering), photographer Mariana Yampolsky captures a native woman against the foothills and architecture of rural Mexico. It is a timeless Mexican scene, and it invites us to share the photographer's commitment to her adopted country.

Yampolsky, born in 1925 in Chicago and now a Mexican citizen, is a distinguished artist with a long career as an engraver, illustrator, editor, curator, and photographer. Her photography continues her early work as a muralist and graphic artist who combines social and political issues through artistic media. Yampolsky seeks to create art that can be seen and shared by a broad population.

She grew up on her grandfather's 123-acre farm in rural Crystal Lake, Illinois, but her family life was enriched by the presence of artists, scientists, and anthropologists, whose collected artifacts introduced her to primitive cultures. It was a free-thinking intellectual environment in which great value was placed on independence, tolerance, education, and ideas. This stimulating childhood created a lifelong passion for books and reading. She had her own library, enlarged with contributions from her German grandmother, who sent her children's books in German. She attended public elementary school and two years of public high school in Crystal Lake. As a child, Yampolsky attended classes at the Art Institute of Chicago. By the age of twelve she was drawing and engraving in every spare moment.

Yampolsky's father, Oscar Yampolsky, a sculptor, introduced her to photography by allowing her to help develop the family portraits he made with an enormous Speed Graflex. She remembers "watching with fascination as the images appeared like magic in the trays, and this sense of amazement is still with me."[1]

Around 1940, Yampolsky entered the University of Chicago, from which she graduated in 1944 with a bachelor of arts degree in the humanities. At that time, the University of Chicago was one of the most exciting yet serious places for education in the United States. Mortimer Adler's "100 Great Books" course was inaugurated under Robert Maynard Hutchins's tenure as president of the University. Football was banned, and there were no sororities or fraternities. Students who chose to be there were dedicated to bettering society. Yampolsky's personal and artistic development was shaped by the university atmosphere and by the events of her time: the Great Depression, social turmoil, war, and displacement of people.

It was in Chicago that she saw John Steinbeck's film about Mexico, *The*

Forgotten Village. She says she "listened entranced" a few weeks later as Max Kahn and Eleanor Coen, two lithographers, described the Mexican mural movement and their experiences at the Taller de Gráfica Popular (TGP; Popular Graphic Arts Workshop) in Mexico City. These two events determined her future; in 1944 she left for Mexico.

Yampolsky joined the stream of artists who by the mid-1940s had been inspired to live and work in postrevolutionary Mexico. The atmosphere of social and economic reform, the inexpensive cost of living, and the nearness of anthropology, art, and folklore attracted expatriate Americans and refugees from World War II. Many people settled in Mexico out of a desire to leave behind an increasingly materialistic society.

In the 1920s, intellectuals, writers, and artists began shifting away from the heavy European influence that had pervaded Mexico's culture since the arrival of European conquerors. Under Minister of Education José Vasconcelos, the Mexican government supported the creation of Mexican art that would unify social sectors fragmented by the Mexican Revolution.[2] Ideas of art for the populace were openly propagandistic. The government supported the monumental public murals executed by Diego Rivera, José Clemente Orozco, and David Alfaro Siqueiros. The government's goal was to promote art that would address Mexico's historical legacy as well as its current social problems. The intent of this art was to encourage awareness and pride in the people; emphasis was on the identity of a Mexican nation.

In the 1930s, graphic artists who were not necessarily sponsored by the government began to record the economic and social plight of the workers and farming people, and to capture a way of life that was authentically Mexican and untainted by foreign influences. During this decade, few foreign photographers were interested in looking beyond the picturesque or idealized Indian. Two prominent exceptions were photographers Anton Bruehl and Paul Strand, who took a more intimate look at the people of

Mexico. Bruehl mainly photographed individuals removed from their historical cultural context. Strand viewed Mexican peasants, ancient walls, and churches with a more critical eye. He also made a politically motivated film titled *The Wave*, which was sponsored by the Mexican government and dealt with social injustice in a Gulf Coast fishing village. Mexican muralist and graphic artist David Alfaro Siqueiros continued the attack upon naive and folkloric depictions of the Mexican Indian that had made their way into American art and the murals of Rivera. Other American painters, like Pablo O'Higgins and Marion Greenwood, undertook mural commissions of workers and political events. Photographer Edward Weston also lived and worked in Mexico during the 1920s. Although he made abstractions of Mexican folk objects and landscapes, he preferred to focus on classical forms, shapes, and textures. Weston was much admired, but his works show little interest in the cultural and social problems of Mexico that Yampolsky would focus upon.[3]

When Yampolsky arrived in Mexico in the mid-1940s she enrolled in the Escuela de Pintura y Escultura (School of Painting and Sculpture), popularly known as "La Esmeralda." The atmosphere at the school was relaxed, and students were left alone to work. In contrast to the more academic or disciplined tradition of teaching, it was an open system.

The most meaningful influence on Yampolsky in Mexico was her participation in the Taller de Gráfica Popular, a cooperative workshop of printers and graphic artists in Mexico City dedicated to social and political issues. It was founded in 1937 by Leopoldo Méndez, Pablo O'Higgins, and Luis Arenal.

The workshop took a strong antifascist stand during the Second World War. Its most active years were part of a tremendously intense period of political ferment in Mexico in which artists played a participatory role. The workshop's heart was shaped by a desire to put its members' creative capacity at the service of the people.[4]

Among her mentors at the Taller were Leopoldo Méndez, whose graphic art illustrated "customs and past times of common folk, re-creation of scenes from the Revolution, and acrid caricaturesque denunciation of contemporary political events,"[5] and the painter Pablo O'Higgins, who used his skills as a muralist and printmaker to illustrate social injustice and to advance the cause of labor and the working class. Both men became her lifelong friends.

Using black-and-white graphics, woodcuts, and linoleum cuts, artists produced posters, pamphlets, leaflets, and illustrations for labor and teachers' unions and farmers' organizations. The aesthetic of the graphic artist was shaped by the muralists; by the expressionist lithographs of George Grosz, Kathe Kollwitz, and master lithographer Jesús Arteaga; and by social realism as a vehicle of political expression. This aesthetic combined political propaganda and artistic expression, a philosophy that continues to be important to Yampolsky. After a six-month apprenticeship, she was accepted as the first female member of the Taller de Gráfica Popular. While working there, she earned her living teaching English literature to high school students, and she went on to teach in the initial foreign language program of the National Polytechnic Institute in Mexico City.

The standards were very high at the Taller, and the work was exacting. Each print had to be approved by all the members. As Yampolsky recalls, "The collective nature also extended to our social role as artists. We were more interested in others than in ourselves."[6]

In 1949, Swiss architect Hannes Meyer, the former director of the Bauhaus, asked Yampolsky to photograph the younger members of the Taller for a book, *The Workshop for Popular Graphic Art: A Record of Twelve Years of Collective Work*. Although she had just begun experimenting with photography, this medium became increasingly important to her work. Mariana was mainly self-taught in photography. While at the Taller she took a short photography course with Lola Alvarez Bravo at the Academy of Fine Arts, San Carlos, Universidad Nacional Autónoma de México (UNAM). Bravo may have introduced Yampolsky to a certain vision, a straightforward formal way of constructing a picture within the lens. Bravo observed painters' technical concerns and photographed the way muralists painted.[7] She encouraged a focus on strong light and shadow; on orderly, elegant shapes; on figures framed in doorways and against walls and other architecture, always with reference to Mexico's historical and natural settings. It was nonconfrontational photography. From making black-and-white engravings, Yampolsky understood the great importance of light, volume, and composition.

At the Taller, Yampolsky served as an engraver, and she was appointed the first female member of the executive committee. As curator of exhibitions, she organized and sent collective exhibits throughout Mexico, the Americas, Europe, Africa, and Asia. Within Mexico, Yampolsky was designer and curator of the twentieth-anniversary retrospective exhibition of the Taller's works. This was held in Mexico City in 1956 at the Palace of Fine Arts under the title *Gran Muestra de la Obra del Taller de Gráfica Popular*. She was illustrator for the magazine *Construyamos Escuelas* (Let's build schools), and she designed a poster for the film *Memorias de un mexicano*, which was among the first documentaries on the Mexican Revolution. She won prizes for a poster in 1952, and for several years was an illustrator in Mexico City for the newspapers *El Nacional* (1956), *Excelsior* (1958), and *El Día* (1962). In 1966, she exhibited in the thirtieth-anniversary show of the Taller at the Museum of Modern Art in Mexico City.

In 1959, two events marked a turning point in Yampolsky's career. There was a schism in the workshop, and she left the organization along with most of the members. She was invited to work with Leopoldo Méndez in editing art books for the Fondo Editorial de la Plástica Mexicana, a publishing house that he had founded. She collaborated with him on a book about the great Mexican illustrator J. G. Posada and was co-editor and photographer for another book, *Lo efímero y lo eterno del arte popular mexicano* (The ephemeral and the eternal of Mexican popular art), later published in 1970 by El Fondo Editorial de la Plástica Mexicana. To produce this two-volume work that described traditional Mexican dances, ceremonies, and objects of folk art, she traveled all over Mexico for three years, visiting collections of popular art. This was the first professional publication of her photographs. But before the book was published, Méndez died and Yampolsky gave up engraving to become a full-time photographer.

At this point, Yampolsky was able to combine all of her interests—editing, curating, and photography—to encourage the production of popular art in the provinces. Working for Mexico's Ministry of Education, she directed graphic design and photography for natural science textbooks used in grade schools. She created and edited a weekly publication for children called *Colibrí*, which used the talents of the foremost writers and painters of Mexico. This gave rise to a radio series that she also directed. Over the years, Yampolsky has edited art books, including *Diego Rivera's Murals in the Ministry of Education*, *Children* (children pictured in art from the pre-Columbian period to the present), *The Imagination of Indigenous Children*, and *Mexican Toys*. She was coordinator of art books on Francisco Toledo, the contemporary painter from Oaxaca, and Pablo O'Higgins, the well-known Mexican painter, lithographer, and muralist.

Experts consider Yampolsky a brilliant curator, and she is widely respected for the exhibitions she has put together throughout the years.[8] The most recent shows she has curated include an international exhibition of Mexican photography for the 150th Anniversary of Photography, *Memoria del tiempo* (Memory of time), in 1989 for the Mexican Museum of Modern Art, and a retrospective of the work of photographer Enrique Díaz for the Mexican National Archives.

The photographers that Yampolsky most identifies with, for enlarging her knowledge of the world and for their concern with aesthetics and social issues, are Dorothea Lange, Paul Strand, Manuel Alvarez Bravo, Brassai, Andre Kertesz, and Henri Cartier-Bresson. Yampolsky says she does not believe women photographers have a distinctive point of view; she thinks that Cartier-Bresson's picture of a father and child, for example, is no less poignant than such a photograph would be if it were taken by a woman. She says that being a woman was never an obstacle within the intellectual and artistic community of Mexico.

In the 1930s and 1940s, women painters, writers, and photographers such as Lola Alvarez Bravo, Frida Kahlo, María Izquierdo, and Lupe Marín (Diego Rivera's first wife) were well known and respected. Women were considered equal to men in this world. She believes Frida Kahlo's popularity abroad has helped Mexican women photographers become better known. She cannot recall ever being discriminated against for being a woman artist. On the contrary, she says she has been encouraged and befriended by men such as Pablo O'Higgins, Leopoldo Méndez, and art historian Francisco Reyes Palma.

The progression of Yampolsky's work from the medium of engraving to the medium of black-and-white photography shows her earnest devotion to the idea of making art available to as many people as possible. Both media allow the artist to make many black-and-white prints. This is important because relatively inexpensive reproduction takes art out of the hands of the elite and makes it more accessible to the larger public. Yampolsky says she is disturbed by numbered prints and restricted editions in photography because these make the images too rare and defeat the potential egalitarianism of the medium.

Like many talented artists, Yampolsky uses her camera as a personal appendage that is always ready to enhance her efforts at writing, editing, publishing, and recording Mexican life. Her books convey themes of and references to history, ancient traditions, and changing culture.

Among these books, *La casa en la tierra* (The house of the earth), with text by Elena Poniatowska in 1981, and *La casa que canta* (The house that sings) and *The Traditional Architecture of Mexico*, written by Chloé Sayer in 1982 and 1993 respectively, are about homes and storage areas of rural Mexico. *Tlacotalpan*, written by Elena Poniatowska in 1987, is a collection of images of a town in Veracruz. *La raíz y el camino* (Roots and paths, 1985), with an introduction by Poniatowska, is a selection of Yampolsky's photographs. *The Forgotten Estates* and *Haciendas of Puebla* explore the old plantation system. *Mazahua* documents a village where the women are left behind when the men go off to work in the cities. *Thinking About Mexico* is a retrospective book of Yampolsky's work published in 1993, with text by Erika Billeter. These publications celebrate Mexico, using Yampolsky's images. She is responsible for monographs on Romualdo García, a turn-of-the-century studio photographer, and on the early-twentieth-century photographer Enrique Díaz.

Throughout her career as a photographer and artist, Yampolsky has been invited to participate in many solo and group exhibitions. In 1976 she exhibited in the first Latin American Photography Colloquium—a significant event that helped create a place for Latin American photographers in the international world of photography. Yampolsky recalls the tough juries and high standards for admission to the exhibitions of the colloquiums. She exhibited in the second colloquium exhibition, *Hecho en Latinoamérica* in Mexico City at the Palace of Fine Arts, and again in 1985 at the third Latin American Colloquium.

Yampolsky's forays into the countryside are reminiscent of the nineteenth-century itinerant photographers who wandered from town to village taking portraits and creating images as if by magic for special occasions. And her work in the countryside continues the tradition of the photojournalists who documented Mexico's revolutionary struggle. She records the present-day events that are rapidly changing the cultural identity of Mexico.

Yampolsky is at ease with rural people and the countryside setting. She says country people are less likely than city people to mask their feelings. She approaches all rural people, from the child to the worker in the field, with respect, concern, and gentleness. Yampolsky says, "Although I try to be unobtrusive, it is not always possible to pass unnoticed. It pleases me when I am taken for an itinerant photographer and not as an intruder utilizing others for my own ends."[9]

She photographs simply and directly and does not manipulate the image. Her subjects fill the lens. She makes large prints that are rich and dense with detail; they are printed by Alicia Ahumada, who, Yampolsky says, "does it better."[10]

In one of her early pictures, *Puesto de naranjas, Axochipan, Morelos,* taken in the 1960s during a two-week trip by foot from the coast of Pinotepa through the mountains, the viewer senses Yampolsky's responsible approach and her identification and sympathy with the common man. A close view of a child sleeping against a man's leg—with the man's calloused hand on the child's head, the rough-textured clothes, the barest glimpse of oranges at their feet, the huarache, grass, and wall—all give us a sense of the man's place in his world. The figures and objects are not exotic or strange, the man is identifiable not simply as a Mexican worker; the image is a universal, human one. Certainly this picture reflects in detail what Yampolsky says interests her most in photography: "People and everything the human hand touches."[11]

Each photograph is like a short narrative sentence—sharp, composed, and tightly focused. In *Crucifixión* from 1991, the viewer first sees in the foreground an ancient religious scene: country women, their heads covered with *rebozos*, gathered near a man portraying Christ on the cross. An automobile intrudes in the background, jarring the viewer back to the present.

The mother and child in *Caricia* (Caress) from 1990 becomes in an instant a poem of the past, the present, and the future.

When asked if her work reflects Mexico today, Yampolsky replies enigmatically that the moment she presses the shutter button it becomes yesterday's. She continues to be imbued with the social conscience of the Taller and remains a conduit for many people in Mexico who have needed public visibility. She has employed photography to record Mexican history and traditions, to depict with honesty and sincerity the struggle for the well-being of the child, the elderly, the artisan, and the people. As an artist she works side by side with the farmer, with the women of Mazahua, who have seen that the artist can be useful and that photography is a worthwhile career. She has collaborated with the people over many years to produce identifiable pieces of a grand photomural of Mexico that gently combines the poetic and the political.

She has participated in many major international group exhibitions in Mexico City and throughout the world, beginning in Mexico City with a collective exhibit for the International Year of the Woman in 1975.

Mariana Yampolsky's photographs are in the permanent collections of the Museum of Modern Art, Mexico City; the Museum of Modern Art, New York; the National Portrait Gallery, Washington, D.C.; the Wittliff Gallery of Southwestern & Mexican Photography, Southwest Texas State University, San Marcos, Texas; the Houston Fine Arts Museum, Houston; The Center for Creative Photography, University of Arizona, Tucson; and in private collections. She is married to engineer and agronomist Arjen van der Sluis.

NOTES

1. Personal communication with artist, October 1993.

2. Ibid.

3. For a greater discussion of this idea, see James Oles's essay "American Artists in Mexico, 1914–1947," in *South of the Border, Mexico in the American Imagination, 1914–1947*, ed. James Oles (Washington and London: Smithsonian Institution Press, 1993): 89.

4. Personal communication with artist, October 1993.

5. From an essay by Karen Cordero Reiman, "Constructing a Modern Mexican Art, 1910–1940," in *South of the Border, Mexico in the American Imagination, 1914–1947*, ed. James Oles, p. 43.

6. Personal communication with artist, October 1993.

7. See essays by Amy Conger and Elena Poniatowska in *Women Photograph Women* (Riverside: University of California, 1990): 47.

8. Personal communication with author-curator James Oles, November 1993.

9. Elizabeth Ferrer, "Encountering Differences," *Photography Center Quarterly* 14, no. 1 (June 1992), 24.

10. Personal communication with artist, October 1993.

11. Ibid.

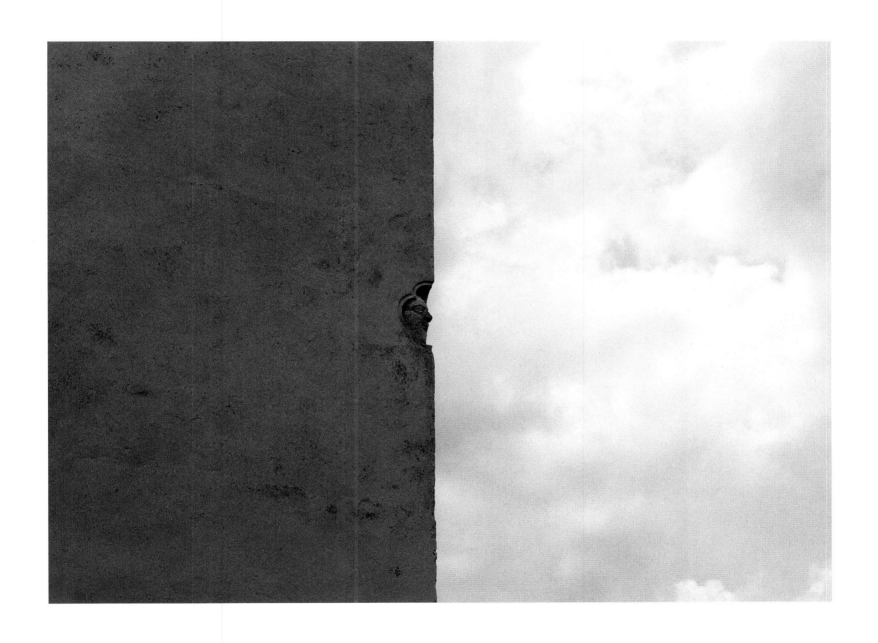

Al filo del tiempo   The Edge of Time

THE PEOPLE

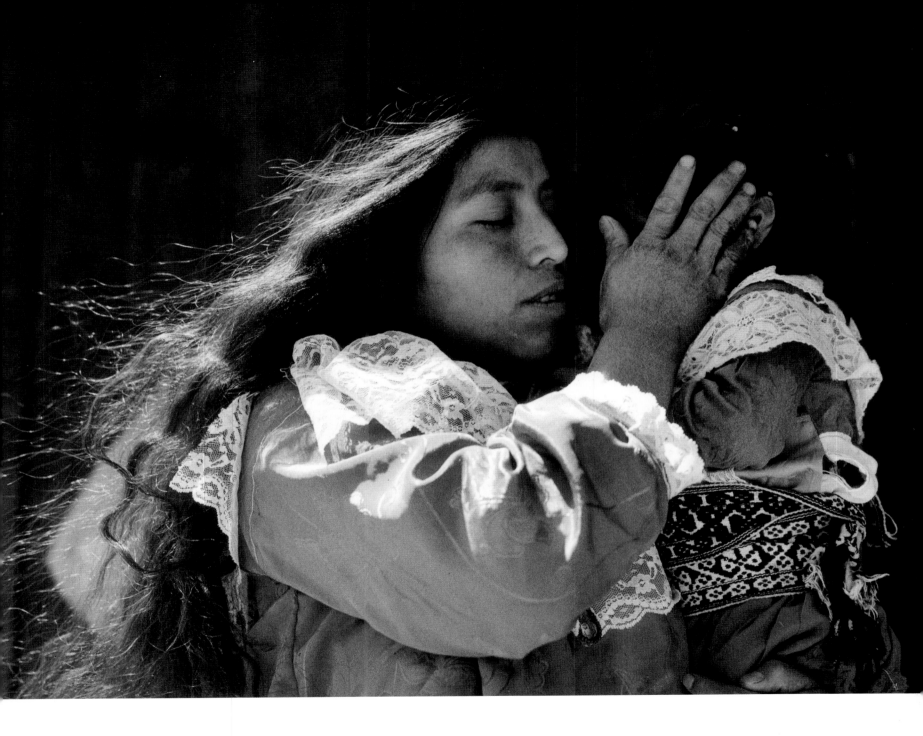

1. *Caricia* *Caress*

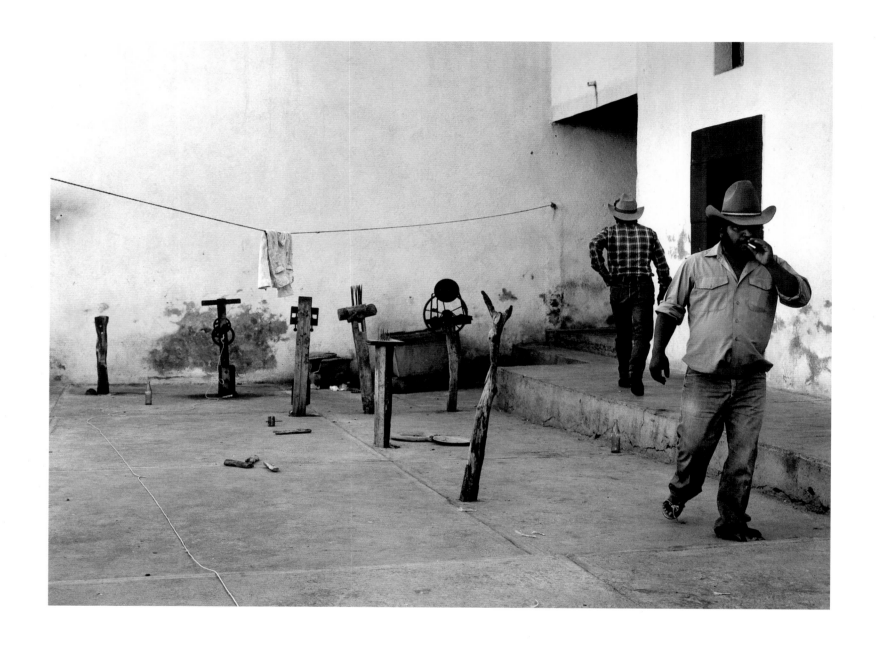

2. Patio de la cárcel   *Jailhouse Patio*

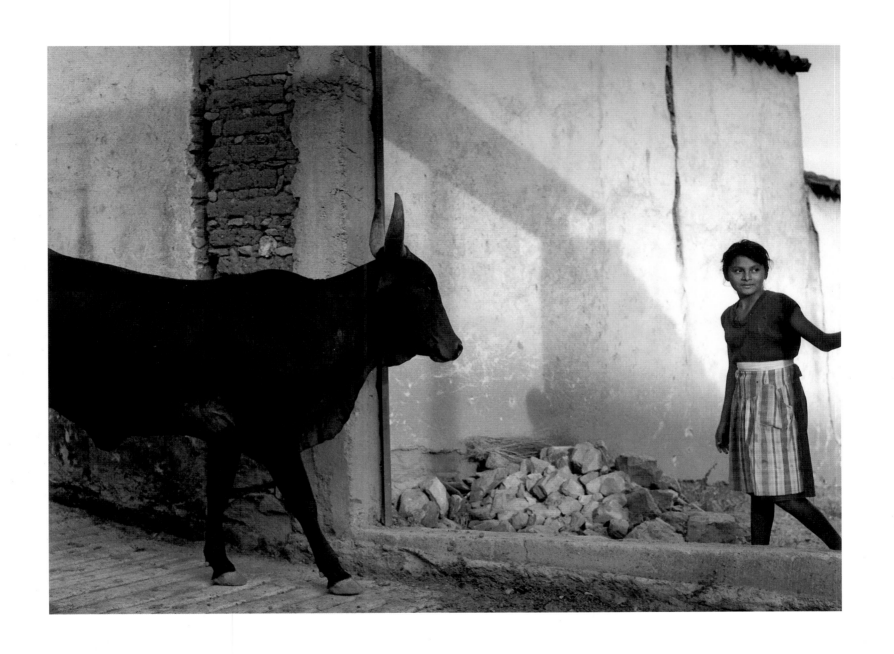

3. *La doncella y el toro*   *The Maiden and the Bull*

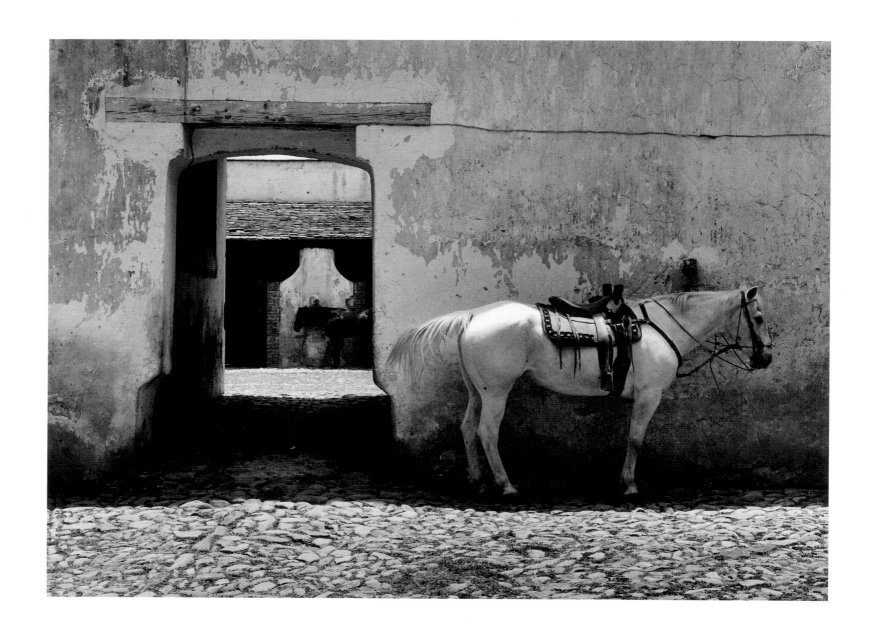

4. Caballeriza *Stable*

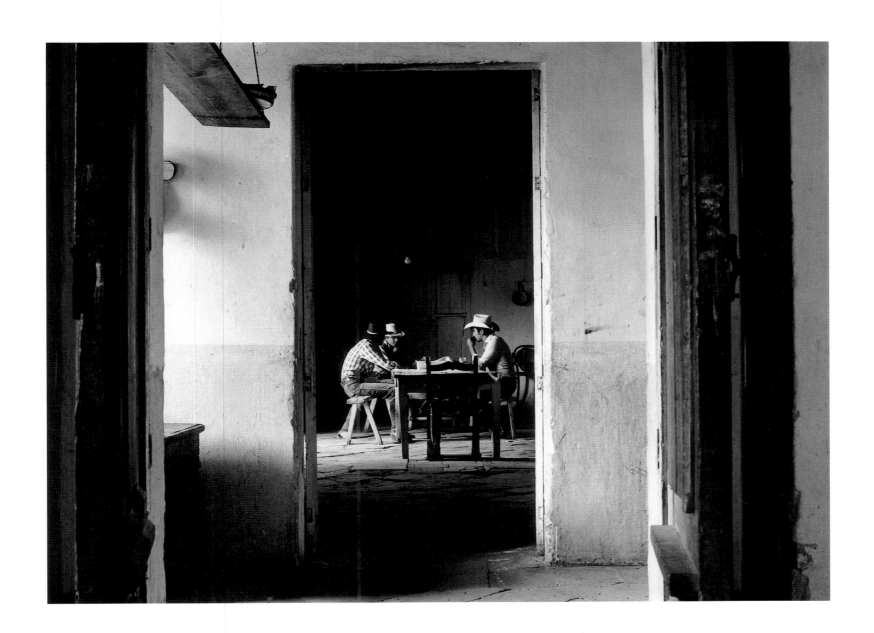

5. El almuerzo *Breakfast*

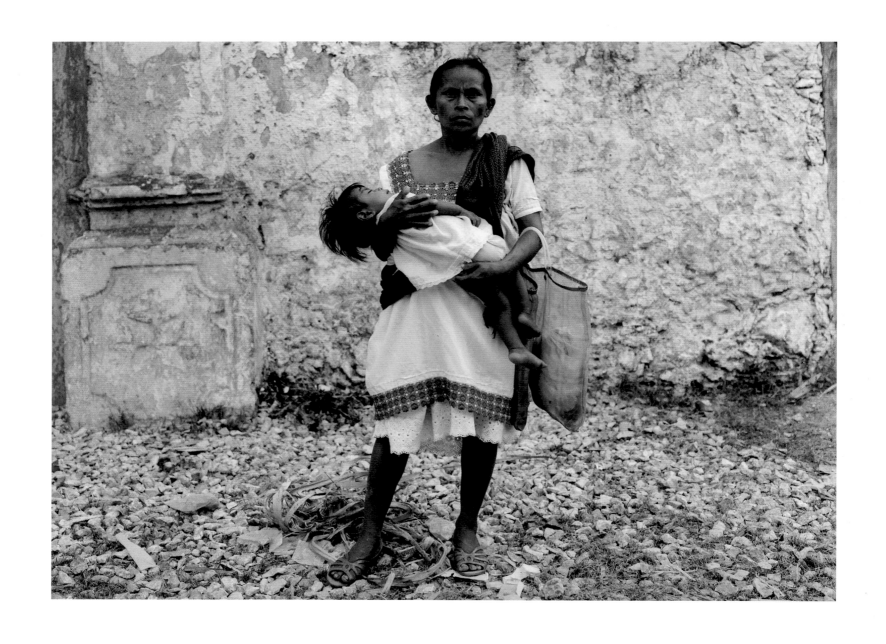

6. *Madre de Campeche*   *Mother, Campeche*

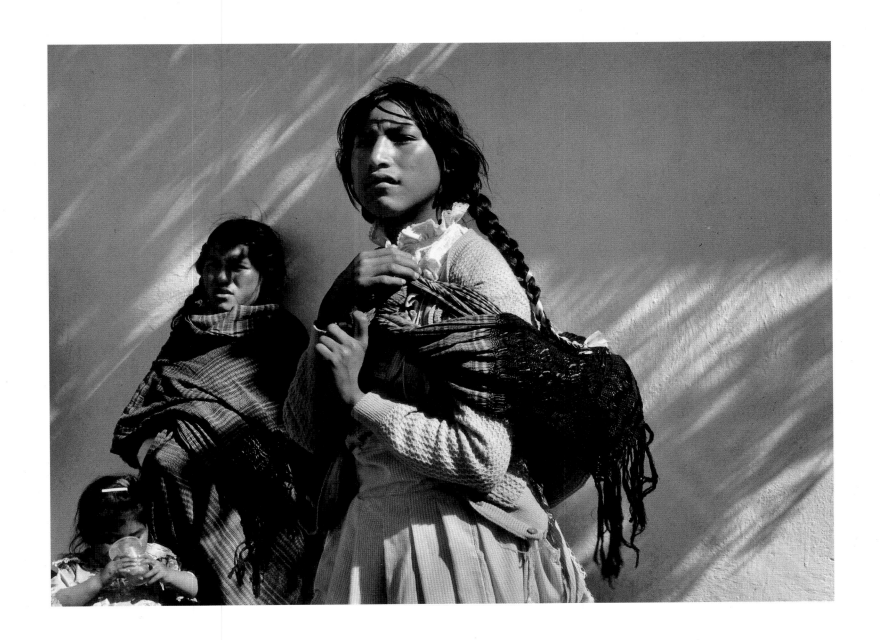

7. *Mujeres mazahua* *Mazahua Women*

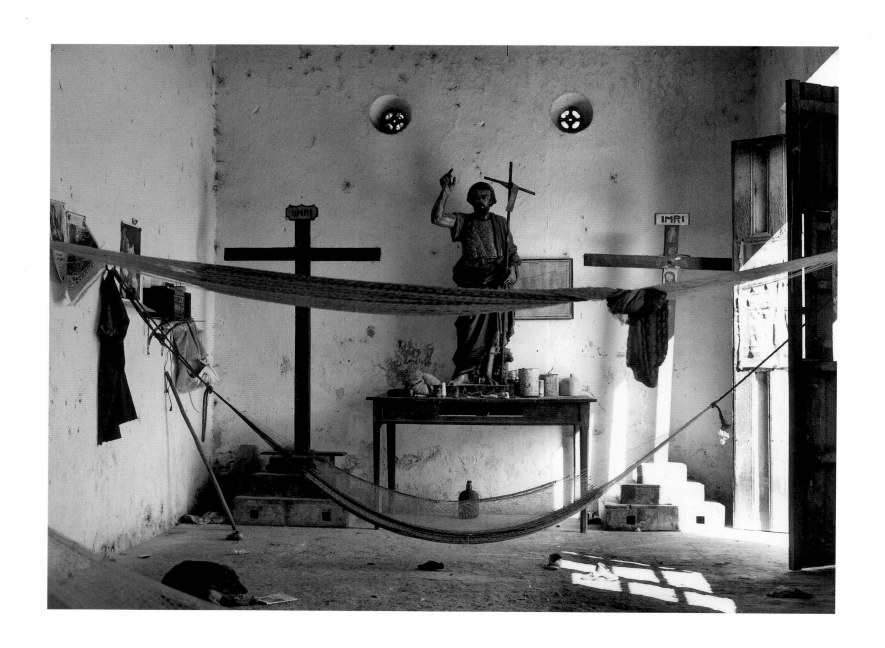

8. Hacienda, Yucatán   *Yucatán Hacienda*

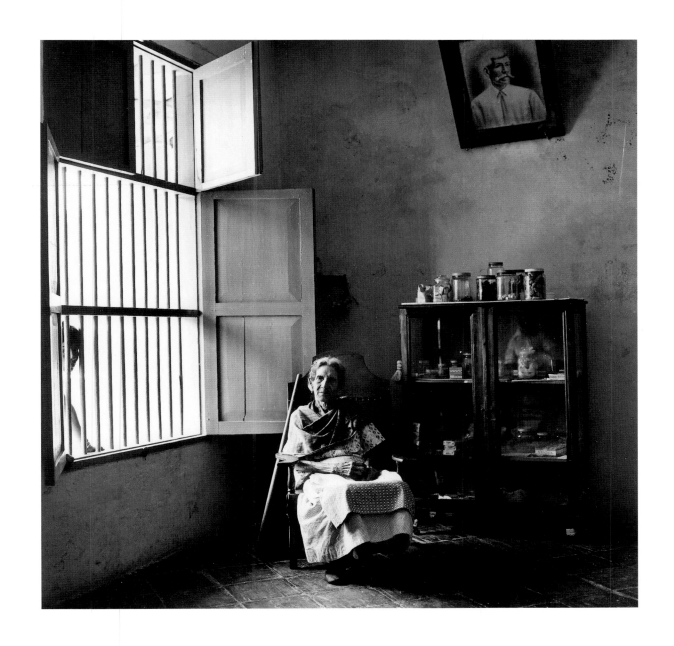

9. *La ciega* The Blind Woman

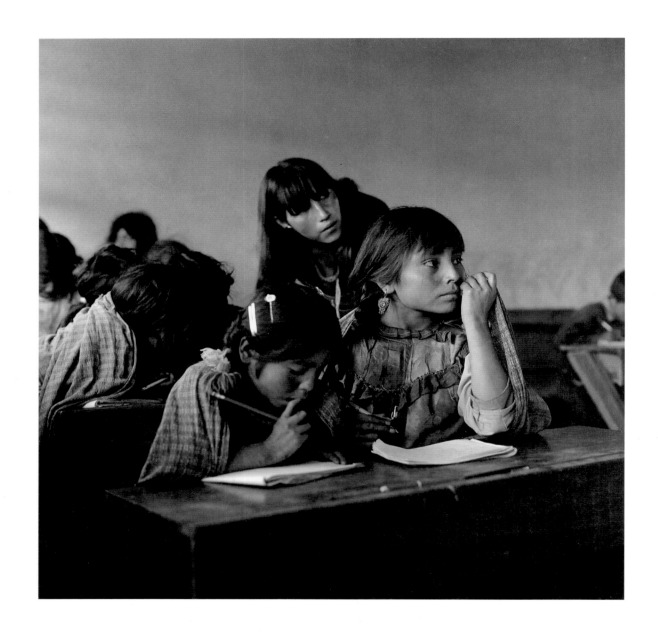

10. *Escuela mazahua*   *Mazahua School*

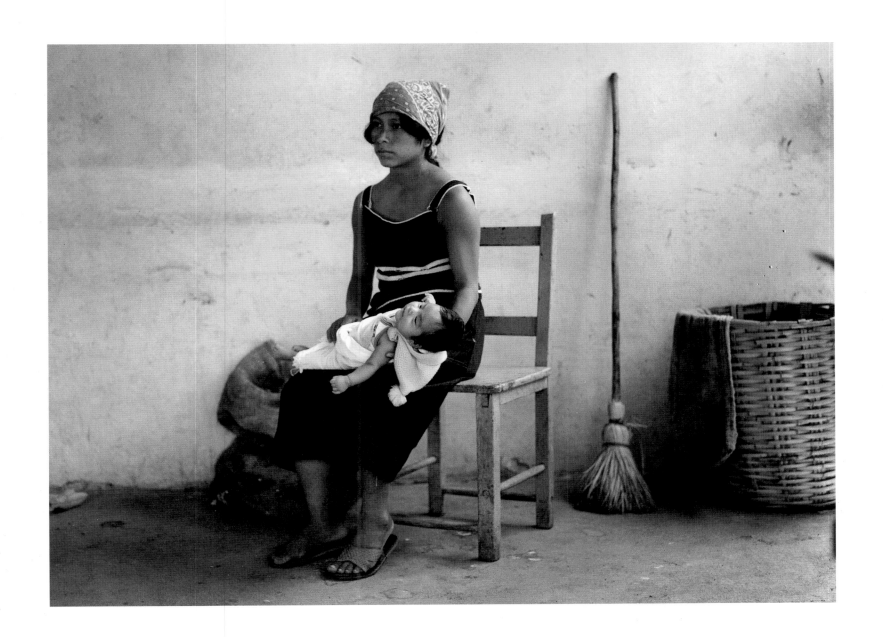

11. *La escoba* The Broom

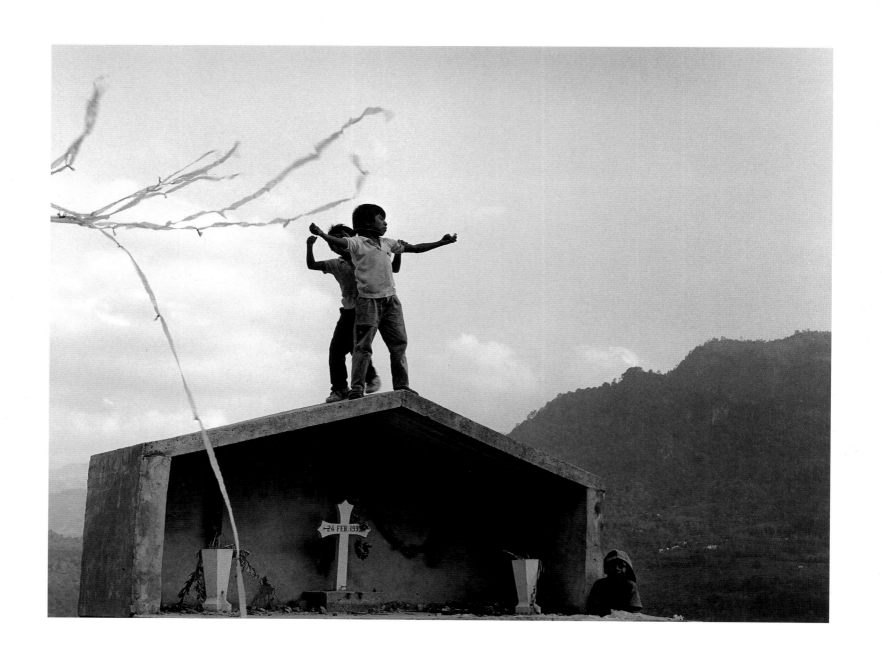

12. La cola del papalote *The Tail of the Kite*

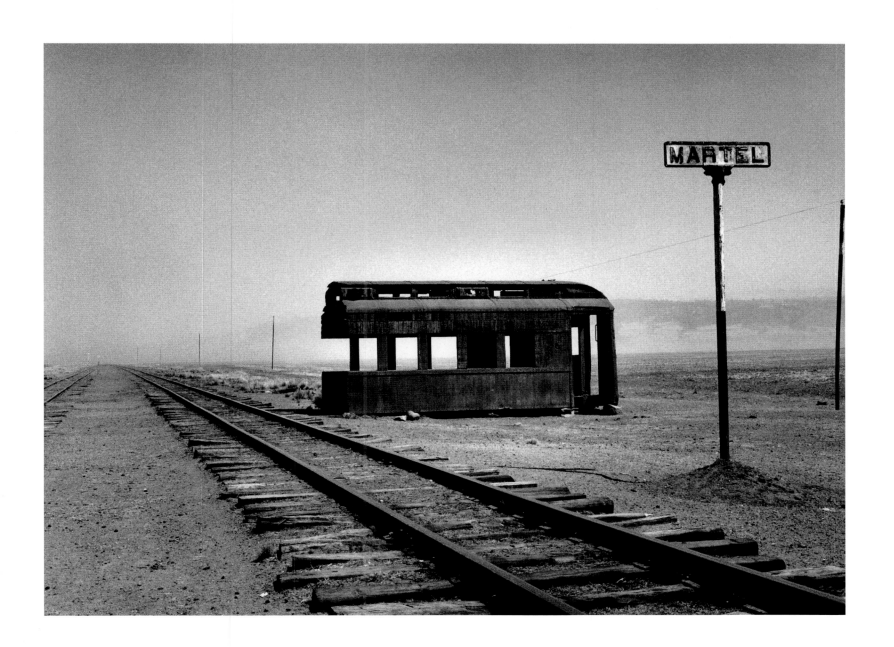

13. *Martel*   *Martel*

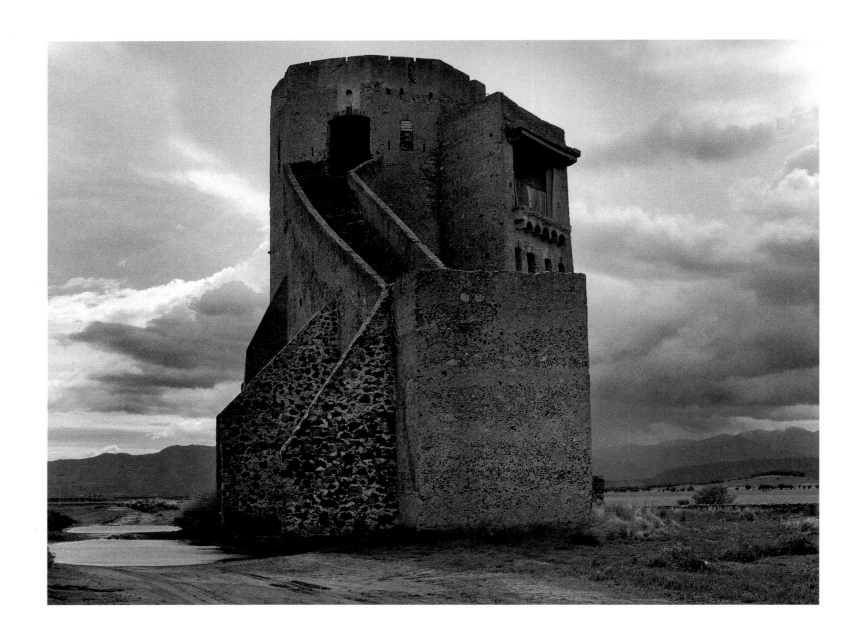

14. *La noria*   *The Water Tower*

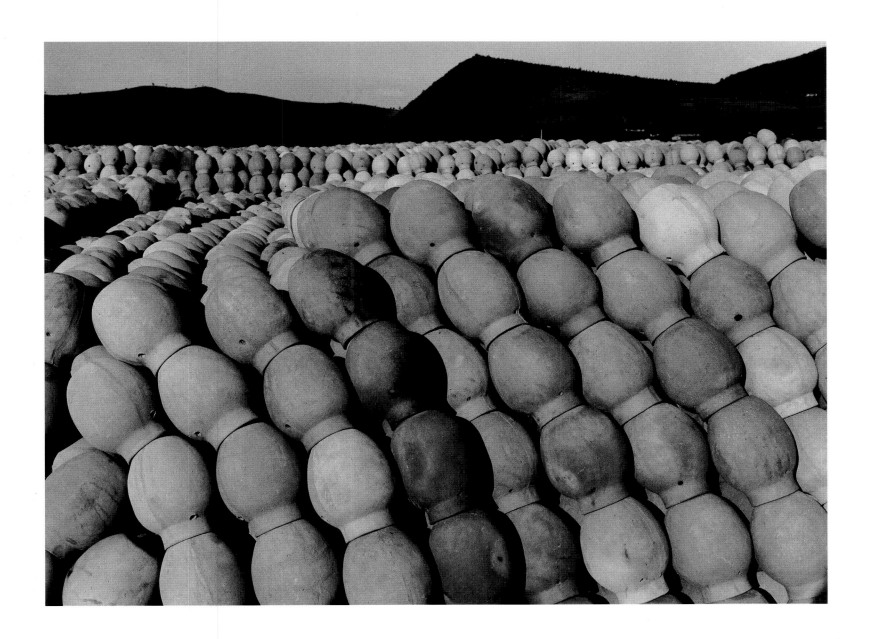

15. *Piñatas apiladas*   *Stacked Piñata Pots*

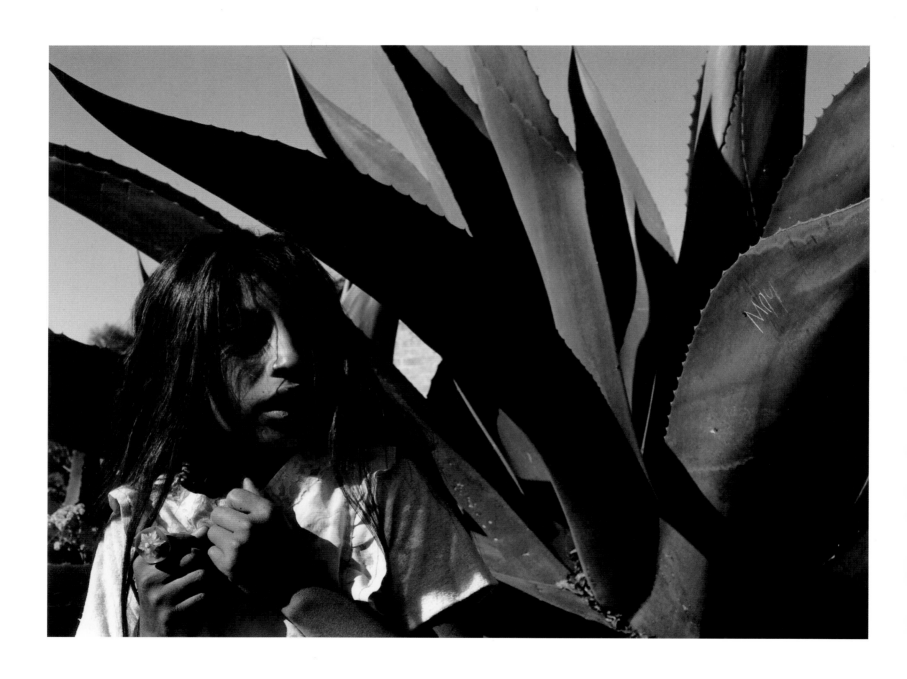

16. Niña con maguey *Girl with Maguey*

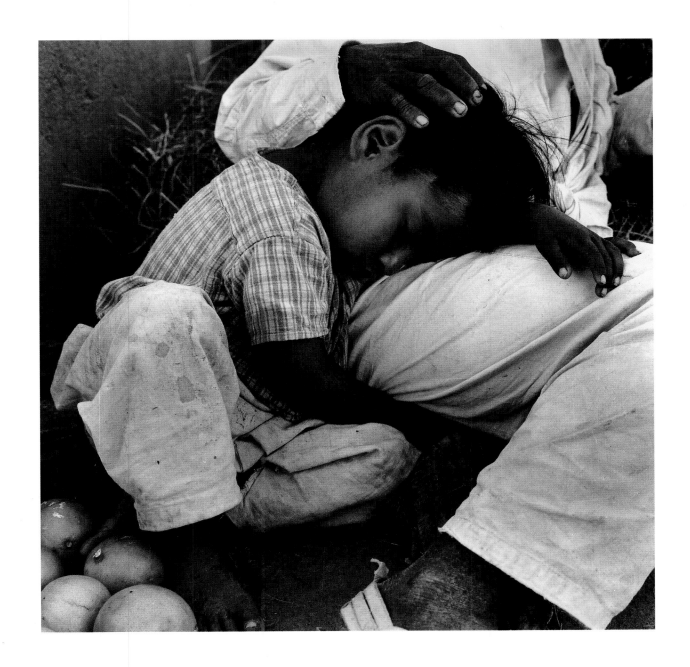

17. *Puesto de naranjas*   *Orange Stand*

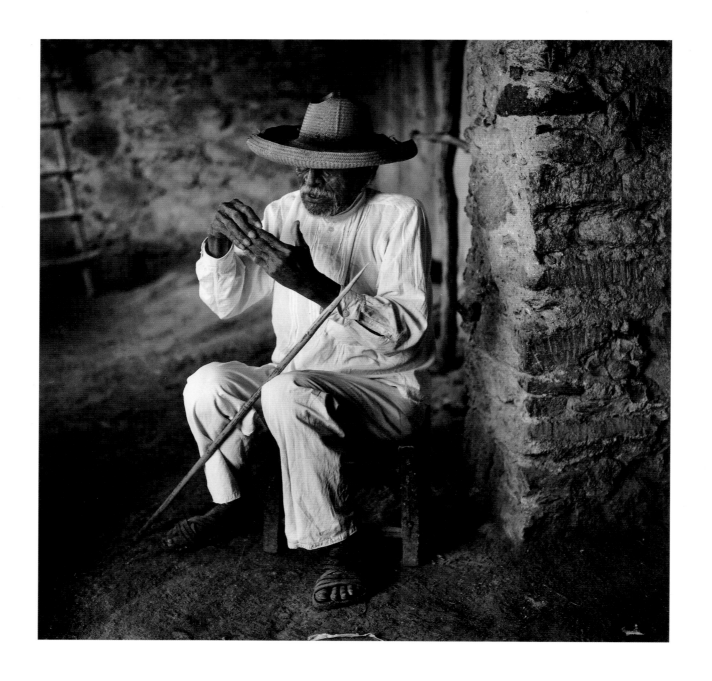

18. *"Así la construí"*   *"This is how I built it"*

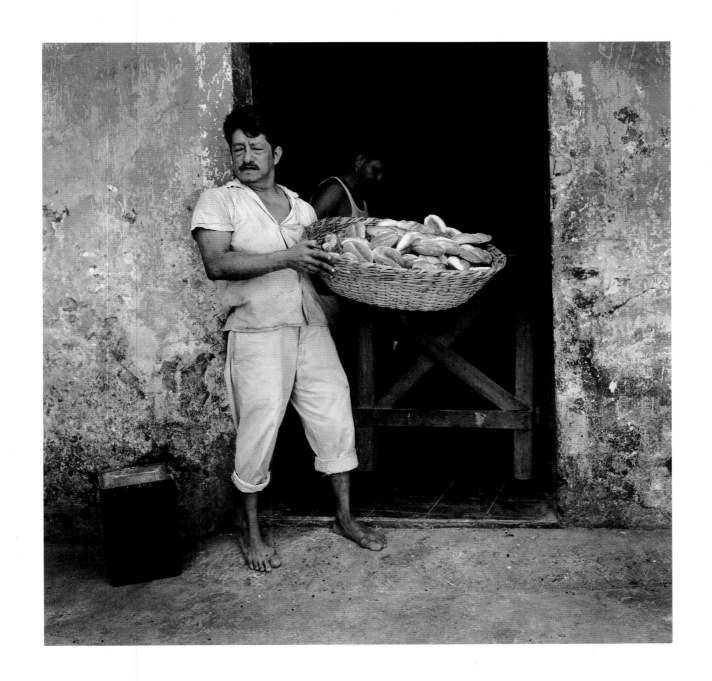

19. El pan   *Bread*

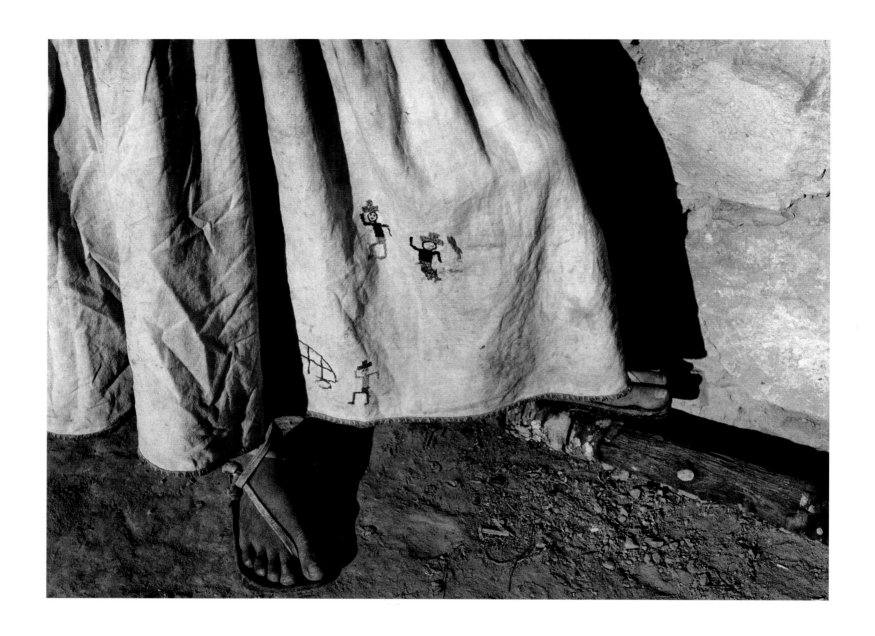

20. *Falda huichola*   *Huichol Skirt*

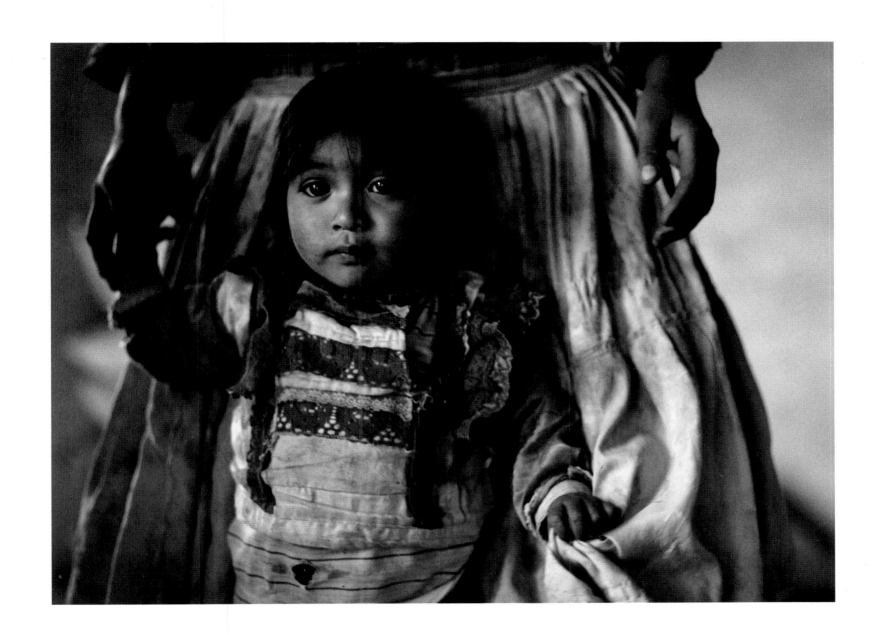

21. *Delantal* *Apron*

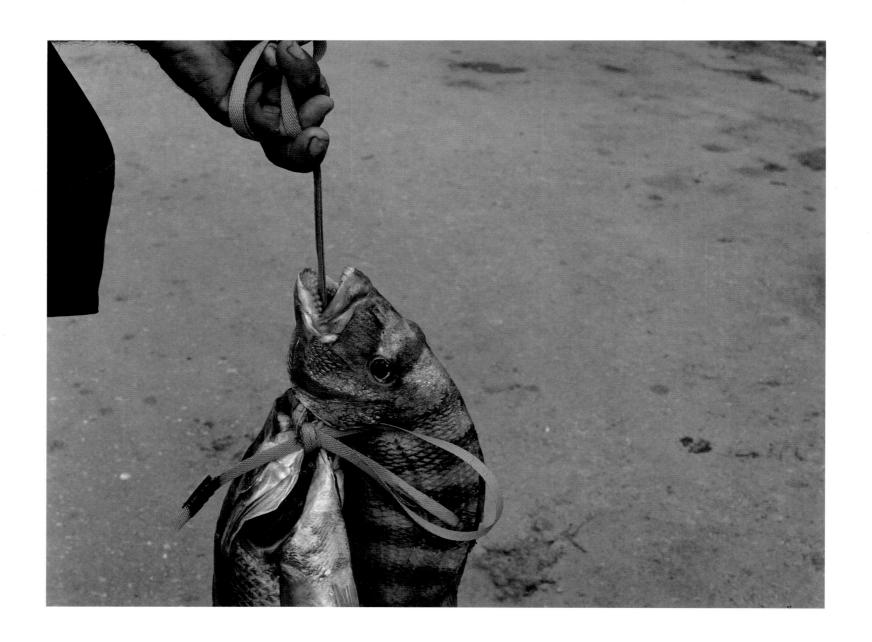

22. *Pescado* *Fish*

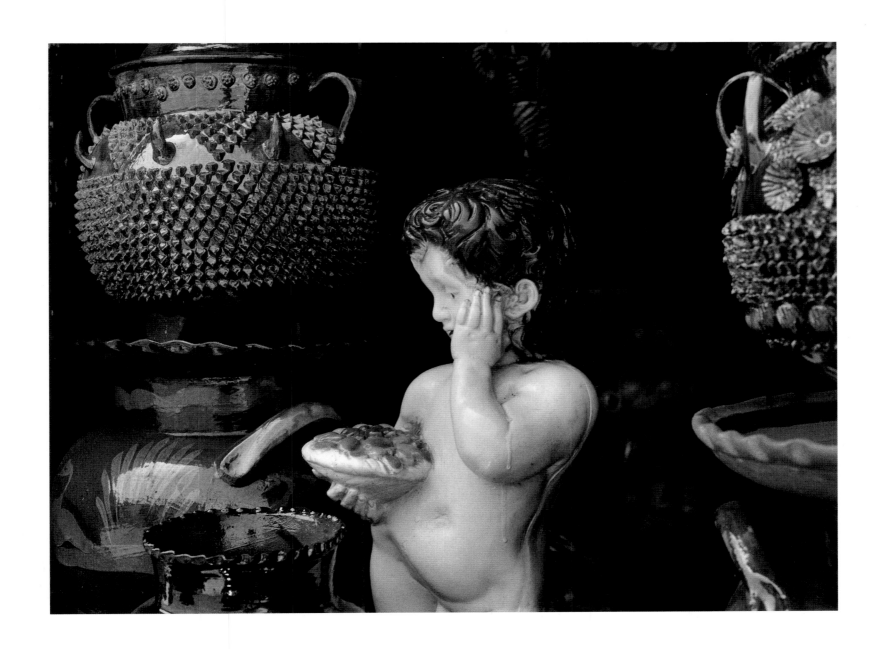

23. *"¿Qué tal?"*   *"What's going on?"*

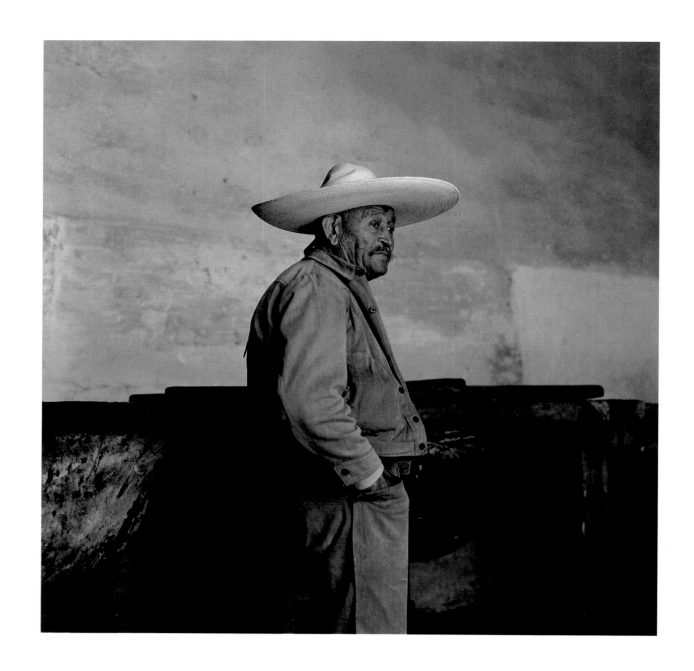

24. *El mayordomo* *The Foreman*

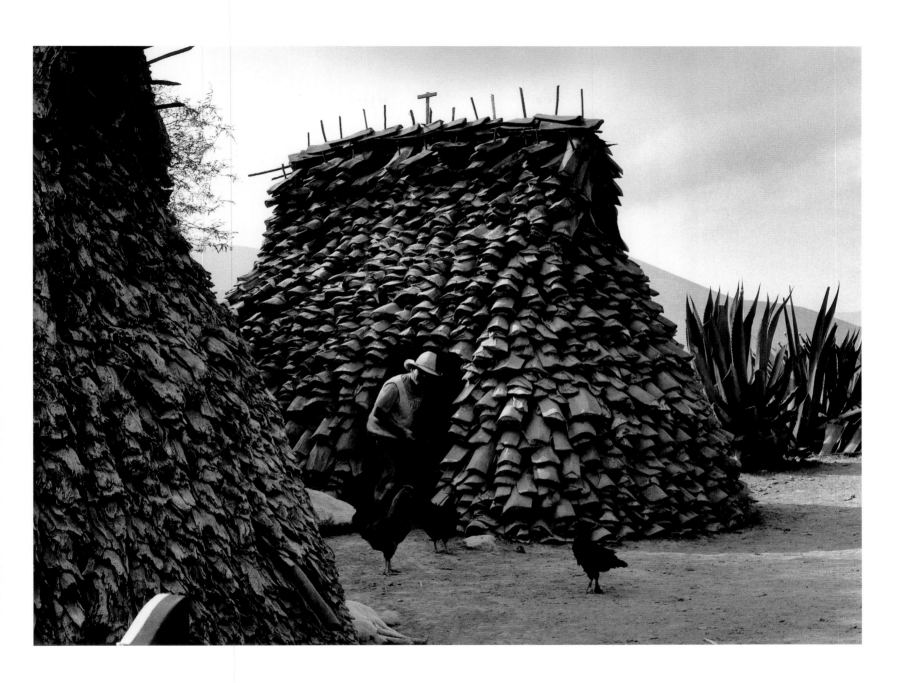

25. *Casa de maguey*   *Maguey House*

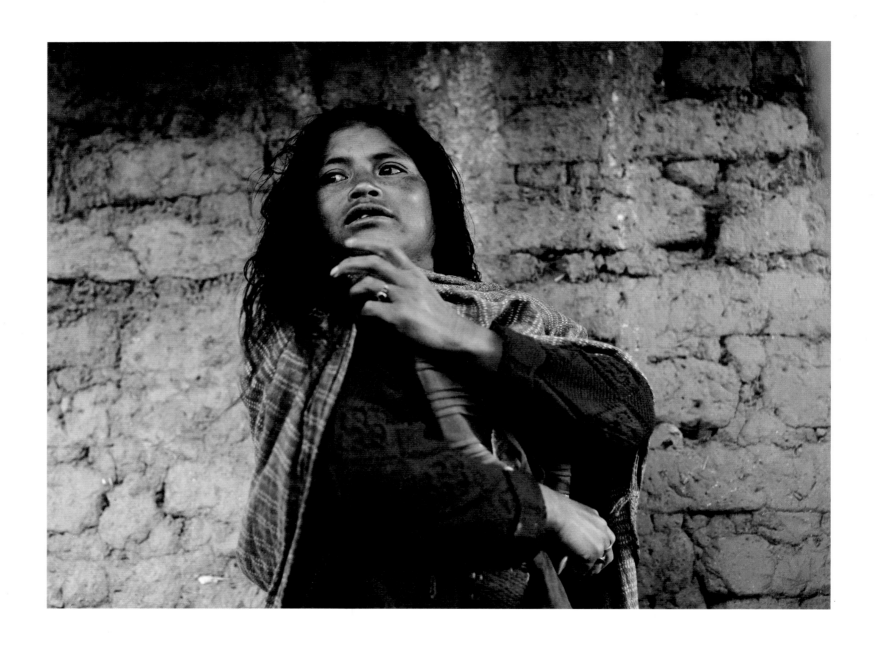

26. *Mujer otomí*   *Otomí Woman*

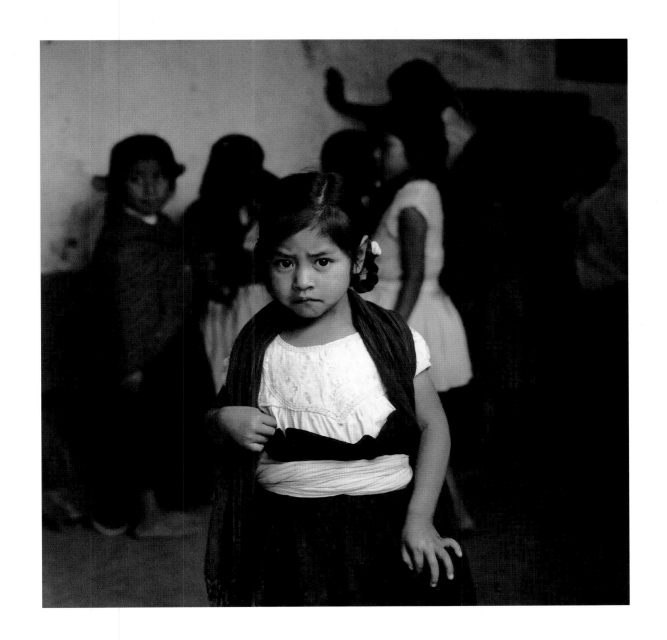

27. *Recreo*   *Recess*

28. *Huipil de tapar* *Headdress*

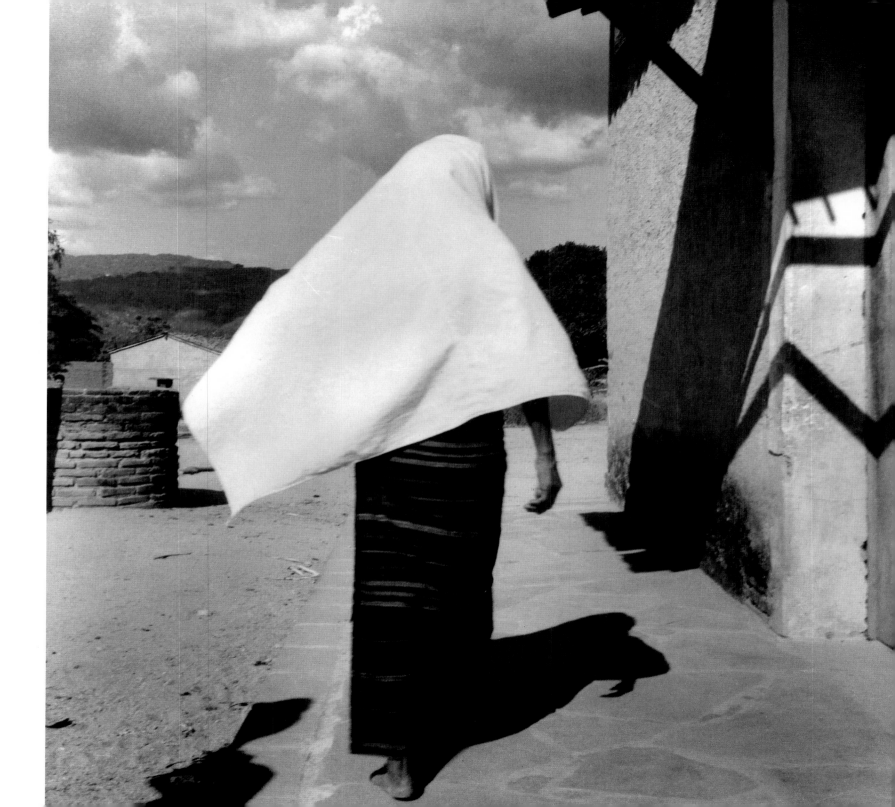

THEIR
CELEBRATIONS

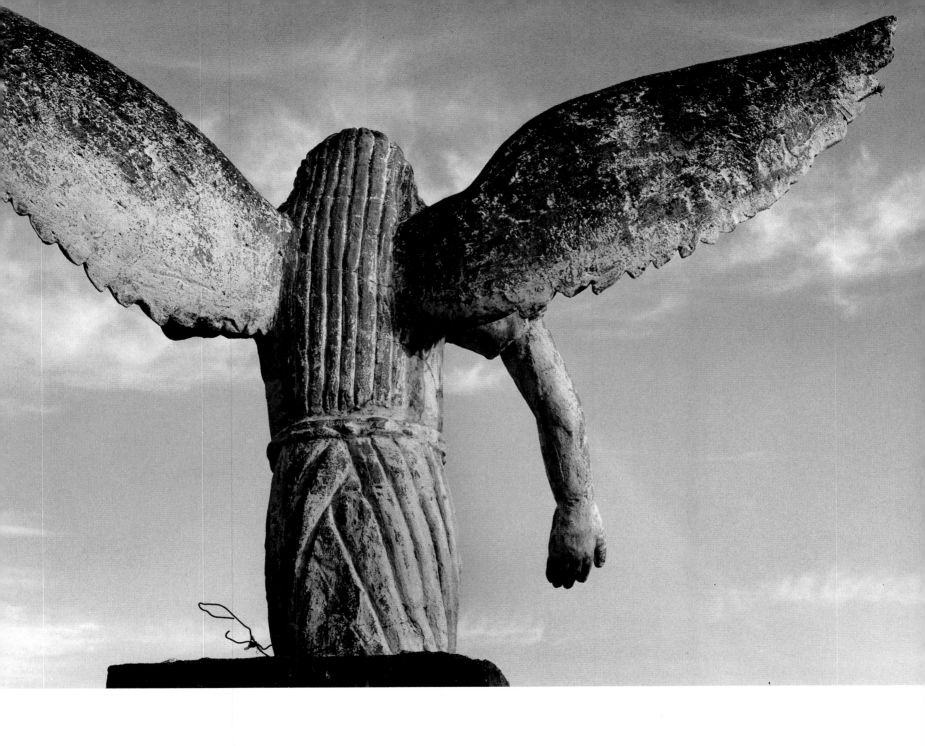

29. El ángel exterminador The Exterminating Angel

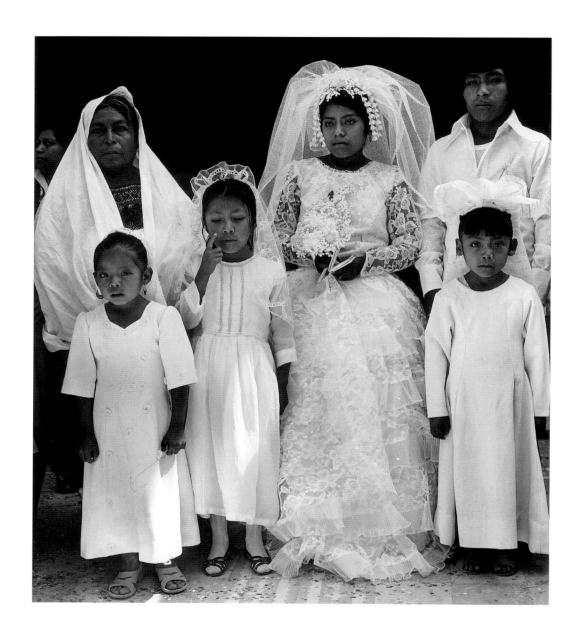

30. Tres generaciones Three Generations

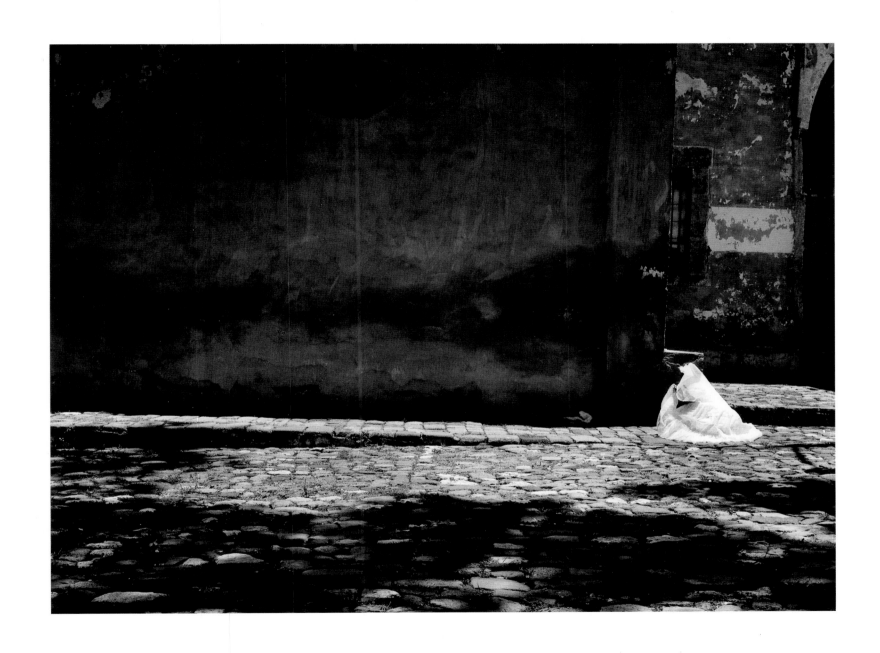

31. *Primera comunión* First Communion

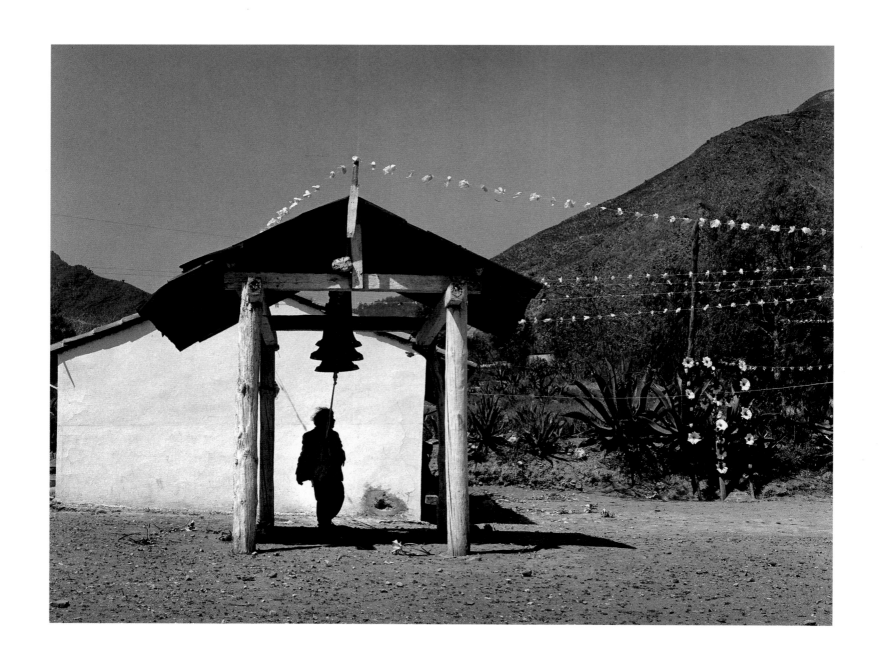

32. *Las campanas*   *Church Bells*

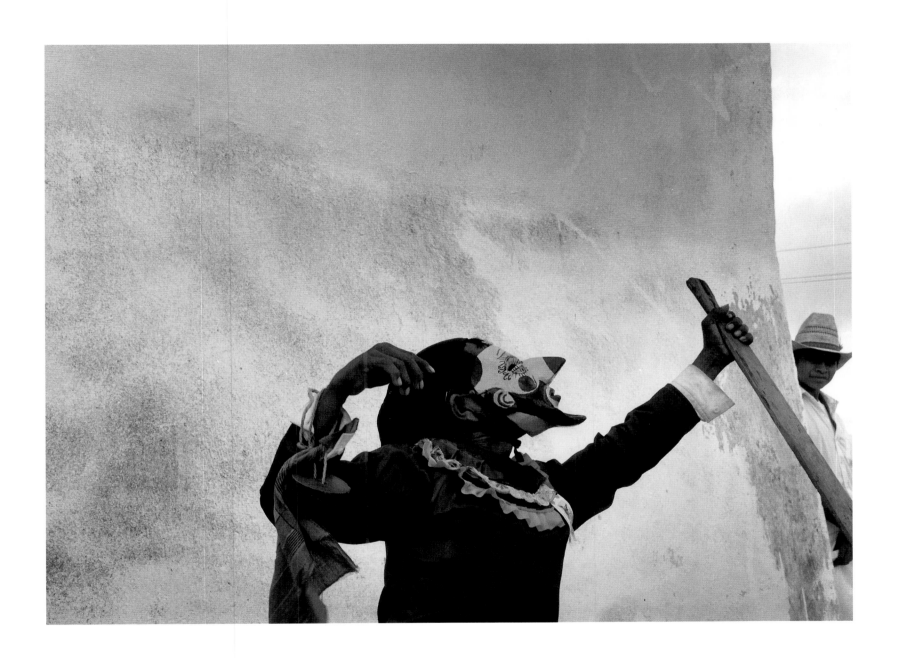

33. La espada *The Sword*

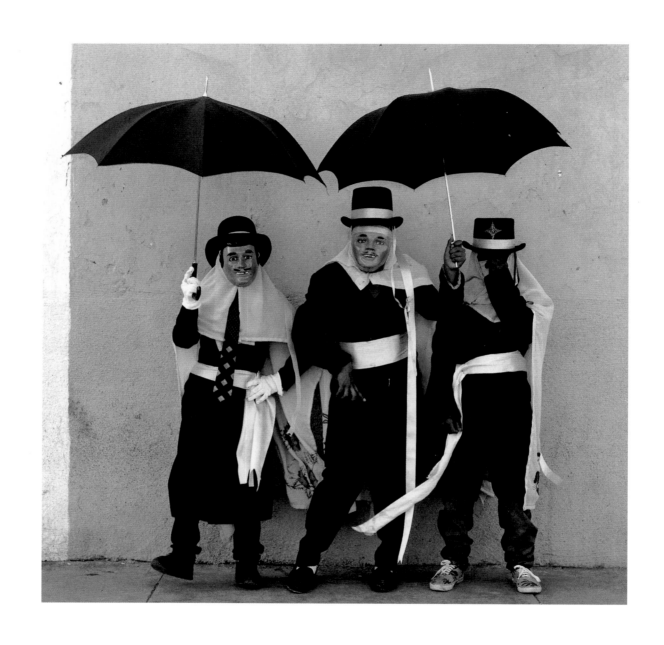

34. Danza de los paragüeros   *Dance of the Umbrella Vendors*

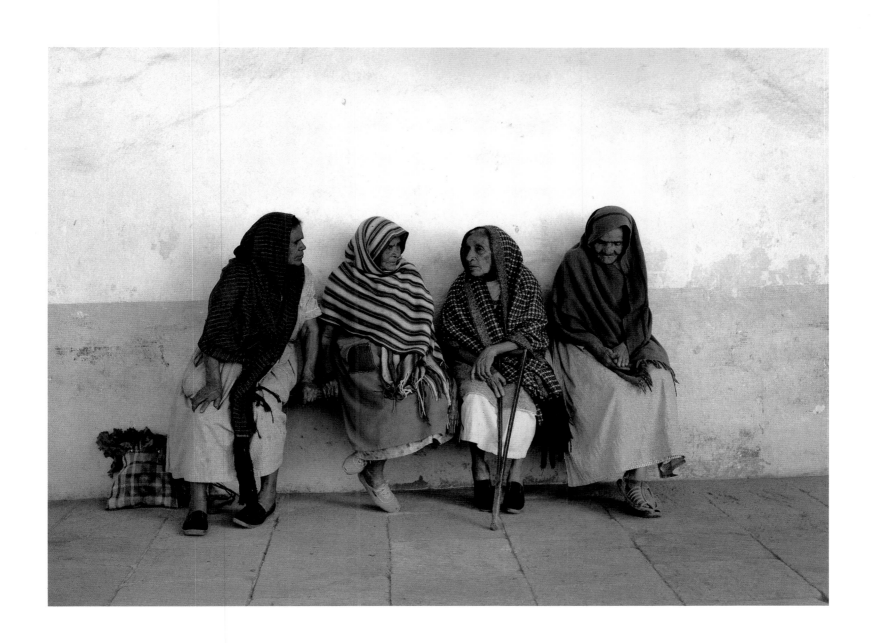

35. *Esperando al padrecito* *Waiting for the Priest*

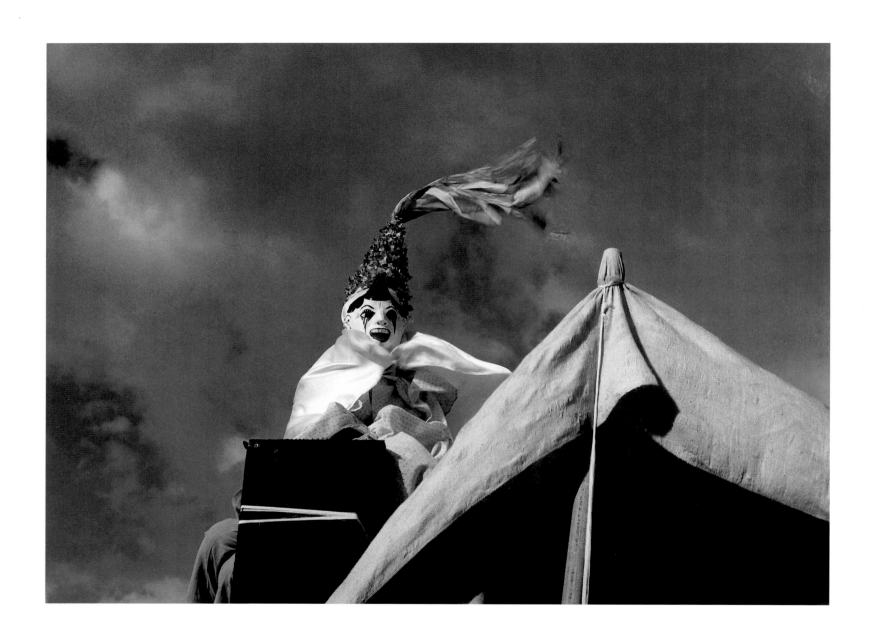

36. *Carnaval*   *Carnival*

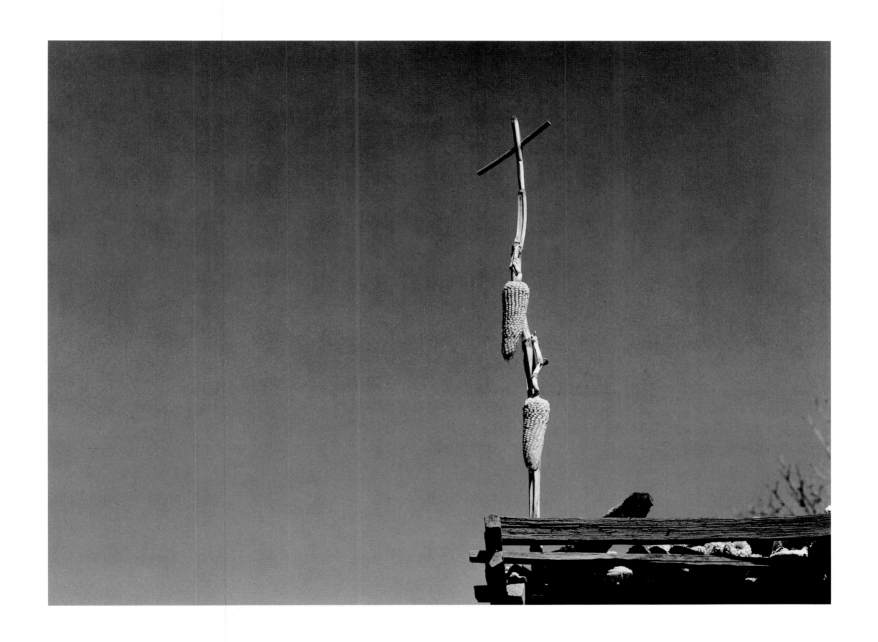

37. *La consagración del maíz*   The Blessing of the Corn

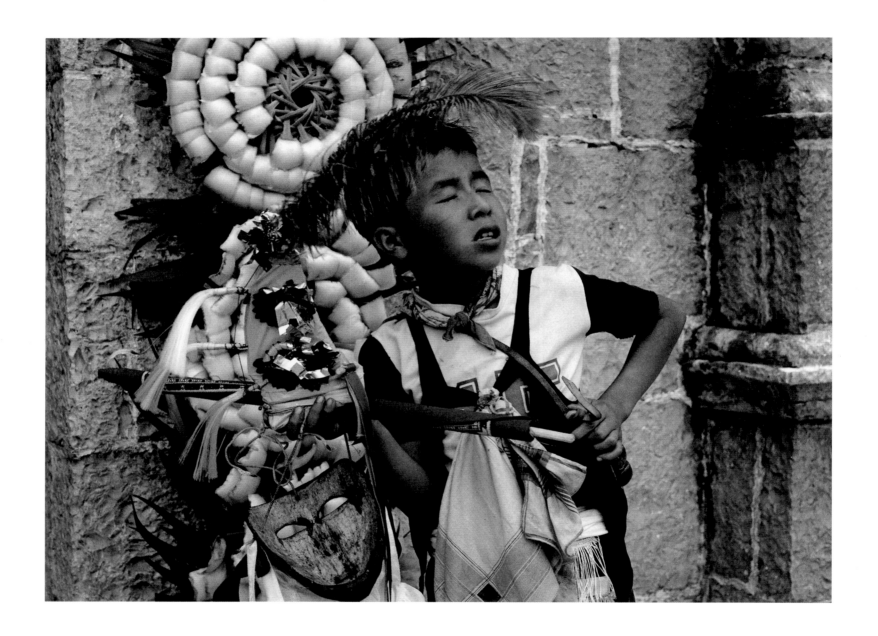

38. Dos máscaras *Two Masks*

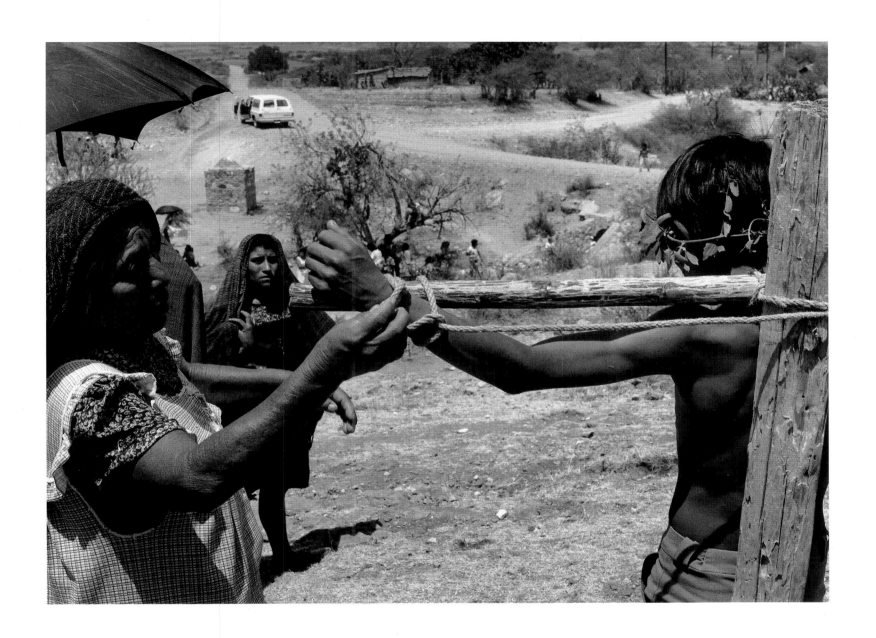

39. *Crucifixión*   *Crucifixion*

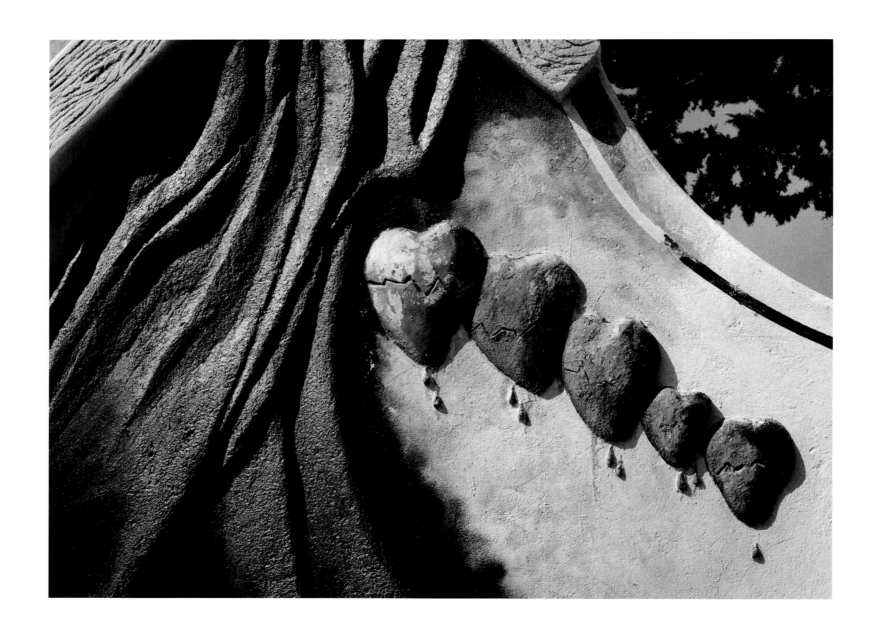

40. *Corazones tristes* *Broken Hearts*

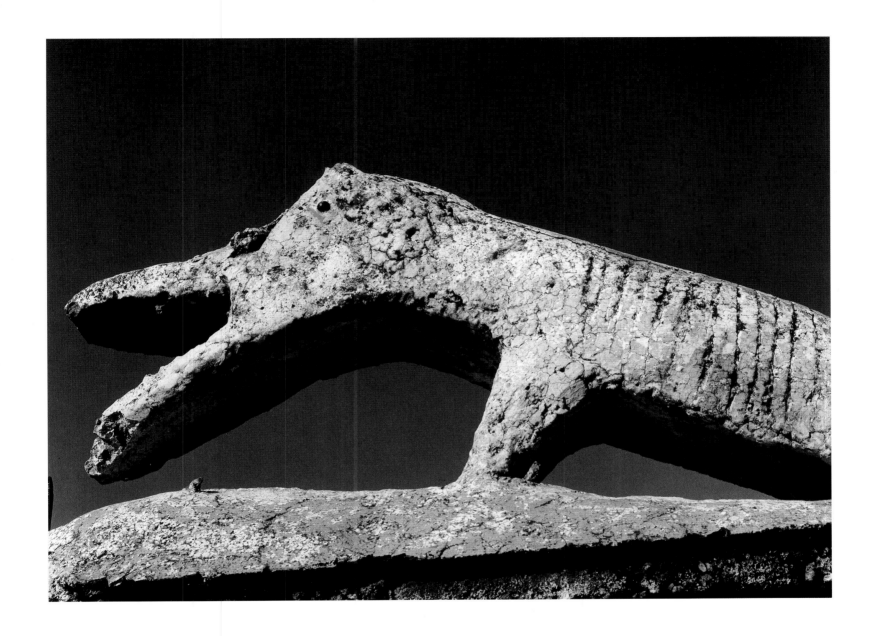

41. *Bestia*   *Beast*

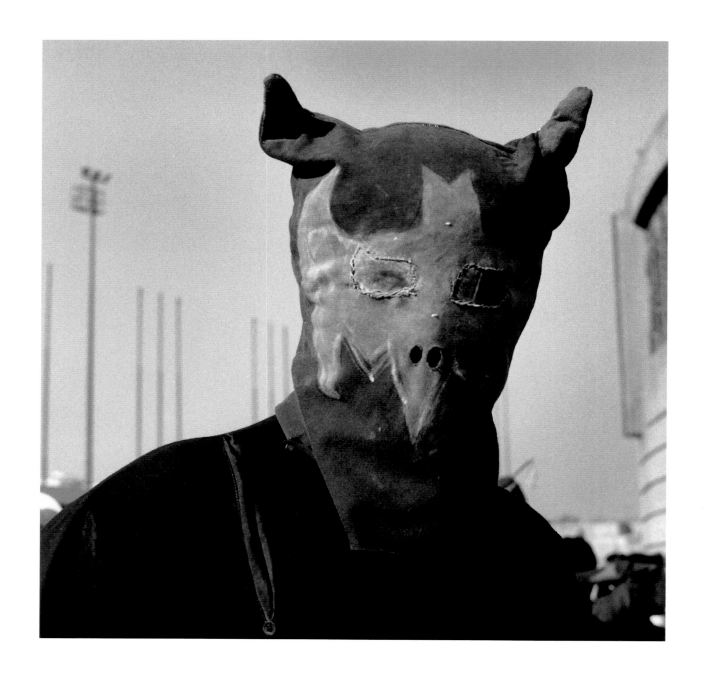

42. *Batman* *Batman*

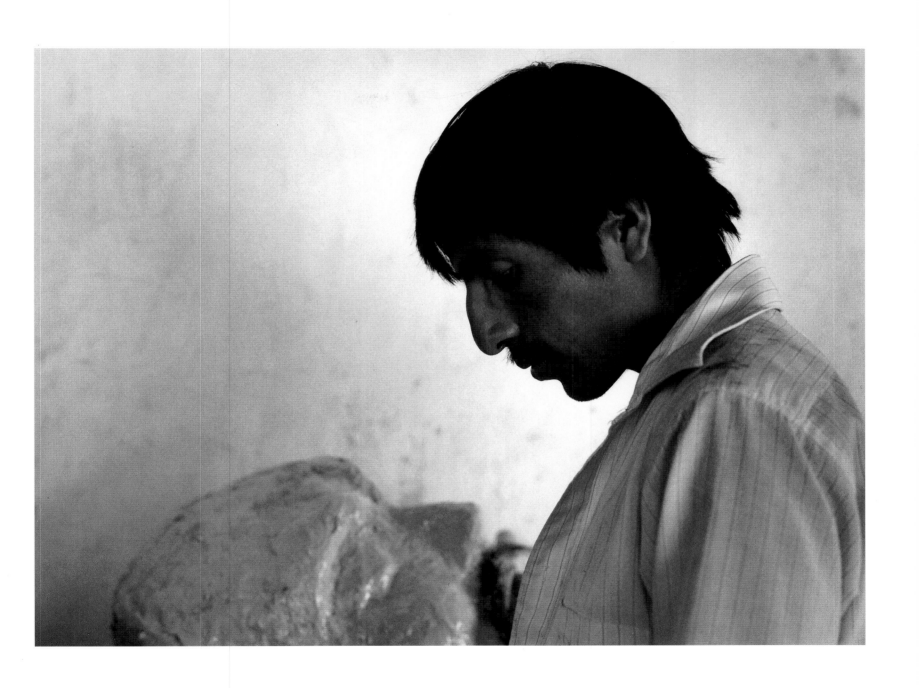

43. *Artesano, Yalalag, Oaxaca* Artisan, Yalalag, Oaxaca

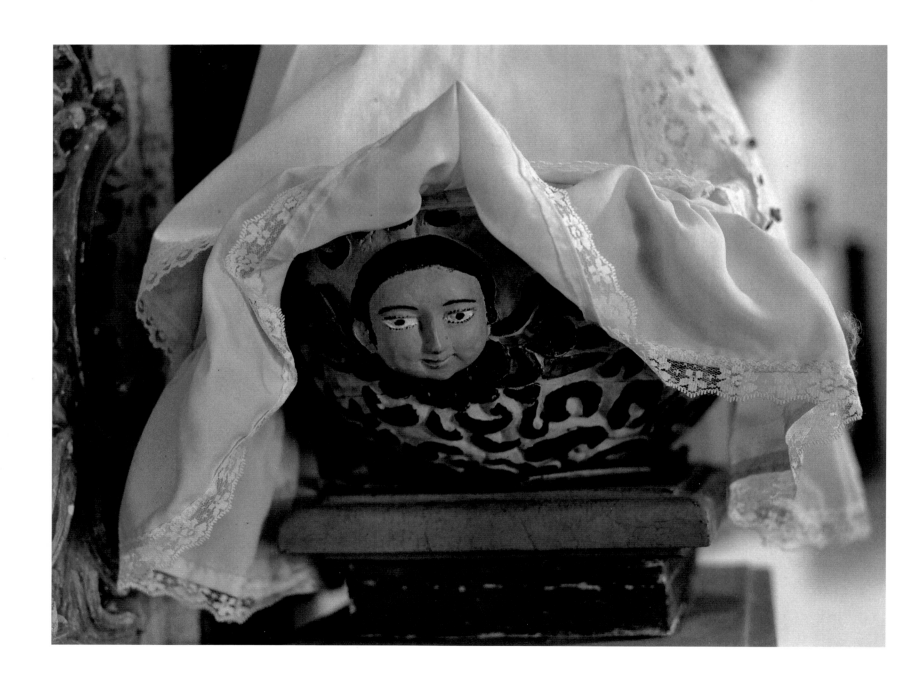

44. Asomando   *Under the Saint's Skirt*

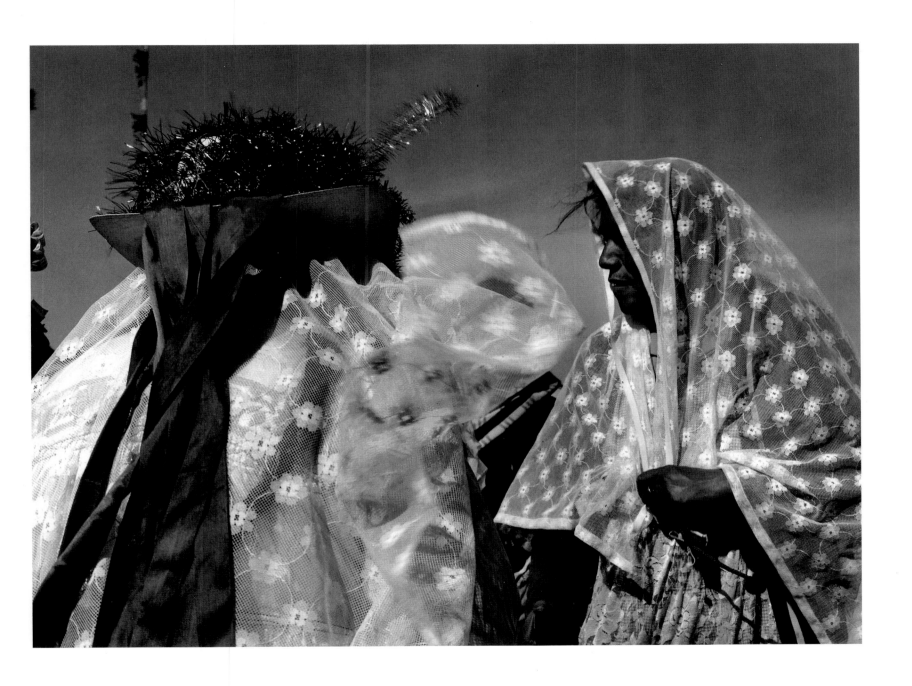

45. Danza de las pastoras   *Dance of the Shepherdesses*

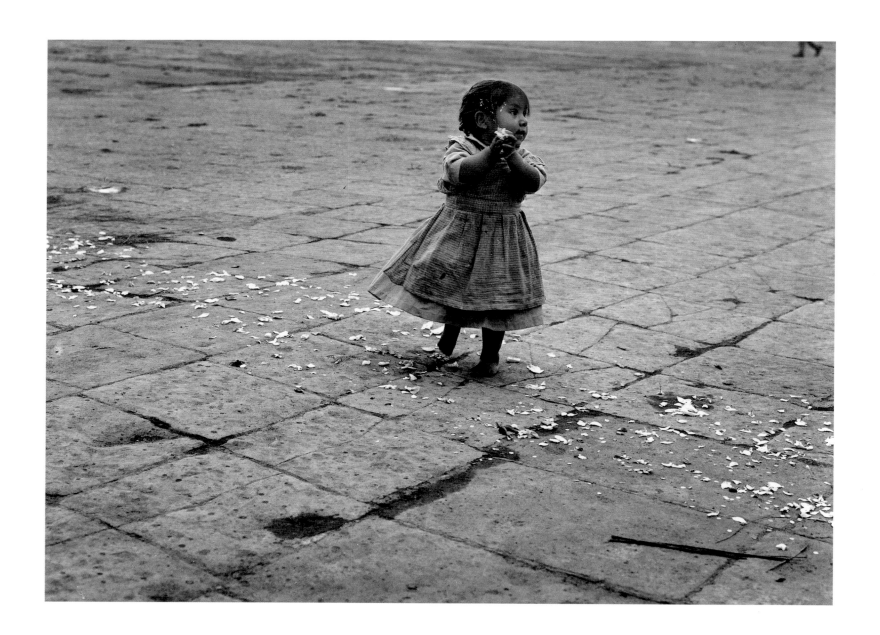

46. Pétalos   *Petals*

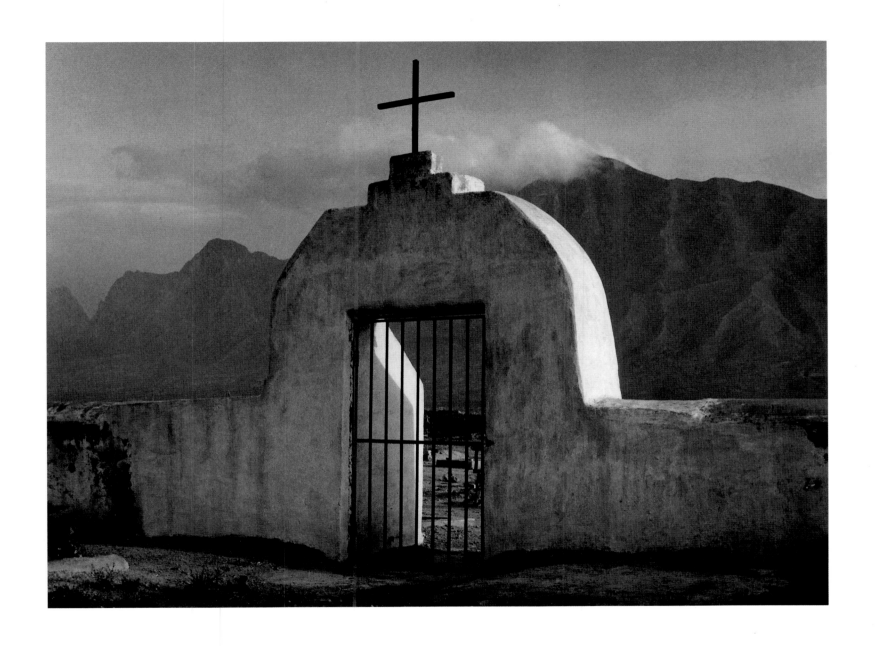

47. Entrada del cementerio   *Entrance to the Cemetery*

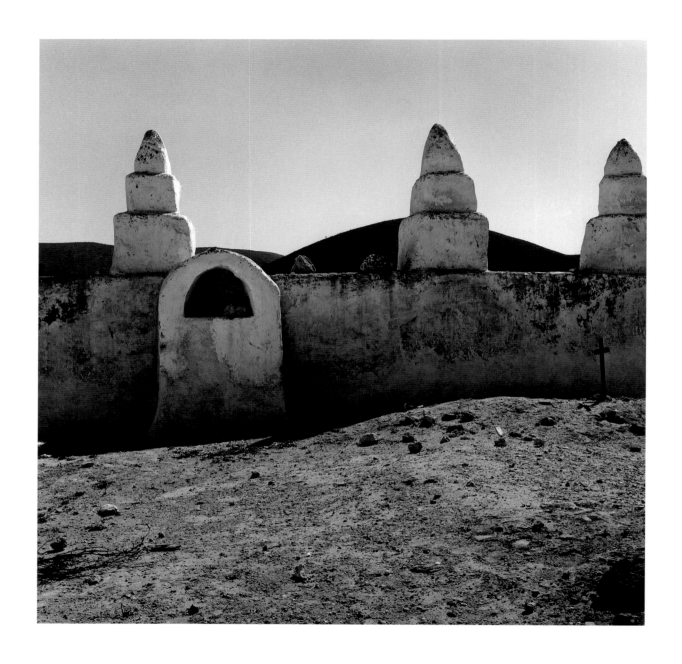

48. *Atrio, Hidalgo*   *Hidalgo Churchyard*

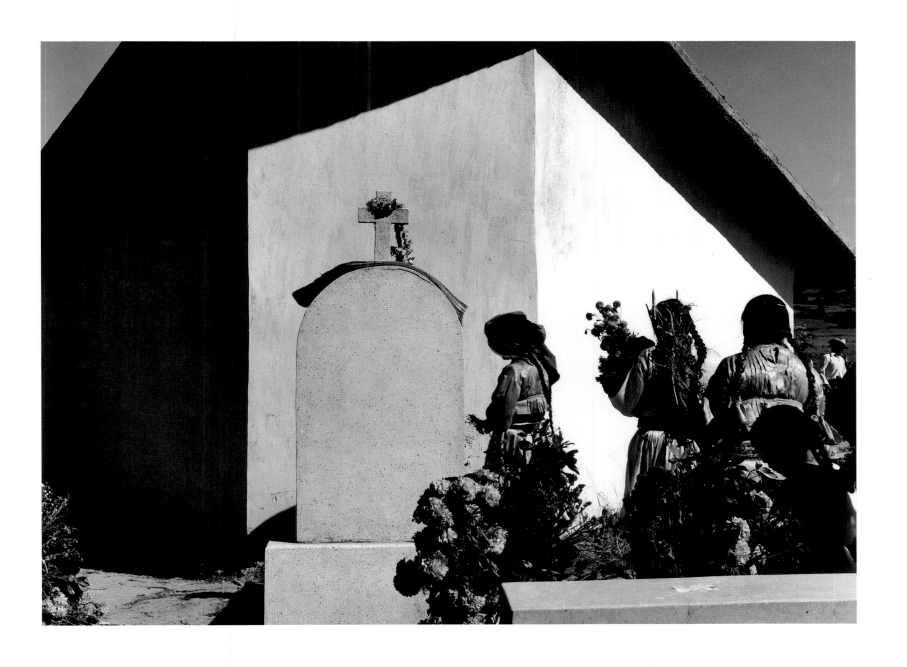

49. Día de los Muertos, Mazahua   Day of the Dead, Mazahua

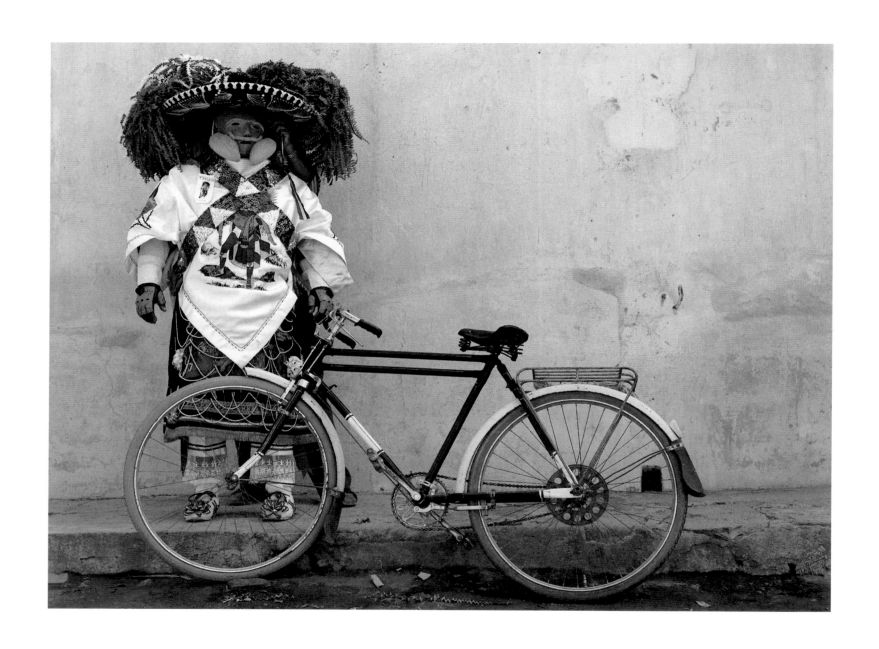

50. *Danzante con bicicleta* *Dancer with Bicycle*

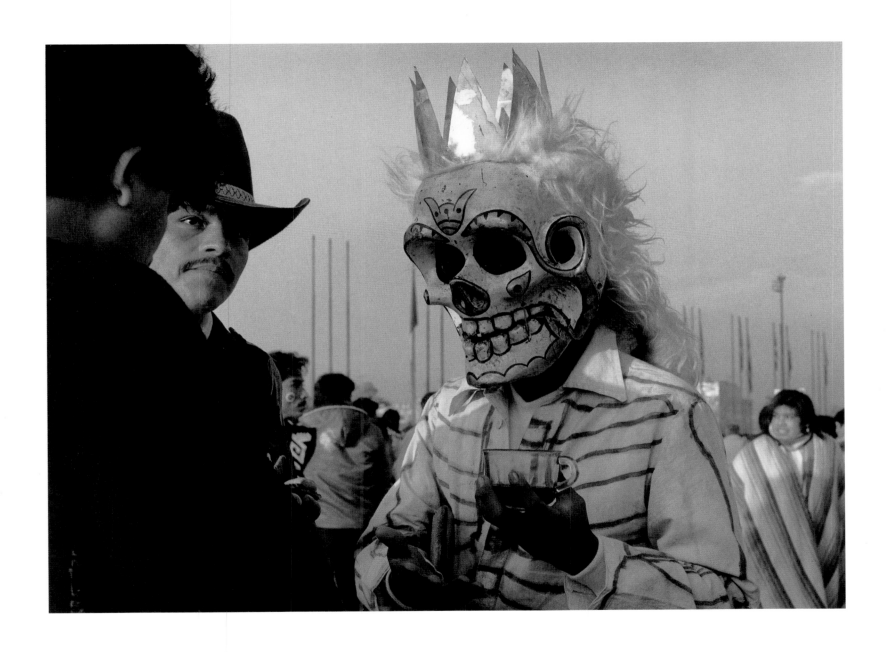

51. *La muerte también bebe café*   Death Also Drinks Coffee

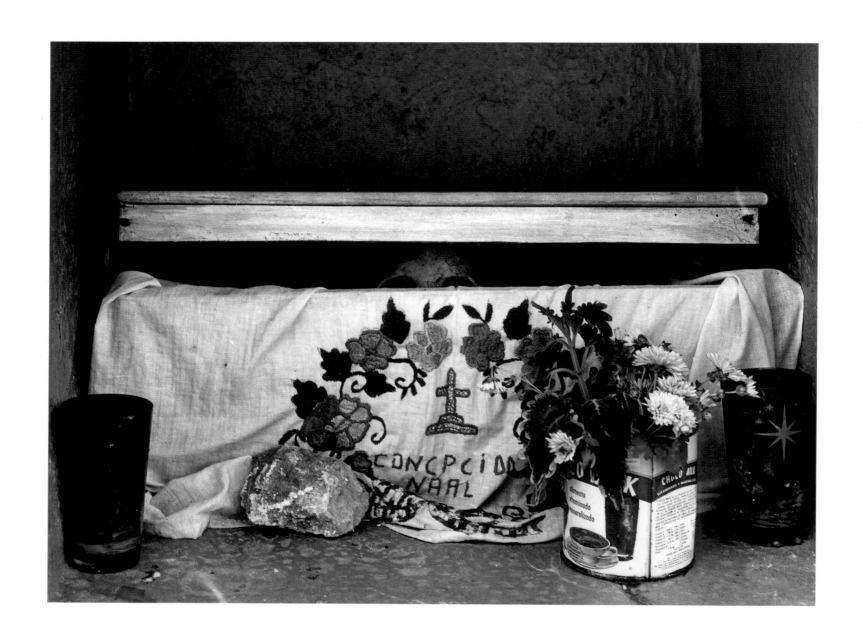

52. *Ultima mirada*   *Last Glimpse*

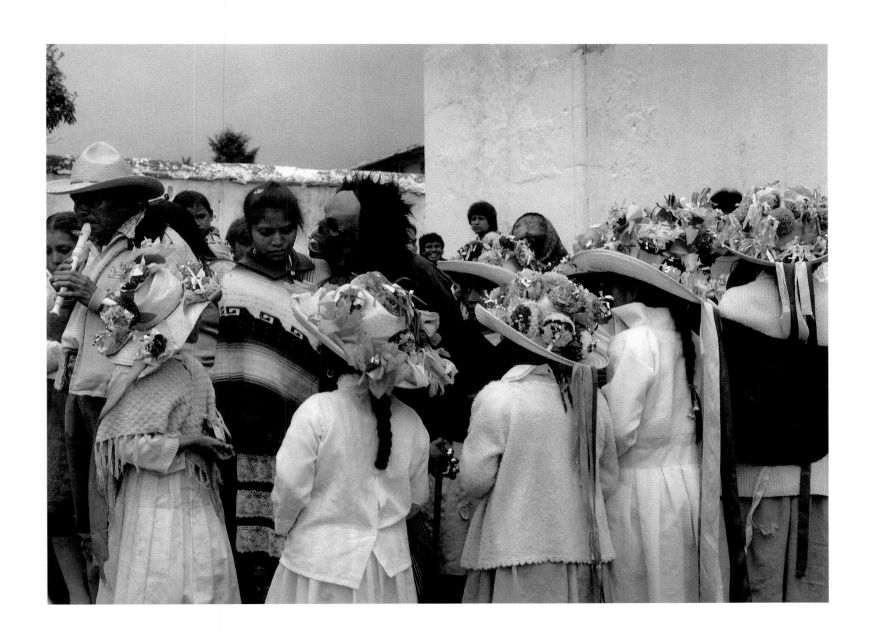

53. *Beso de la muerte*   *Kiss of Death*

54. *Osario* *Pauper's Grave*

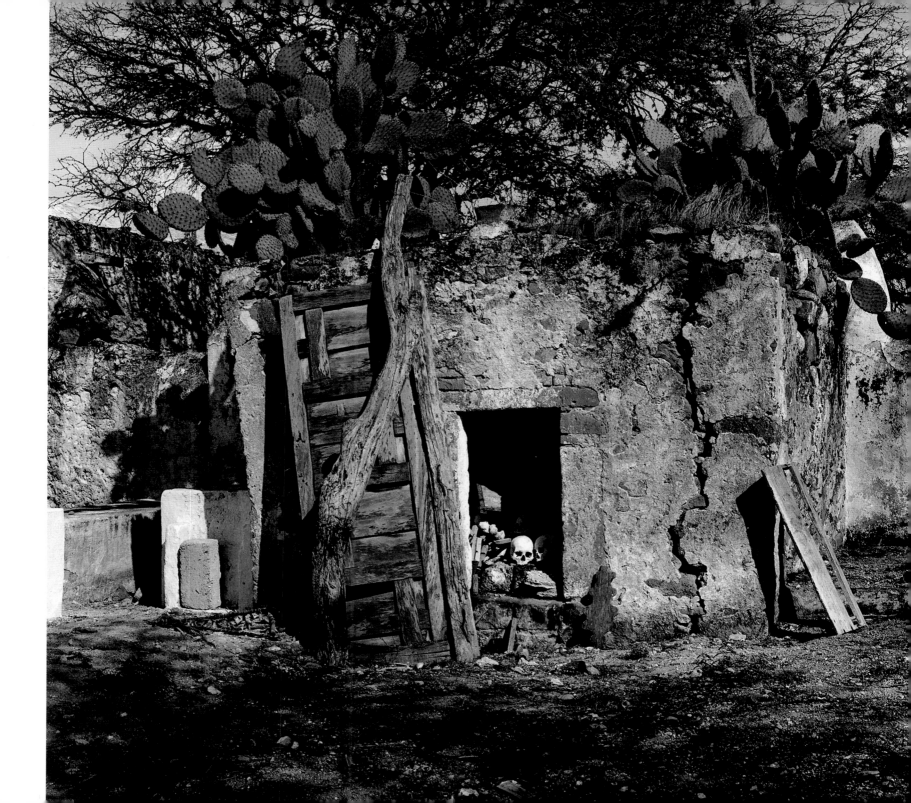

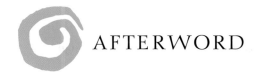 AFTERWORD

And Thus We Resist Death: The Photographic Cycles of Mariana Yampolsky

BY FRANCISCO REYES PALMA

Photography is born of a depredatory gesture and saturated with a violence that has its origin in the act of subtracting an image from the visible universe.

This is only the beginning of a practice which, in spite of its 150-year metropolitan history, has attempted to colonize and subjugate the image of the Other, making that which is photographed exotic by masking or estheticizing it. Mariana Yampolsky knows this and acts accordingly. She never puts the capture of her images above the innate integrity of her subjects. For her, even constructed objects are subjective forms and deserve respectful treatment.

She realizes, moreover, that her medium places her in a paradoxical modality of power that is capable of fixing a fragment of life and, at the same time, saving it as memory. She uses the actualizing potential of the medium in such a way that the ethical and the esthetic are inseparable.

During childhood, Yampolsky absorbed her family's tradition of tolerance and love of knowledge. She internalized the principle of cultural equality held by her great-uncle, anthropologist Franz Boas, who believed that cultural difference is not a stigma, but can be an enriching aspect of human experience.

Yampolsky gave her first book of photographs the title *La raíz y el camino* (Roots and paths; 1985), two words in apparent opposition: one implying permanence, the other movement, creating a dialectic of ceaseless wandering through the realm of identity.

As a young artist of nineteen, Yampolsky came to Mexico City in 1944 to join the Taller de Gráfica Popular (Popular Graphic Arts Workshop), a small republic of printmakers whose members shared a concern for the inner lives and aspirations of the Mexican people. There she began to treasure the diverse and complex cultures of Mexico, a country she soon made her own.[1]

But in 1959, concerned that the Taller had lost its original spirit, Yampolsky left it, as did a number of its other members, foremost among them Leopoldo Méndez, who had been the mainstay and guide of the collective.[2] A decade later, Méndez, Yampolsky, and the photographer Manuel Alvarez Bravo published a definitive book on Mexican folk art.[3] As co-editor, Yampolsky was in charge of visiting museums and private collections to select objects to be included in the book. She also traveled throughout the country to photograph costumes and ceremonies, houses and objects.

Her extensive contact with varied artistic manifestations strengthened her appreciation of the individual effort as an expression that validates the collective whole, as opposed to a system that exalts individualism while producing social asymmetry and human stereotypes.

In choosing photography as her medium in the 1960s, Yampolsky discovered a new kind of artistic process. The first stage is centered in subjectivity; this liminal moment comes with the first click of the shutter when the gaze, the gesture, and the sound become one: at that very instant Yampolsky feels an incommunicable inner joy, a moment of astonishment—of discovery—that determines her obsession with the photographic act. Then there follows a latent phase in which she distances herself to some degree: the revealed image ceases to carry that first emotion; once the image is fixed she has no interest in its critical fortune or its success. Finally the photographer reaffirms her sense of service, so important to the ideals of her formative years, unfolding the image in the book, multiplying it to constitute her pragmatic space. She supports this imperative of the medium in opposition to the aureatic cult of original, limited editions, made fashionable by the reverential spaces of the museum or the mercantile spaces of the gallery.

Yampolsky has based the logic of her production on a series of photographic investigations with recurrent themes. The most extensive of her studies concerns architecture and is distinguished by its valorization of cultural aspects capable of resisting the seduction of the machine. She redeems the principle of craftsmanship on a human scale in dialogue with the natural world. Vernacular architecture, Indian and mestizo, distillations of secular knowledge enriched through time, appears in *La casa en la tierra* (1981) and *La casa que canta* (1982). Later she followed the traces of the haciendas of Mexico from the earliest years of New Spain to the nineteenth century in *Estancias del olvido* (1987) and *Haciendas poblanas* (1992). In these books Yampolsky plays with the contrasts between the lordly delirium of castles, palaces, fortresses, and mansions, with their strange, hybrid models, and the presence of the modest dwellings of the common people. *The Traditional Architecture of Mexico* (1993) sums up these endeavors.

In recent years, the photographer has made another ongoing study of buildings that defy the homogenizing dictates of the constructive canon. The thematic repertory of her photographs is as dynamic as the world toward which she directs her camera, dedicated to capturing the shifting identities of heterogeneous signs. Yampolsky's gaze has become familiar with hybridization, with the movement of objects through time, without harboring a purist nostalgia for that which changes or disappears or taking a primitivist approach dictated by financial or touristic impositions. She does not promote either a return to the past or a vision of progress, only an active present, the point of emergence of which is the encounter between the photographer and the creative signs of the Other.

In her daily tasks, the photographer makes use of her lifelong artistic training. Among her childhood memories she finds the magic of her artist-father's darkroom and the guessing games they played in which she identified Impressionistic juxtapositions of colors.

Her sharp eye was trained, by years in the Taller, to the chromatic scale of black and white, with its infinite range of intermediate tones. Her personal inclination lies in her system of composing through the lens, which she does with a sense of equilibrium and completeness that places her images both in the realm of art and in the sphere of life. She adheres to the tenets of straight photography, but not in a search for Truth, because the emotional intensity of the world around her overrides any need to construct the photograph from a pose or in the laboratory.

A second series of investigations focuses on the strength of the feeling of community: *Tlacotalpan* (1987) and *Mazahua* (1993). Opposed to an ethic of accumulation, Yampolsky prefers the notion of lavish celebration in the ecstatic sense of imagination and shared ceremony. In contrast to an art that represents a simulation of the Self, this photographer's path is heterodox, honoring the direct image and thereby keeping alive the referent, inseparable from its material, affective, ceremonial, and esthetic world. Her poetics of everyday life invert the mandates of power, which deny the visibility of cultures that have long and profound traditions. Her photography encompasses forms that overflow their boundaries, and forms that express visual syntheses; she moves with equal freedom between the realistic and the abstract. Yampolsky harvests traces of vitality, traces which in the moment of being viewed recover their force and move the spirit.

With the carefulness of an investigator, Yampolsky assigns genealogies and ancestries to the rich experience of humankind, and creates archives that preserve the subtle and irreducible gaze of the people. Thousands of images await their turns to occupy those places in the conceptual weave that will put them in published form.

She is currently working on a book about death as an imaginary domestic presence: habitats that aspire to eternity (cemeteries, flower-bedecked tombs, colossal crypts, shelters for melancholy sculptures); skeletons painted on bakery windows; breads sprinkled with a red reminiscent of cinnabar, as used in ancient burials; sugar skulls, toys, and innumerable effigies. The celebration of death and the act of photographing it seem to merge into the same ritual. In the camera's mechanical image we find death's multiple countenances, evidence of a physical reality, live absences that remind us of that which was once there, or a symbolic representation that casts a spell to protect us from the fragility of existence. To photograph is, in brief, a strange way to *be* death and to resist it.

Yampolsky's work can be defined as an anthropology of the emotions, a politics of memory leading to the creation of contexts capable of reconstructing experience and reclaiming possible futures. For Mariana Yampolsky, photography corresponds to a rite of initiation through which a community transmits that which it most treasures: a modern shamanic practice, mediated by optical technologies and chemical processes. Through this ritual the act of photography is consummated in the moment that ancestral knowledge is transmitted to the viewer, so that memory returns with the intensity of a metaphor of life.

—TRANSLATION BY DEBORAH CAPLOW

NOTES

1. Mariana Yampolsky always claimed to have been born in Mexico; to make it official she became a Mexican citizen in 1954. In this act of creating her own mythic origins, the photographer put an end to a tradition of dispersion and found her place. Her paternal grandparents had emigrated from Russia to the United States at the end of the century because of anti-Semitic persecution. Her German mother left Berlin upon marrying Yampolsky's father, an artist who came to Europe from the United States to study after winning a Prix de Rome. The rest of the German side of the family emigrated to Brazil at the beginning of the Second World War. Mariana was born in Chicago in 1925, but she grew up in an ambiance of European culture, of free thinkers, in the rural world of her grandfather's farm. Upon the death of her father in 1944, Mariana started off on the last of these exoduses, putting down her roots in Mexico City, which became the base of her activity.

2. Through printmaking, Yampolsky developed an ethic of service that later manifested itself in her work as an editor. In the field of educational publishing she coordinated the illustration of free textbooks and a series of art books published by the Ministry of Education, and edited the *Enciclopedia Infantil Colibrí*. In addition, she has been a curator of important exhibits such as *Memoria del tiempo*, which commemorated the 150 years of photography in Mexico, and *Bailes y balas*, which brought attention to one of the most significant photographic archives of the postrevolutionary period.

3. *Lo efímero y lo eterno del arte popular mexicano*. Mexico City: Fondo Editorial de la Plástica Mexicana, 1971.

NOTES ON CONTRIBUTORS

Sandra Berler is an art dealer in the Washington, D.C., area who specializes in the acquisition and exhibition of twentieth-century fine photographic prints and is a member of the Association of International Photography Art Dealers, Inc. (AIPAD). She is a researcher, lecturer, writer, and curator of photography.

Elena Poniatowska, a leading Mexican writer, has written over twenty books, among which *Massacre in Mexico, Dear Diego,* and *Tinísima* are translated into English. She has received honorary doctorates from the New School for Social Research and Florida Atlantic University. Her special interest in photography as an art and a documentary force has led her to write about Mariana Yampolsky's work in numerous books and other publications.

Francisco Reyes Palma, an art historian specializing in twentieth-century Mexico, has conducted research at the Centro Nacional de Investigación de Artes Plásticas of the Instituto Nacional de Bellas Artes since 1980, serving as research coordinator there from 1984 to 1989. He is a frequent contributor to various art journals and has been a curator of exhibitions such as *Memoria del tiempo: 150 Years of Mexican Photography* at the Museo de Arte Moderno in Mexico City in 1989, and *Modernidad y modernización en el arte mexicano, 1920–1960* at the Museo Nacional de Arte in 1991. Reyes Palma is the author of various books, the most recent of which is *Leopoldo Méndez, el oficio de grabar* (ERA-CONACULTA, 1994).

LIST OF PHOTOGRAPHS

Frontispiece: *Al filo del tiempo* / The Edge of Time / *1992*

CURRICULUM VITAE:
MARIANA YAMPOLSKY URBACH

BIRTH DATE: September 6, 1925

NATIONALITY: Mexican

EDUCATION: Bachelor of Arts in Humanities, University of Chicago, 1944
Studied in the School of Painting and Sculpture, known as
"La Esmeralda," Mexico City, 1945–1948.

ENGRAVER

1945–1958

Member of the Taller de Gráfica Popular (TGP), the Popular Graphic Arts Workshop, founded in Mexico by artists (Leopoldo Méndez, Pablo O'Higgins, and Alfredo Zalce) to produce and promote art for urban and rural masses and to benefit the progressive and democratic interests of the Mexican people, especially in the fight against fascism. Through broadsheets, book illustrations, posters, and exhibitions, the TGP reached a wide popular audience, not only in Mexico, but also abroad.

The first female member of the Executive Committee, as Curator of Exhibitions, she organized and sent monthly collective exhibitions of the Taller's works throughout Mexico, the Americas, Europe, Africa, and Asia. In Mexico, she was the designer and curator of the 20th Anniversary Retrospective Exhibition of the Taller's works in the *Gran Muestra de la Obra del*

Taller de Gráfica Popular at the Palace of Fine Arts, Mexico City. The following is a selective list of some of the shows of the Taller's engravings, including those of Mariana Yampolsky:

1950   *Mexikansk Grafik*. Kungshallen, Stockholm, Sweden.

1951   *Mexikanische Druckgraphik*. Kunstgewerbemuseum der Stadt, Zurich, Switzerland.

1952   *International Peace Congress Exhibit*. Vienna, Austria.

1953   *Eleventh National Exhibition of Prints Made During the Current Year*. Library of Congress, Washington, D.C., U.S.A.

1954   *Print Exhibition*. Charlottenburg, Germany.

1955   *Mexican Art*. National Museum, Tokyo, Japan.
        Canadian Freedom Committee Exhibit. Hart House, University of Toronto, Canada.

1956   *Mostra d'Arte Grafica Messicana*. Trieste, Italy.
        Mexicke Vytuarné Umenie. Slovenská Narodná Galéria, Prague, Czechoslovakia.

1957   *Deuxième Exposition Internationale de Gravure*. Moderna Galerija, Ljubljana, Yugoslavia.

1958   *Contemporary Mexican Engravings*. Musée Galliéra, Paris, France.

1947   Illustrator for the magazine *Construyamos Escuelas* (Let's build schools), under the direction of Hannes Meyer, former head of the Bauhaus group.

1950   Designer of poster for the film *Memorias de un mexicano*, among the first documentaries on the Mexican Revolution.

1951   Founding member of the Salón de la Plástica Mexicana, an artists' association formed to promote contemporary Mexican art.

1952   Third prize in poster competition sponsored by the Ministry of Hydraulic Resources, Mexico City.

1953   Third prize in children's book illustration competition sponsored by the Pan American Round Table, Mexico City.

1954   In the first *Print Salon Exhibition*, Palace of Fine Arts, Mexico City.

1955   Illustrator for the Sunday section of the newspaper *El Nacional*, Mexico City.

1958   Illustrator for the cultural section of the newspaper *Excelsior*, Mexico City.

1958–1959   Illustrator for *Annals*, put out by the Ministry of Communications and Public Works. Study trips to the Pacific coast of Mexico and the Yucatán peninsula.

1962   Illustrator for newspaper *El Día*, Mexico City.

1966   Exhibited in the 30th Anniversary Show of the Taller, Museum of Modern Art, Mexico City.

PHOTOGRAPHER

Books of Her Photographs

1981   *La casa en la tierra* (The house of the earth), text by Elena Poniatowska. Mexico City: Instituto Nacional Indigenista, Fonapas. A book on Mexican Indian architecture.

1982   *La casa que canta* (The house that sings), text and photos by Mariana Yampolsky. Mexico City: Secretaría de Educación Pública. A book on vernacular architecture of rural Mexico showing living, working, and ceremonial spaces.

1985   *La raíz y el camino, fotografías de Mariana Yampolsky* (Roots and paths, photos by Mariana Yampolsky), text by Elena Poniatowska. Mexico City: Fondo de Cultura Económica. A selection of her photographs.

1987   *Tlacotalpan*, text by Elena Poniatowska. Veracruz, Mexico: Instituto Veracruzano de Cultura. A book on the town of Tlacotalpan, Veracruz, Mexico.

Estancias del olvido (Forgotten haciendas), text by Elena Poniatowska. Mexico, Estado de Hidalgo: Educación Gráfica. Documents the dying tradition of the pulque-producing hacienda.

1992   *Haciendas poblanas* (Pueblan haciendas), text by Ricardo Rendón. Mexico City: Universidad Iberoamericana.

1993   *Mazahua*, text by Elena Poniatowska. Toluca, Mexico: Gobierno del Estado de México. Mazahua Indian women cope in the absence of men who have gone to the cities in search of work.

        The Traditional Architecture of Mexico, text by Chloé Sayer. London: Thames and Hudson.

        Nachdenken über Mexiko (Reflections on Mexico), text by Erika Billeter. Bern, Switzerland: Benteli Verlag.

1994   *La fotografía en México, Mariana Yampolsky*. Mexico City: Litográfica Turmex. A collection of postcards.

Background

1948   Began experimenting with photography. Published photos (e.g., El T.G.P./ The Popular Graphic Arts Workshop, 1949).

1964–1967   Photography for book *Lo efímero y lo eterno del arte popular mexicano* (see Editor and Educator section)

1968   Assigned to photographic pool for the Olympic Games for intensive coverage of sporting and cultural events. Published in the *Annals of the Mexican Olympic Committee*.

Solo Exhibitions

1960   *Imágenes del Medio Oriente*. José María Velasco Gallery, Mexico City.

1977   *Mariana Yampolsky, Fotografías*. Galería de Fotografía, Casa del Lago, Mexico City.

1978   Madurodam, The Hague, Holland.

1979   University of Manchester, England.

1980   *Images of Mexico*. La Tortolita Galleries, Tucson, Arizona, U.S.A.

Idaho State University, U.S.A.

Portrait from Mexico. Hospital Diakonessenhuis, Holland.

1982   Casa de Artesanías, Pachuca, Hidalgo, Mexico.

1983   Galeria Cannon, Milan, Italy.

1985   Photographer's Gallery, London, England.

1986   Bayly Art Museum, University of Virginia, Charlottesville, Virginia, U.S.A.

Las Estancias del Olvido. Chopo Museum, Universidad Autónoma de México, Mexico City.

1988   *Mariana Yampolsky*. Washington Arts Center, Washington, England.

Eternal Mexico: Photographs by Mariana Yampolsky. Queens College, The City University of New York, Flushing, New York, U.S.A.

1988–
1994   *La Mujer Mazahua*. Toluca, Mexico: Museo de Arte Moderno and Centro Cultural Mexiquense; Gobierno del Estado de Oaxaca; Mexico City: Instituto Mexicano del Seguro Social, UNAM, Eco, Universidad Iberoamericana, Centro Cultural del ISSSTE, FOVISSSTE, Infonavit; Coordinadora del TNI, Mérida, Yucatán; Guadalajara, Jalisco: Casa Jalisience de las Culturas Indígenas and the Delegación Estatal del INI; various venues in the state of Oaxaca.

1989   *La Raíz y el Camino*. Richland College, Dallas, Texas, U.S.A.

Mazahua. Galería del Arte Contemporáneo, Mexico City.

1990   *Estancias del Olvido*. Universidad Iberoamericana, Mexico City, and Galería del Arte Contemporáneo, Tlaxcala, Tlaxcala, Mexico.

Emancipación e Identidad de América Latina 1492–1992. Centro Artes, Quito, Ecuador.

1991   *Mariana Yampolsky*. Galería Sin Fronteras, Austin, Texas, U.S.A.

México Es una Sola Luz. Club Fotográfico de México, A.C., Mexico City.

1992 *Haciendas de Hidalgo*. Fototeca, Instituto Nacional de Antropología e Historia, Pachuca, Hidalgo, Mexico.

Casas Acariciadoras. On rural houses, with plans and scale models by Oscar Hagerman. Museo Nacional de Antropología, Mexico City; Museo Amparo, Puebla, Puebla, Mexico.

1992–1993, 1995 *Constructores de Sueños*. Curare, Espacio Crítico para las Artes, Mexico City, and Metro Pino Suárez as part of Fotoseptiembre, Mexico City; Galería Universitaria Ramón Alva de la Canal, Universidad Veracruzano, Xalapa, Veracruz, Mexico.

1993 *Mariana Yampolsky, A Retrospective*. Zelda Cheatle Gallery, London, England.

Mariana Yampolsky. Hafnarfjordur International Art Festival, Hafnarfjordur, Iceland.

Mariana Yampolsky. Ibero-Amerikanisches Institut, Preussischer Kulturbesitz, Berlin, Germany.

Mazahua. Museo Mural Diego Rivera, Mexico City.

1993–1994 *Casas Acariciadoras* (selected version of 1992 exhibition). Universidad Iberoamericana, Mexico City; Werklund, Berlin, Germany; Museo de Arte Moderno, Oaxaca, Oaxaca, Mexico; Casa de las Américas, Havana, Cuba.

1994 *A Collection of Photographs by Mariana Yampolsky*. Art Center, Brown University, Providence, Rhode Island, U.S.A.

México Indígena. III Festival Mexicano, ANA Hotel, Sydney, Australia.

1995 *Mariana Yampolsky*. University of Salamanca, Salamanca, Spain.

Mariana Yampolsky, Photographs. Lafayette College, Williams Center for the Arts, Easton, Pennsylvania, U.S.A.

Mariana Yampolsky. Centro Cultural de Belen, Lisbon, Portugal.

1996 *The Edge of Time: Photographs of Mariana Yampolsky*. Stephen L. Clark Gallery, Austin, Texas, U.S.A.

Collective Exhibitions

1975   Exhibit for the International Year of the Woman, Mexico City.

1976   Exhibit for the First Mexican–Central American Symposium on Women, Alvar Carrillo Gil Museum, Mexico City.

1977   Graphic Art Biennial, International Salon of Fine Arts, Mexico City.

Blanco y Negro. Paintings by Pablo O'Higgins, photos by Mariana Yampolsky, Museo de la Alhóndiga de Granaditas, Guanajuato, Guanajuato, Mexico.

Exhibition on the Day of the Dead, Circle Gallery, Mexico City.

1978   First Latin American Photography Colloquium, Mexico City.

1979   *El Retrato Contemporáneo en México.* Alvar Carrillo Gil Museum, Mexico City.

Carifesta, Havana, Cuba.

1980   *El Desnudo Fotográfico.* Casa del Lago, Universidad Nacional Autónoma de México, Mexico City (with catalogue).

Sección de Fotografía. Salón de la Plástica Mexicana, Mexico City.

México-Berlin, La Creación Femenina. Sponsored by the Goethe Institute, Mexico City and Berlin, Germany.

Hecho en Latinoamérica. The second show of the Latin American Photography Colloquium, Palace of Fine Arts, Mexico City.

1981   *Latin American Photography.* Kunsthaus, Zurich, Switzerland.

Artists of Mexico. Kunstlerhaus Belhanien, Berlin, Germany.

1982   *Hecho en Latinoamérica I.* Quito, Ecuador.

Artists in Mexico. Galerija Bih, Sarajevo, Yugoslavia.

10 x 10. Ten works by ten contemporary Mexican photographers, Austin, San Francisco, Los Angeles, and New York, U.S.A.

Five Women Photographers in Mexico. Mexican Council of Photography, Mexico City.

Mexican Photography. Stockholm, Sweden, and Oslo, Norway.

Photographs published in *Women in the Magic Mirror, 1842–1981*, presented in the Civiche Raccolte d'Arte, Milan, Italy.

1983 *Photography as Photography 1950–1980*. Museum of Modern Art, Mexico City. Permanent Gallery of Contemporary Mexican Art, Museum of Modern Art, Mexico City.

1984 *Photo America '84*. Genoa, Italy.
Woman Artists/Artists Women. Sponsored by the Museum of Fine Arts, Toluca, Mexico, Mexico.
Presences. Anglo-Mexican Institute of Culture, Mexico City.
Portrait of a Distant Land, Aspects of Contemporary Latin American Photography. Australian Center for Photography, Australia.

1985 *La Fête des Morts au Mexique*. Musée d'Art Moderne de la Ville and Musée des Enfants, Paris, France.
Exhibition on architecture, sponsored by the Ministry of Public Education in Baja California, Mexico.
Third Latin American Photography Colloquium, Havana, Cuba.

1986 *Inside Mexico*. Pierre Paolo Pasolini Center, Sicily, Italy.
Retrato de lo Eterno. Museo de Arte Moderno, Bogotá, Colombia.
Exhibition for the inauguration of the Salón de la Plástica Mexicana, Mexico City.
Photos of popular architecture for a series of posters for the Architecture Department, Universidad Autónoma de México, Mexico City.

1987 *Mexican Photographers*. Long Island, New York, U.S.A.
10 Mexican Photographers. Sponsored by the Mexican Ministry of Foreign Affairs, sent to New Delhi, India, and China.
New Vistas, New Voices: The Contemporary Art of Mexico. New Orleans, Louisiana, U.S.A.

1987–1988 *Manos a la Obra*. Mesa Southwest Museum, Mesa, Arizona, and South Mountain Community College, Phoenix, Arizona, U.S.A.

1988   *Images of Mexico*. Frankfurt, Germany; Vienna, Austria; Dallas, Texas, U.S.A.

El Desnudo. Foro de Arte Contemporáneo, Mexico City.

Diverse Images of Mexico. Mexican Fine Arts Center, Chicago, Illinois, U.S.A.

1988   *Mexico: A Century of Indian Photographs*. Museum of Popular Culture, Mexico City.

III Mes de la Fotografía Iberoamericana. An exhibition of photos by Lola Alvarez Bravo, Flor Garduño, and Mariana Yampolsky, Huelva, Spain.

É ora de messico! Il Diaframma, Milan, Italy.

Contemporary Mexican Photography. Gallery 44, Toronto, Canada.

Réalités magiques. Hotel de Ville de Nivelles, Brussels, Belgium.

Soucasná Mexická Fotografie. Prague, Czechoslovakia.

Retrato de lo Eterno. Museo del Carmen, Mexico City.

1989   *Polo Donna*. Galleria Civica d'Arte Moderna, Palazzo dei Diamante, Padiglione d'Arte Contemporanea, Palazzo Massari, Ferrara, Italy.

Mujer x Mujer. Twenty-two women photographers, Museo San Carlos, Mexico City; Instituto Cultural Mexicano, San Antonio, Texas, U.S.A.

Two-Woman Exhibition. Museo de Antropología, Xalapa, Veracruz, Mexico.

Artistas por la Vida, Compartiendo el Desafío. El Juglar, Mexico City.

Querida Frida. M.A.Q. Galería, Mexico City.

1989–   *Pinta el Sol*. Collective exhibition of nine women photographers, Sala Ollin
1990   Yoliztli, Mexico City; Veracruz, Mexico; Mérida, Yucatán, Mexico.

1989–   Head curator of the exhibition *Memoria del Tiempo: 150 Years of Mexican*
1993   *Photography*. Museo de Arte Moderno, Mexico City. It traveled to the following venues: Mussarnok Museum/Exhibitions Palace, Budapest, Hungary; Gallery of the Union of Photographic Artists, Varsovia, Poland; Photo Gallery, International Photographic Center, Berlin, Germany; Museum of Popular Arts and Traditions, Rome, Italy; Exhibition Hall of the Monument to Portuguese Discoverers, Lisbon, Portugal; Alesund Art Association, Reykjavik, Iceland; International Photographic Biennial,

Tenerife, Canary Islands; Musée de l'Élysée, Lausanne, Switzerland; Anthropological Museum, Amsterdam, Holland; Cankarjev Dom. Ljubljana House of Culture, Slovenia, Yugoslavia; Museum of Photography, Helsinki, Finland; Jerusalem Museum, Israel; National Museum of Photography, Film and TV, Brandford, Great Britain; Austria; Spain; China.

1990   *What's New: Mexico City*. The Art Institute of Chicago, Chicago, Illinois, U.S.A.

Día de los Muertos. Mexican Fine Arts Center, Chicago, Illinois, U.S.A.

Mujer x Mujer. New Brunswick Craft School, Federicton, New Brunswick, Canada.

Nature. Lithuania.

Muestra de Fotografía Ambientalista. Museo Carrillo Gil, Mexico City.

Niños de México. Quinta Colorada in the Primera Sección del Bosque de Chapultepec, Mexico City.

Nuestra América. Salón de la Plástica Mexicana, Mexico City.

1990–1991   *Compañeras de México: Six Mexican Women Photograph Women*. Gallery of the University of California at Riverside; Ventura County Museum of History and Art, Los Angeles, California, U.S.A.

Women in Mexico. National Academy of Design, New York, New York, U.S.A.; Centro Cultural/Arte Contemporáneo, Mexico City; Museo de Monterrey, Monterrey, Nuevo León, Mexico.

1990–1992   *Between Worlds: Contemporary Mexican Photography*. Impressions Gallery, York, and University of East Anglia, England; Camden Arts Centre, London, England; International Center for Photography, New York, New York; San Antonio Art Museum, San Antonio, Texas; Santa Monica Museum of Art, Santa Monica, California; Nexus Contemporary Art Center, Florida; University of Colorado, Boulder, Colorado; Museum of Photography, California; Bass Museum, Florida; Photographer's Gallery, Dublin, Ireland; Limerick City Gallery, Limerick, Ireland.

Other Images, Other Realities: Mexican Photography since 1930. Sewall Art Gallery, Rice University, Houston, Texas; Art Museum of South Texas, Corpus Christi, Texas; Vassar College Art Gallery, Poughkeepsie, New York; Visual Studies, Workshop Galleries, Rochester, New York; Stephen F. Austin State University, Nacogdoches, Texas; Lowe Art Gallery, Syracuse University, Syracuse, New York; Grand Rapids Art Museum, Grand Rapids, Michigan.

1991   *Mexican Contemporary Photography*. Il Diaframma, Milan, Italy.
Festival of Photography, Arles, France.
Altars and Idols. Exhibition on the life of the dead in Mexico, University of Essex, England.

1992   *Mexico-Myte og Magi*. Charlottenborg, Denmark.
El Hechizo de Oaxaca. Exhibition on the state of Oaxaca, Palacio de Bellas Artes, Mexico City; Marco Museum, Monterrey, Nuevo León, Mexico.
I Encuentro de Antropología Visual. Auditoria, Instituto de Investigaciones Antropológicas, Universidad Nacional Autónoma de México, Mexico City.
Latin American Photography. Institute of Philology and History, University of Genoa, Italy.
Culture and Colonization in North America. Collective of Edward S. Curtis (U.S.A.), Harlan I. Smith (Canada), and Mariana Yampolsky (Mexico), Rijksuniversiteit, Groningen, Holland.
Las Artes Plásticas y la Identidad Nacional. Museo de San Carlos, Mexico City.

1992–   *Mexikanische Fotografen, Die Schrift, 13 x 10, La Escritura, Fotografías*
1993   *Mexicanas*. Frankfurt Book Fair, Frankfurt, Germany; International Book Fair, Bogotá, Colombia.

1992–   *Encountering Difference*. Photos of Graciela Iturbide, Pablo Ortiz Monasterio,
1994   Carlos Somante, and Mariana Yampolsky. The Center for Photography, Woodstock, New York; Falkirk Cultural Center, San Rafael, California; Center for Photography, Pittsburgh, Pennsylvania; Northlight Gallery, Arizona State University, Tempe, Arizona.

1993   *Photographie, 1920–1992*. Europalia. Belgium: DeMarkten, Brussels; Bibliothèque Plantin Moretus; Namur; Galerie CGER, Liege; Provinciaal Hof, Bruges; Cultureel Centrum, Hasselt; Musée des Beaux-Artes, Mons; and Holland; Luxembourg; Germany; France; Spain.

Oaxaca, Magia de México. Europalia. Hunsthal Museum, Rotterdam, Holland.

A Woman's View. Musée d'Art Moderne, Liege, Belgium.

On the Elbow, A Group Show of Photographs. The Witkin Gallery, New York, New York, U.S.A.

Through Mexican Eyes. Colette Alvarez, Flor Garduño, Graciela Iturbide, and Mariana Yampolsky. Sandra Berler Gallery, Chevy Chase, Maryland, U.S.A.

Contemporary Mexican Photography. El Paso Museum of Art, El Paso, Texas, U.S.A.

Encuentro de Fotografía Latinoamericana, 1993. Caracas, Venezuela.

Canto a la Realidad, Fotografía Latinoamericana, 1860–1992. Casa de América, Madrid, Spain.

Al Filo del Tiempo. UAM-Azcapotzalco, Mexico City.

Grabadores y Fotógrafos. Galería del Salón de la Plástica Mexicana, Mexico City.

1994   *Si muero lejos de aquí . . . fotógrafos mexicanos en el extranjero*. Museo Nacional de las Culturas, Mexico City.

Selections from the Permanent Collection. Center for Creative Photography, University of Arizona, Tucson, Arizona, U.S.A.

México de las Mujeres. Galería Arvil, Mexico City.

Flowers. The Witkin Gallery, New York, New York, U.S.A.

1995   *Women Photographers*. Beijing, China.

What We've Discovered: Images of Our Cultural Identities. Artists' Alliance, Lafayette, Louisiana, U.S.A.

1996   *Inaugural Exhibit*. The Wittliff Gallery of Southwestern & Mexican Photography, Southwest Texas State University, San Marcos, Texas, U.S.A.

Represented in the Following Major Collections:

The Museum of Modern Art, New York, New York, U.S.A.

Museo de Arte Moderno, Mexico City.

Centro Cultural/Arte Contemporáneo, Mexico City.

Fototeca del Instituto Nacional de Antropología e Historia, Pachuca, Hidalgo, Mexico.

The National Portrait Gallery, Washington, D.C., U.S.A.

The Center for Creative Photography, University of Arizona, Tucson, Arizona, U.S.A.

The Wittliff Gallery of Southwestern & Mexican Photography, Southwest Texas State University, San Marcos, Texas, U.S.A.

Winten Bell Gallery, Brown University, Providence, Rhode Island, U.S.A.

Houston Fine Arts Museum, Houston, Texas, U.S.A.

St. Petersburg Art Museum, St. Petersburg, Florida, U.S.A.

Museo de Arte Contemporáneo de Puerto Rico, San Juan, Puerto Rico.

Bert Hartkamp Collection, Holland.

Photographic Museum of San Diego, San Diego, California, U.S.A.

EDITOR AND EDUCATOR

1963   Editorial advisor on book *José Guadalupe Posada*, about a nineteenth-century Mexican engraver, published by the Fondo Editorial de la Plástica Mexicana.

1964–1967   Co-editor with Leopoldo Méndez of *Lo efímero y lo eterno del arte popular mexicano* (The ephemeral and the eternal of Mexican popular art), published in 1970 by the Fondo Editorial de la Plástica Mexicana. This two-volume work deals with traditional Mexican dances, ceremonies, and objects of folk art.

1967	Teacher in the initial foreign languages program (CENLEX) of the National Polytechnic Institute, Mexico City.
	Planner and initiator of the school museum program, founded by the National Institute of Anthropology and History under the direction of Iker Larrauri.
1972– 1976	Planner, coordinator, designer, and co-author of natural science textbooks for the primary school education program, Ministry of Public Education, Mexico City.
1974	Designer of books for adult education (CEMPAE), Ministry of Public Education, Mexico City.
1978– 1980	Coordinator of the *Enciclopedia Infantil Colibrí*, a collection of weekly magazines for children. First of its kind, it was illustrated by leading Mexican artists and published by the Ministry of Public Education.
1979	Creator and coordinator of *La imagen de Zapata* (The image of Zapata), a book of drawings by children from Emiliano Zapata's home town.
1980	Coordinator and editor of *El ciclo mágico de los días* (The magic cycle of days), a book illustrated by a native painter from Guerrero who describes in words and images the customs and ceremonies of his village throughout the year.
	Creator and coordinator of *Imaginación y realidad* (Imagination and reality), a book of Indian children's paintings, visually and textually illustrating the child's role within the community.
	Co-author and coordinator of *Niños* (Children), a lavishly illustrated art book published by the Ministry of Public Education on the child's life cycle in paintings, sculpture, drawings, engravings, and photographs from pre-Hispanic to modern times.
	Coordinator of the book *Diego Rivera y los frescos en la Secretaría de Educación Pública* (Diego Rivera and the frescoes in the Ministry of Public Education), published by the Ministry of Public Education.

1981   Coordinator of *Juguetes mexicanos* (Mexican toys), published by the Ministry of Public Education. A book on the often overlooked, ephemeral, inexpensive, and popular toys and games of modern-day Mexico.

Coordinator of *Francisco Toledo*, an art book on the contemporary Mexican painter from Oaxaca, published by the Ministry of Public Education.

1985   Coordinator of *Pablo O'Higgins*, an art book on the well-known Mexican painter, lithographer, and muralist, published by the Fondo Editorial de la Plástica Mexicana.

Photographer for *Cuide a sus hijos* (Take care of your children), published by the Social Security Institute for Government Workers.

1987   Co-author of the eight-volume series *...y la comida se hizo* (. . . and food was made), published by the Social Security Institute for Government Workers.

1988   Editor of *Goitia*, on the painter Francisco Goitia from Zacatecas, published by the Social Security Institute for Government Workers.

1989   Editor of *Romualdo García, Portraits*, on the photographer García, who worked in Guanajuato from about 1866 to 1914, published by Educación Gráfica.

Exhibition curator and editor of *Memoria del tiempo* (Memory of time), catalogue for an exhibition of Mexican photography commemorating the 150th anniversary of the history of photography, Museo de Arte Moderno, Mexico City, with a European tour.

1991   Exhibiton curator and editor of *Bailes y balas: Ciudad de Mexico 1921–1931* (Dances and bullets in Mexico City, 1921–1931), catalogue for an exhibition at the Archivo General de la Nación on photos from the archives of Enrique Díaz.

CONFERENCES/TALKS

1990   On Mexican photography. Museum of Mankind, London, England.

1991   Commentary at the presentation of the books *Papantla* and *Tuxpan*, III
Congreso de la Colección Veracruz, Imágenes de su Historia, Veracruz,
Mexico.

Segundo Encuentro Nacional de Escuelas de Diseño Gráfico, Pátzcuaro,
Michoacán, Mexico.

On photography, at the Séptima Semana de Diseño in the seminar
"Retrospectiva Fotográfica," Universidad Iberoamericana, Plantel Golfo
Centro, Puebla, Puebla, Mexico.

On children's book illustration, Museo José Luis Cuevas, Mexico City.

1992   Commentary at the presentation of the book *Testigos del tiempo, photographs by
Flor Garduño*, Museo de Arte Moderno, Mexico City.

Segundo Encuentro de Escritores Mexicanos, Instituto Tecnológico y de
Estudios Superiores de Monterrey, Monterrey, Nuevo León, Mexico.

On architecture, at the Semana Iberoamericana de Arquitectura del Nuevo
Mundo al Mundo Nuevo, Universidad Iberoamericana, Mexico City.

1992   Participated in the round table of "La Fotografía en la Encrucijada," Museo
de Monterrey, Monterrey, Nuevo León, Mexico.

1993   On photography, at the Primer Coloquio Universitario de Fotografía,
Universidad Autónoma Metropolitana, Azcapotzalco, Mexico City.

On architecture, at Arquidiálogos, Museo Rufino Tamayo, organized by the
Colegio de Arquitectos de México, Mexico City.

Round table on "Lo Gráfico en lo Fotográfico," Museo Mural Diego Rivera,
Mexico City.

"Observations on Contemporary Mexican Photography," El Paso Museum of
Art, El Paso, Texas, U.S.A.

On photography and printed media, for a course sponsored by the newspaper *El Financiero*.

1994   On Mexican photography, Rhode Island School of Design, Providence, Rhode Island, U.S.A.

Round Table, Archivo General del Estado de Hidalgo, Pachuca, Hidalgo, Mexico.

On photography, at the symposium "El Color," sponsored by the Instituto de Investigaciones Estéticas, Universidad Nacional Autónoma de México, Mexico City.

Symposium "The Artist Is a Woman," Brown University, Providence, Rhode Island, U.S.A.

1995   Television interview, "Con los ojos de Mariana Yampolsky, fotógrafo," Channel 11, Mexico City.

On photography, at the conference "En Foco" at the University of the Sacred Heart, San Juan, Puerto Rico.

1995   Brown bag lecture, Williams Center for the Arts, Easton, Pennsylvania, U.S.A.

BIBLIOGRAPHY

Agosín, Marjorie. "Reading the Gaze." In *Mexico: The Artist Is a Woman*. Thomas Watson Jr. Institute for International Studies, Brown University, Occasional Paper no. 19, pp. 21–28, 1995.

——, ed. *Surviving Beyond Fear: Women, Children, and Human Rights in Latin America*. Human Rights Series. Fredonia, N.Y.: White Pine, 1993.

Berler, Sandra. "Mariana Yampolsky: An Artistic Commitment." In *Mexico: The Artist Is a Woman*. Thomas Watson Jr. Institute for International Studies, Brown University, Occasional Paper no. 19, pp. 29–42, 1995.

Billeter, Erika. *Fotografie Lateinamerika 1860–1993, Canto a la realidad*. Bern: Benteli Verlag, 1994.

——. *Nachdenken über Mexiko: Fotografie von Mariana Yampolsky*. Vol. 2 of *Fotografie Lateinamerika*. Bern: Benteli Verlag, 1993.

——. "Photographen, Die Geschichte Belegen." *Imagen de México: Der Beitrag Mexikos zur Kunst des 20. Jahrhunderts*. Frankfurt: Schirn Kunsthalle, 1987.

——. *The World of Frida Kahlo, The Blue House*. Photographs by Mariana Yampolsky, pp. 33–47. Seattle: University of Washington Press, 1993.

Brittan, David. "Mariana Yampolsky: Drinking from the Roots." *Creative Camera* 5, 1989, pp. 9, 16–21.

Castañón, Adolfo. *Retratos de mexicanos, 1839–1989*. Colección Río de Luz. Mexico City: Fondo de Cultura Económica, 1991.

Cohen, David, ed. *Images from the Circle of Life*. San Francisco: Harper, 1992.

Conger, Amy, and Elena Poniatowska. *Compañeras de México: Women Photograph Women*. Exhibition catalogue. Riverside: University Art Gallery, University of California at Riverside, 1990.

Connor, Celeste. "Images of Identification." *Artweek* 24 (August 19, 1993): 18.

Coronel Rivera, Juan. "Mariana Yampolsky: El acto fotográfico." *Artes de México* 12 (1991): 117.

Encountering Difference. Center Quarterly #53. Exhibition catalogue. Woodstock, N.Y.: The Center for Photography, 1992.

Eternal Mexico: Photographs by Mariana Yampolsky. Exhibition catalogue. New York: Queens College, 1988.

Ferrer, Elizabeth. "Encountering Differences." *Photography Center Quarterly* 14, no. 1 (June 1992): 24.

——. "Masters of Modern Mexican Photography." *Latin American Art* 2, no. 4 (Fall 1990): 61–65.

Fotografía latinoamericana: Tendencias actuales. Serie catálogos. La Rábida: Universidad Hispanoamericana Santa María de la Rábida (Universidad de Sevilla), 1991.

Franco, Jean. *Plotting Women: Gender and Representation in Mexico*. New York: Columbia University, 1989.

Giese, Lucretia. "Women Photographers in Historical Context." Paper presented at the symposium "Mexico: The Artist Is a Woman: A Symposium on Contemporary Film and Photography," held at Brown University, 1994.

Glancey, Jonathan. "Architecture: Humble Huts and Vast Haciendas." Review of *The Traditional Architecture of Mexico* (London: Thames & Hudson, 1993), text by Chloé Sayer, photographs by Mariana Yampolsky. *The Independent*, March 9, 1994.

Goldman, Shifra. *Dimensions of the Americas*. Chicago: University of Chicago Press, 1994.

Heggelin-Schwager, Susanna and Michael. "Mexican Photography: The Power of Astonishing Light." *Swiss Review of World Affairs*, April 1993.

Hopkinson, Amanda. "All's Well down Mexico Way." *British Journal of Photography* 136 (November 30, 1989): 10–13.

Johnson, Patricia C. "Mexican Art: Photography Exhibit Spans 20th Century." *Houston Chronicle*, May 10, 1992.

Kunsterinnen aus Mexiko. Berlin: Neue Gesellschaft für Bildende Kunst, 1981.

La mujer en México: Tina Modotti, et al. Exhibition catalogue. Mexico City: Fundación Cultural Televisa, Centro Cultural/Arte Contemporáneo, 1990.

Niccolini, Dianora, ed. *Women of Vision: Photographic Statements by Twenty Women Photographers*. Verona, N.J.: Unicorn, 1982.

Oles, James, ed. *South of the Border: Mexico in the American Imagination, 1914–1947*. Washington and London: Smithsonian Institution Press, 1993.

Olivares Larraguivel, Jorge. "Hagerman y Yampolsky." *Enlace, Arquitectura y Diseño* 4, no. 1 (1994): 114–116.

Ollman, Arthur. *Other Images, Other Realities: Mexican Photography since 1930*. Houston: Rice University Press, 1980.

Parada, Esther. "Río de Luz." *Aperture* 109 (Winter 1987): 71–78.

Photography 1975 / The Female Eye. Ottawa: Still Photography Division of the National Film Board of Canada (Clarke Irwin), 1975.

Rabago Palafox, Gabriela. "Mariana Yampolsky, the Singing Camera." *Voices of Mexico* 27 (1994): 57–61.

Reyes Palma, Francisco. *Al filo del tiempo*. Exhibition catalogue. Mexico City: Curare, 1992.

Schaefer, Claudia. *Textured Lives: Women, Art, and Representation in Modern Mexico*. Tucson: University of Arizona Press, 1992.

Stathatos, John. "Mariana Yampolsky-Urbach." *Creative Camera* 245 (May 1985): 8.

Tibol, Raquel. *Episodios fotográficos*. Mexico City: Libros de Proceso, 1989.

Tucker, Anne, ed. *The Woman's Eye*. New York: Knopf, 1973.

Wiesenfeld, Cheryl, et al., eds. *Women See Woman*. New York: Crowell, 1976.

Women of Photography: An Historical Survey. San Francisco: San Francisco Museum of Art, 1975.

Yampolsky, Mariana. *La casa en la tierra*. Text by Elena Poniatowska. Mexico City: Instituto Nacional Indigenista, Fonapas, 1981.

———. *La casa que canta: Arquitectura popular mexicana*. Text and photos. Mexico City: Secretaría de Educación Pública, 1982.

———. *Estancias del olvido*. Text by Elena Poniatowska. Mexico City: Educación Gráfica, 1987.

———. *Haciendas poblanas*. Text by Ricardo Rendón. Mexico City: Universidad Iberoamericana, 1992.

——. *Mazahua*. Text by Elena Poniatowska. Toluca, México: Gobierno del Estado de México, 1993.

——. *La raíz y el camino*. Text by Elena Poniatowska. Mexico City: Fondo de Cultura Económica, 1985.

——. *Tlacotalpan*. Text by Elena Poniatowska. Veracruz, México: Instituto Veracruzano de la Cultura, 1987.

——. *The Traditional Architecture of Mexico*. Text by Chloé Sayer. London: Thames & Hudson, 1993.

——, ed. *Bailes y balas: Ciudad de México 1921–1931*. Text by Elena Poniatowska. Exhibition catalogue. Mexico City: Archivo General de la Nación, 1991.

——, co-editor. *Lo efímero y lo eterno del arte popular mexicano*. Mexico City: Fondo Editorial de la Plástica Mexicana, 1971.

——, coordinator. *Memoria del tiempo: 150 años de fotografía en México*. Exhibition catalogue. Mexico City: Consejo Nacional para la Cultura y las Artes, Instituto Nacional de Bellas Artes, Museo de Arte Moderno, 1989.

Ziff, Trisha, ed. *Between Worlds: Contemporary Mexican Photography*. New York: New Amsterdam, 1990.

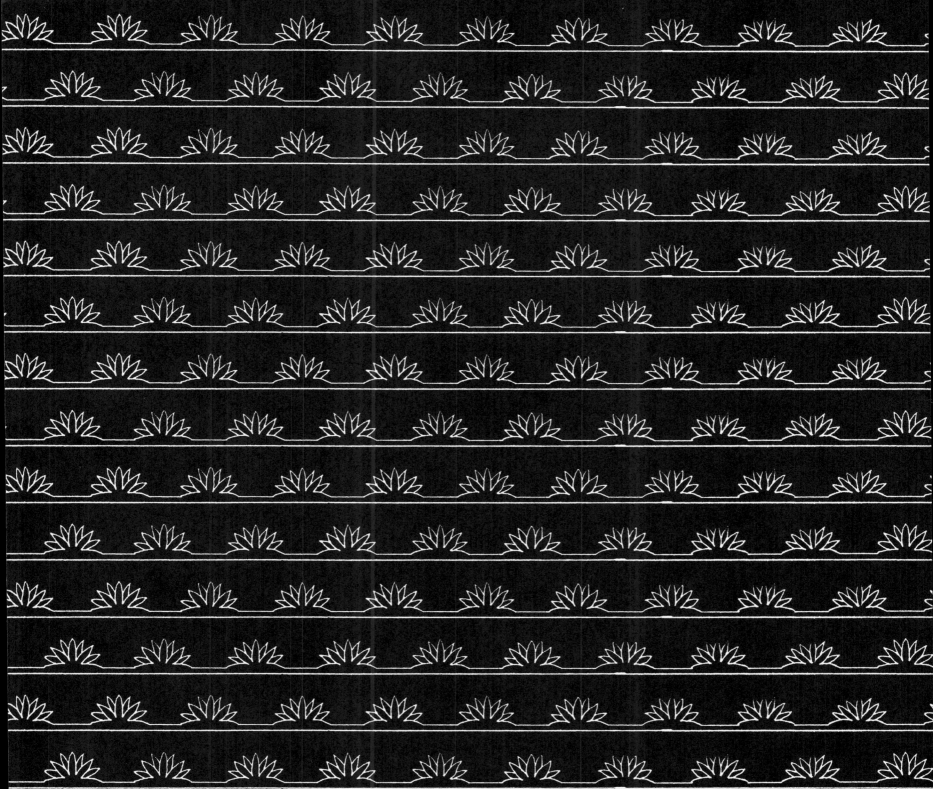